The Medical Management of Menopause and Premenopause

THEIR ENDOCRINOLOGIC BASIS

1984

J. B. LIPPINCOTT COMPANY
Philadelphia

LONDON   MEXICO CITY   NEW YORK   ST. LOUIS   SÃO PAULO   SYDNEY

Acquisitions Editor: Lisa Biello
Sponsoring Editor: Darlene Pedersen
Manuscript Editor: Pamela W. Fried
Indexer: Pamela W. Fried
Design Coordinator: Earl Gerhart
Designer: Susan Caldwell
Illustrator: Caroline Meinstein
Production Supervisor: Carol Kerr
Production Assistant: Pamela W. Fried
Compositor: McFarland Graphics and Design
Printer/Binder: R.R. Donnelley & Sons, Inc.

6 5 4 3 2 1

Library of Congress Cataloging in Publication Data

Cutler, Winnifred Berg.
    The medical management of menopause and premenopause.

    Bibliography: p.
    Includes index.
    1. Menopause.   2. Hormone therapy.   3. Hormone
therapy—Complications and sequelae.   I. García, Celso-
Ramón.   II. Title.   [DNLM: 1. Menopause.   WP 580 C989m]
RG186.C927   1984   618.1′72   84–5785
ISBN 0–397–50631–7

The authors and publisher have exerted every effort to ensure
that drug selection and dosage set forth in this text are in
accord with current recommendations and practice at the time
of publication. However, in view of ongoing research, changes
in government regulations, and the constant flow of
information relating to drug therapy and drug reactions, the
reader is urged to check the package insert and research
publications for each drug for any change in indications and
dosage and for added warnings and precautions. This is
particularly important when the recommended agent is a new
or infrequently employed drug.

Let us remember always that whatever truth we may get by scientific study about ourselves and our environment is always relative, tentative, subject to change and correction and that there are no final answers.

Chauncey D. Leahe
New York State Journal of
Medicine 60: 1496, 1960

Preface

The human female has a very intricate reproductive physiology that continually is called upon to function in so many different ways during the various epochs of life. The female system is vastly more complex than that of the male. Although the two systems start from similar embryologic origins, they begin to differentiate early. The complexity of the female system becomes more apparent with the onset of puberty, through the era of mate selection, the period of procreation and child rearing, and the menopause and probably later than we presently understand.

Potentially the beginning of a whole new career for women starts when the offspring become self-sufficient. In many women, this time of potentially high productivity can be confounded by a sequence of changes. These changes relate to alterations that are secondary to the varying degrees of conversion of ovarian activities—alterations from those of the younger ovulating organ to those of the mature menopausal structures. The effects of these changes on the vasomotor system and on the vascular system in general are becoming clearer. The effects of ovarian alterations on the integument, the immune system, and the mucosal structures of the body have been poorly studied and offer a less satisfactory level of their assessment. The interrelationship of the ovarian hormones, e.g., estrogen, whose premenstrual levels continue to depreciate during the climacterium culminating, in the long term, in the cessation of ovarian function, is critical to the support of numerous vital functions. Some of the estrogen production may in part be taken over by the adrenals, although this has not yet been clearly defined. The interplay of estrogens with cardiovascular disease, with bone metabolism, and with fat deposition and the interrelationships of estrogen secretion with physical and sexual activity and of vasomotor instability with emotional attitudes all comprise relevant issues for the clinician.

In recent years, the technology has so improved that measurements could be made where they were previously unavailable. The literature abounds with reviews, studies, and a variety of confusing and perhaps at times, diametrically opposing views. These differences are often due to the limitations of the technology that was available, as well as to the lack of comments about or awareness of this limitation as a cause for the different conclusions. Most people can barely keep up with the literature that comes across their desk in their own areas of competence. A few reach further, through review articles or participation in conference presentations. The management of the climacterium is encompassed in an enormity of literature, which makes it difficult, nigh impossible, for any one person with active health care responsibilities to personally make such a review and appraisal. To do so would require devoting an onerous amount of time and effort.

Herein, we present an encompassing attempt to clarify the facts and their potential interpretations. The state of the art of biomedical discovery is moving rapidly. By combining the efforts of a biologist with those of a gynecologist, we hope to have overcome many of the inherent research–review difficulties. Both authors are active scientific investigators with special interests in the care and concerns of menopausal women. After systematically reviewing, critically evaluating, and cross-referencing the data from over 2000 published studies and corresponding with the original researchers whenever questions arose, we formed some tentative conclusions concerning how to optimize health care for women in the 1980s. We find an overall cohesiveness in the various pieces of the puzzle.

We wish to express our deep appreciation to the many people consulted who guided the studies that proved necessary to reach the conclusions that have been expressed in this monograph. We particularly thank the following individuals who have contributed significantly: Dr. Luis Blasco, Dr. Julian Davidson, Dr. Lawrence Dubin, Dr. Richard Edgren, Dr. David Edwards, Dr. Erika Friedmann, Dr. Don Gambrell, Dr. David Goodman, Dr. Gilbert Gordan, Dr. Gilbert Greenwald, Dr. Emmet Lamb, Dr. Eberhard Lotze, Dr. Purvis Martin, Dr. John Morley, Dr. Santo Nicosia, Dr. Alan Ominsky, Dr. Harry Reiss, Dr. Norman Rosenblum, Dr. Richard Sherins, Dr. Jerome Strauss III and Dr. Richard Tureck. Without the help of these individuals, who in many cases acted as sounding boards, the development of this monograph would have taken much longer and perhaps would not have achieved fruition. Help in retrieving numerous articles and referencing is also appreciated: Mrs. Kathy Kelly, Ms. Peggy Lorenski, Mr. Michael Rissinger, and Mrs. Helen Springer. We are also grateful to Lisa Biello, Pamela Fried, and all of the other Lippincott staff for their invaluable support.

This compendium should be of use to the internist, the gynecologist/obstetrician, the general surgeon, the psychiatrist, or, in fact, to anyone who comes in contact with and treats the problems of the maturing female.

Traditionally, the male has been called upon throughout his gainful years to provide not only for himself but for his mate and offspring. Social changes are apparent. Women often feel a need to develop their own area of competence. To achieve this effectively and more easily, both the support of the family and the guidance of her physician(s) are needed. Quality medical care requires a well-thought-out approach that provides support to the whole woman. Our hope in presenting this monograph is to add to that capacity.

Winnifred Berg Cutler, Ph.D.
Celso-Ramón García, M.D.

Contents

The Medical Management of Menopause and Premenopause

The Menopausal Transition and Beyond

Caring for the menopausal woman is enhanced when the clinician retains a focus on the basic biology of healthy development from birth through senescence. These developmental patterns must be incorporated into our thought processes concerning the management of the maturing woman.

Aging in the human is the composite of endocrine actions on the general cellular milieu and of behavioral and general maturational processes. However, no clear or definitive research has defined what relative influence each component has. Moreover, normal age-related changes often cannot be separated from those that are secondary to pathology. Finch has divided the mammalian life span into four stages, listing particular characteristics for each:

1. The postnatal period, which is characterized by puberty, chemical maturation, and collagen maturation
2. Maturity, which is characterized by the achievement of adult body size, maximum immunologic responses, maximum levels of thyroid activity, maximum muscular strength, minimum reaction time, and, in the male, maximum sex drive
3. Middle age, which is defined by female reproductive senescence, increasing incidence of noninfectious disease, abnormal growth, autoimmune phenomena, declining resistance to temperature stress, and onset of osteoporosis, reduced sex drive in the male, and disturbed sleep patterns in both the male and the female
4. Senescence, the last of the developmental stages

In addition, some perception of cellular aging is useful. Calkins, in describing aging of cells and of people, expresses a current view that aging involves a gradual accumulation of both intracellular and extracellular complex molecules that undergo crosslinking. These crosslinks become increasingly less degradable, leading to a loss of flexibility.[16] Not only do Finch's four stages and the alterations in cellular and molecular structure show developmental changes throughout the life span, but in the female the influence of the ovary is also apparent.

The maturational changes in the ovary throughout life appear to exert the most critical influence of all of the factors that control the maturation of the female. Further attention to these details will be reviewed in terms of ovarian maturation through the reproductive years and on to senescence. Specific attention is focused on the following points:

Morphology, histochemistry, and steroidogenesis of the ovaries including the implications of oophorectomy

The interrelationship of these factors with adrenal gland secretions and the relationship of the estrogens to the androgens

The influences of the environment

The influences of the endocrine system on obesity (and obesity on the endocrine system)

The reproductive target organ effects of both pre-, peri-, and postmenopause

Other target organ changes that represent the hormonal measure of the importance of ovarian maturation

The osteoporotic process

The integumental changes

Sexual changes in women and impotence in the male partner

These reviews present the intertwining, modifying influences of the ovary in the menopausal transition.

OVARIAN MATURATION: THE REPRODUCTIVE YEARS THROUGH SENESCENCE

Greenblatt, among others, suggests that the human female is the only species known to live beyond her reproductive years. Improved environmental conditions permit her 25 or more productive years after procreational exhaustion.[56] However, it has not been established that the human female is unique in living productively beyond her procreative years. In fact, two studies suggest the opposite. For example, in 1787, Hunter reported that in the sow females appeared to have only a limited portion of the *midstage* of their lives allotted to reproduction.[70] More recently, Nelson and co-workers published the first extensive longitudinal study of a nonhuman mammalian species (C57BL/6J mice). They established that only the midportion of the life span is devoted to reproductive function in this species.[117] Nonetheless, the question of continuity across species remains unresolved. This review focuses on human studies. The complexity of ovarian function and procreation requires that these must be evaluated by a variety of methodologies. Each has information to offer, and when the methodologies are taken together, they present a consistent picture. Both morphological observations in the ovary and in target tissue combine to reveal a cohesive picture of ovarian function.

The potential approaches for evaluating the ovary are unlimited. The capacities that do exist are constrained by available technology and the ingenuity of the investigator. Therefore, these individual and combined studies must be interpreted within the context of the limitations of each technique. Each technique is further constrained by the sampling vis-à-vis age of the subject, timing in the cycle, and so forth. Moreover, none of the physiological events is static.

MORPHOLOGICAL OBSERVATIONS

The maturing ovary has long been known to differ from the younger ovary. Hertig, among others, has commented about the undeniably low number of oocytes found in the older ovary.[68] The density of different structures also varies with age. The older ovary presents relatively more tissue devoted to corpora albicantia and stroma and less to follicles.[157] Moreover, with advancing years, there is a progressive decrease in the number of germ cells (oocytes).[120,145]

In a classic study, Tervila demonstrated the changes in ovaries and adrenals as a function of age. The increase in ovarian size is paralleled by an increase in adrenal size during early development; after age 35, the adrenal maintains its size whereas the ovary tends to lose weight precipitously (Fig. 1–1). This gradual diminution in mass accelerates after age 45, when ovarian shrinkage increases more rapidly.[158] The size of the ovary varies during pregnancy as well.[158] In the first trimester there is a clear increase in ovarian size. In the latter trimesters there is a reversal—below that of nonpregnant, age-matched controls.[158] The adrenal glands do not change in size as a function of pregnancy.

Photomicrographs (Fig. 1–2) have provided a clear visual comparison of ovarian cellular tissue at different ages. The ovarian sections from a recently delivered newborn show orderly follicular maturation attributed to maternal hormonal influence in utero. The differences among the ovary of the newborn, that of the 30-year-old, and that of the 55-year-old woman are striking. With age, a general decrease of the population density of follicular structures and a relative increase of the stroma are evident. Nonetheless, some older ovaries continue to function. Novak has reported a study in which 23% of the women past the age of 50 who underwent abdominal hysterectomy and salpingo-oophorectomy showed at least one corpus luteum estimated to be less than 6 months old.[120] He concluded that the sixth decade should not necessarily be considered a stage of functionless atrophic ovarian demise because it is apparent that there are a significant number of women who continue to ovulate after age 50. Nonetheless, the general age trends are clearly directed toward ovarian follicular atrophy. The stromal activity is less appreciated.[48]

There is an unambiguous trend toward a gradual diminution of primordial follicles that contain normal oocytes. There were some healthy-looking primordial follicles but there was a clear decline in their number in the studies of Costoff and Mahesh.[28] They noted that the more advanced differentiating follicles of old ovaries were undergoing atretic change. The only corpus luteum present was an unhealthy one, and numerous

FIG. 1-1. Age-related changes in ovarian and adrenal size (Tervila L, 1958, Ann Chir Gynaecol Fenn 47:232–244)

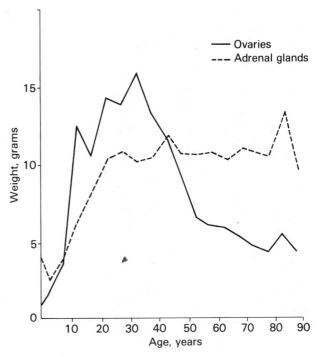

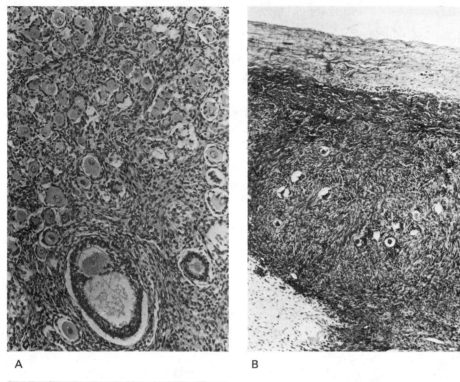

A

B

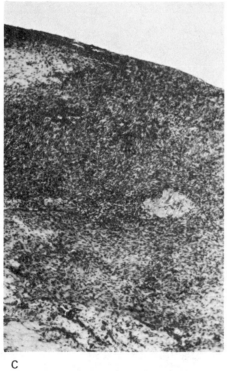

C

FIG. 1-2. Ovarian cross sections of (*A*) newborn (×220), (*B*) 30-year-old (×130), and (*C*) 55-year-old (×130). Courtesy S.V. Nicosia, M.D.

atretic follicles were seen in that ovary. These atretic follicles had clear granulosa cells without the well-developed polysomes, mitochondria, or endoplasmic reticulum that are characteristic of the younger follicular tissue. Changes in the ovarian cortex were also pronounced with the passage of time. With the relative exhaustion of the postnatal supply of germ cells, definite atrophic changes could be noted in the ovarian cortex.[28] However, the ovarian medullary region was filled with stromal or interstitial cells that increased in number as age advanced.

Thus, the ovary does change with age, and, although total exhaustion of primordial follicles is rarely seen, the general declining trend is unmistakable. Likewise, the changes in follicular development parallel these other effects. Although the ovary retains a capacity for some (small) primordial development, these small follicles are destined for rapid atresia. The rate-limiting step in the process appears to be a loss of the ovarian capacity to respond to gonadotropin.[28]

The morphological evidence suggests that the aging ovary is different from the younger ovary but that the human postmenopausal ovary is not the completely inert, nonfunctional fibrous mass that many formerly thought it to be.[61] The implications of the ovarian stromal and interstitial increases have been dwarfed by the focus on the apparent follicular demise. Morphological studies, though valuable, do not permit the actual assay for hormone that the in vitro studies of ovarian tissue have allowed. Sections through tissues with microscopic review of histochemical approaches have likewise added to our knowledge regarding the ovarian morphology.

HISTOCHEMICAL EVIDENCE

As the ovary ages, a general loss of granulosa cells ensues as well as a tendency toward less-ordered follicular structures. At the same time, there is an increased conversion of thecal cells into stromal cells that accumulate lipids. This results in the formation of a lipid band. This band was not seen at all prior to age 33.[48]

The lipid band and the thecal stroma cells show a striking inverse relationship to each other, suggesting that the lipid band is formed *from* the stromal thecal tissue as a function of increasing age.[48] With the recent use of ultrasonography for determination of ovarian morphology and volume, investigators have added *in vivo* studies to our perspective. Using real-time ultrasound mechanical sector scan, Campbell and co-workers studied both the ovaries of 11 climacteric women and also confirmed their findings by use of laparotomy the next day. Ovarian volumes were highly related to each other. A correlation coefficient between laparotomy and ultrasound of 0.97 showed that ultrasound, in competent hands, produces volume results equivalent to those obtained by evaluation at laparotomy. Elsewhere, 31 healthy postmenopausal women were evaluated by ultrasound. A mean volume difference of about 43% between the left and the right ovary is common and is considered to reflect normal variation.[17]

Histochemical studies have revealed that the lipid band is positive to cholesterol and related steroids, but devoid of the oxidative enzyme activity (glucose-6-phosphate and 3-B-ol dehydrogenases) found in the stromal theca as well as theca interna cells.[48] These missing enzymes are required for steroid hormone synthesis. However, others have reported frequent evidence of enzymatic activity in the hilus region as well as in the stromal cells.[121] Apparently, ovaries may vary in their stromal enzymatic capacity.

STEROID PRODUCTION IN OVARIES

Follicular Content

During the active reproductive years, it is the time in the cycle as well as the size of the follicular structures that determines the quantity and concentration of hormone. Reports of steroid levels in aspirated fluid from particular ovarian compartments have been revealing. The earlier researchers attempted to locate the site of origin of androgenic and estrogenic steroids in the normal human ovary.[12,118,137]

Early on, it was appreciated that the steroids produced by follicular tissue included progesterone, androstenedione, and estradiol. By 1969, it was known that follicular tissue produces progesterone, androstenedione, estradiol, estrone, and testosterone and that the stromal tissue produced little or no estrogens.[147] Further studies began to distinguish steroid concentration differences in different sized follicles. For example, testosterone concentration is higher in the less ripe follicles.[81] That there was an interaction between the granulosa and the thecal cells in the production of estradiol was clear and for a while the exact nature of these cellular dynamics was vigorously debated.

Stromal Content

Stromal production of androgens, testosterone, and dehydroepiandrosterone was observed by Mattingly and Huang in 1969.[100] The postmenopausal ovary, with its predominance of stromal tissue, provides an obvious site of androgen production in older women. Tissue incubation studies indicate that estradiol and progesterone are also present.

In Vitro Incubation Studies

In vitro studies in which thecal cells were bathed in a solution lacking gonadotropin indicated that thecal cells produce androgen and cyclic AMP (cAMP). The addition of human chorionic gonadotropin (HCG) induces an increase in androgen and cAMP activity although follicle-stimulating hormone (FSH) does not have these stimulating effects.[165] The thecal cells respond differently from the granulosa cells. Granulosa cells produce no androgen, either with or without stimulation of FSH, HCG, or cAMP. However, the failure of granulosa cells to produce androgen was considered to suggest immaturity of the granulosa cells rather than the inability to synthesize hormone.[165] The steroidogenic biochemical pathways starting from cholesterol, represented in Figure 1–3, show the formation of the estrogens. Recently, McNatty has shown that postmenopausal stroma functions differently from premenopausal stroma as expressed by the *in vitro* analysis of the production of progesterone, androgens and estrogens by granulosa cells, thecal tissue and stromal tissue by human ovaries.[102] All of the ovarian compartments had the capacity to produce all the steroids, but the quantities varied as a function of the developmental stage of the follicle and the developmental period in the life of the ovary.

In the young ovaries, stromal tissue has lower levels of cellular activity, mitotic activity, and cell hypertrophy than thecal tissue. In the postmenopausal ovaries the situation reverses. The level of cellular activity in the stroma is high and considerable hypertrophy is observed.[102] Other evaluations of steroid production and responsiveness to gonadotropin in isolated postmenopausal stromal tissue show that cortical stroma produce measurable amounts of androstenedione, estradiol, and progesterone *in vitro*[35] whereas hyperplastic stromal tissue yields even greater amounts of androstenedione and

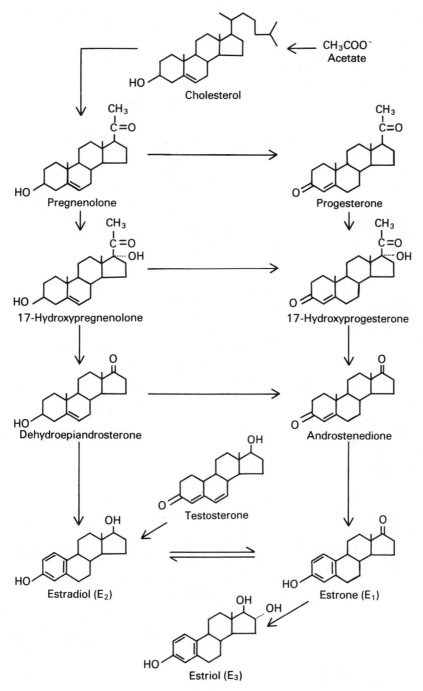

FIG. 1-3. Derivation of estrogens from cholesterol

estradiol. Androstenedione is the predominant steroid in both of these stromal tissues. Hyperplastic stromal tissue responds to human chorionic gonadotropin by producing significant increases in cAMP.

Combining the evidence from morphological, histochemical, and *in vitro* steroidogenic observations confirms the ovarian developmental pattern; with increasing age, there is a greater appreciation of relative mass toward stromal tissue, and this increase of stromal tissue results in an increase in the capacity to synthesize androstenedione.

OVARIAN SECRETION OF STEROIDS: CATHETERIZATION STUDIES

Several investigators have compared steroid levels in the peripheral circulation to those obtained from ovarian vessels during gynecological surgery. Differences between the ovarian and peripheral concentration levels of steroids can provide useful information. However, a significant portion of the blood supply to the ovary derives from the uterine vasculature through complex anastomoses. Thus plasma obtained from the ovarian vein may only partially reflect the true secretion rate of ovarian production of hormones. Because of the complexity and the magnitude of the uterine blood flow relative to the ovarian vasculature, investigators who wish to get a direct measure of ovarian hormone secretion are placed in a somewhat restricted position. Nonetheless these studies offer a valuable relative perspective about ovarian maturational changes in steroid production.

Mikhail evaluated the hormone secretion of ovaries at hysterectomy and noted that menopausal ovarian vein is righ in dehydroepiandrosterone and estrone ($1 \mu g/100$ ml of plasma).[109] After such an observation, it is obvious that the term "quiescent ovary" for a menopausal gonad is truly a misnomer. Other reports of postmenopausal women undergoing bilateral oophorectomy supplied further data.[79] Measurements of ovarian and peripheral vein concentrations showed significant differences as seen below and in Figure 1–4.

Hormone	Ovarian:Peripheral Vein Concentration
Testosterone	15:1
Androstenedione	4:1
17B Estradiol	2:1
Estrone	2:1

Some, but not all, postmenopausal ovaries secrete estrogens and androgens, which suggests that there is a spectrum of ovarian function in postmenopausal women that is variable from one woman to the next.[92] Among those women studied, 36% were estrogen producers, 38% were androstenedione producers, 50% produced abundant testosterone, whereas only 7% produced abundant dehydroepiandrosterone. Of special note is the observation that, in those cases in which the ovary was abundantly producing testosterone, the testosterone gradient was equal to that of premenopausal ovaries whereas the estrogen gradient was smaller. This suggests a real decline in estrogen while potentially the aging ovary can continue to secrete abundant androgens.

OVARIAN SECRETION OF STEROIDS: PERIPHERAL PLASMA STUDIES PRE-OOPHORECTOMY AND POST OOPHORECTOMY

Several investigators have studied the ovarian secretion of steroids by measuring peripheral plasma levels before and then at some short period after surgery. The ovarian

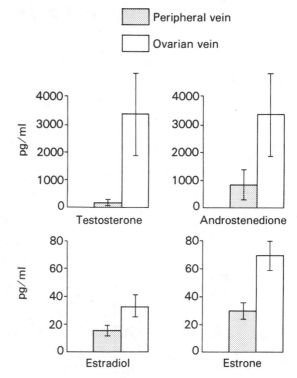

FIG. 1-4. Endocrine function of postmenopausal ovary: estimated by peripheral vs. ovarian vein plasma assays of T, A, E_2, E, (Judd HHL, Judd GE, Lucas WE, Yen SSC, 1974, J Clin Endocrinol Metab 39:1020)

production of dehydroepiandrosterone, androsterone, estrone, and estradiol as reflected in pre- and postoophorectomy values is clearly different four years earlier than later in the postmenopausal period. Figure 1-5 shows these changing relationships in the ovarian role in peripheral hormone levels.[169] The most obvious change in the transitional years from early to late postmenopause lies in the estrogen production of these ovaries. The early postmenopausal stages show severe reduction of the average plasma level of estrogen following ovariectomy. In the later postmenopausal years, when circulating estrogens are much lower, oophorectomy has a minimal influence on the further reduction of peripheral estradiol levels. The picture for estrone is similar. In contrast, testosterone concentrations are reduced by oophorectomy both early and later in the postmenopausal years.

The gonads of menopausal women have been suggested to contribute about 50% of the testosterone and 30% of the androstenedione, but the adrenal cortex in the late postmenopausal years is considered to be the almost exclusive source of plasma estradiol, estrone, progesterone, and 17-hydroxyprogesterone and the most important source of dehydroepiandrosterone.[76,83,168]

Thus, a cohesive understanding of the menopausal ovary becomes apparent from the composite observations of morphological, histochemical, and *in vitro* studies of ovarian tissue as well as of ovarian vs. peripheral vein studies and pre- and postoophorectomy plasma steroid evaluations. As the ovary ages, it continues to contribute to the steroidal milieu of the menopausal women albeit in a declining fashion. Although not appreciated universally, this ovarian presence represents a significant contribution when compared to the deprivation of the castrate.

ADRENAL CONTRIBUTION TO SEX HORMONES AT MENOPAUSE

The adrenals show no tendency for diminution in size with age. Further, according to ACTH infusion studies, the adrenal glands are not the site of a sensitive and rapid regulation of the steroid sex hormones in women; the concentration of androstenedione and of DHA as well as that of cortisol rises rapidly, but the concentrations of testosterone, estrone, and estradiol do not change.[41] Somewhat contradictory findings have been

FIG. 1-5. Endocrine function of early vs. late postmenopausal ovary: estimated by pre- vs. postoophorectomy levels of $D_1 A_1 T_1 E_2, E_1$ (redrawn from Vermeulen A, 1980, Maturitas 2:81–89)

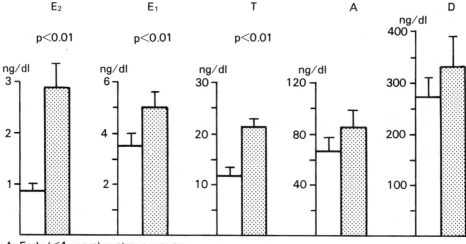

A. Early (<4 years) postmenopause

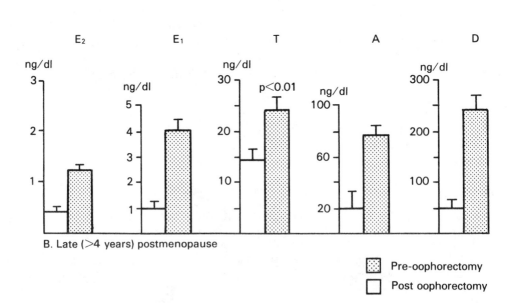

B. Late (>4 years) postmenopause

Pre-oophorectomy

Post oophorectomy

reported elsewhere.[8] ACTH stimulation increases estradiol production after ovariectomy for carcinoma of the breast.

A highly significant fall in plasma androstenedione occurs between ages 51 and 55.[31,93] Such a sharp drop caused Crilly and co-workers to suggest an "adrenopause." The idea of an adrenopause is interesting since it is startling, is not related to ovaries (these women were oophorectomized), and corresponds to the reverse phenomenon of increased adrenal androgen at puberty. The changing hormone status of the aging woman has been a subject of considerable investigation. Regardless of the source of secretion of these hormones (see, *e.g.,* reference 94), changes in peripheral levels are apparent.

CHANGING ENDOCRINE MILIEU

PLASMA STEROIDS

Estrogens

From the many estrogen studies, it is obvious that a single plasma reading of estradiol concentration can be misleading. Fluctuations can be observed within the same woman of about twice the level from one sample to the next obtained within minutes of each other.[71] Therefore the use of repeated measures is essential. Furthermore, episodic adrenal secretion of estrone occurs when androstenedione levels are suppressed.[72] Since androstenedione is the precursor for most postmenopausal estrone, this estrone pulsing is unexpected. Because of this potential for a rapidly occurring fluctuating pulse of plasma estrogen levels, one's evaluation of any study should consider the sampling procedure used.

Hormonal characteristics in the human menstrual cycle appear to change from one stage of ovarian development to the next. Only two studies have been published assessing these changes in a meticulous way. Sherman and Korenman in 1975 presented hormonal characteristics of the human menstrual cycle; they superimposed on these the hormonal characteristics of the late or perimenopausal woman who was still menstruating. Figure 1–6 shows their data.[143] One notes that after age 45 there was a tendency for a lower level of estrogen at any given time of the cycle. In direct contrast to these results is a more recent report by Reyes and co-workers.[129] Figure 1–7 arrays the estrogen levels of women grouped by age from the youngest group in their 20s to the oldest group approaching 50. Early follicular, late follicular, and luteal phase estrogen levels are shown. If one were to connect the average level of estrogen at any stage of the cycle with its matched cycle-stage in another age group, certain trends become apparent. Early follicular estrogen levels hardly vary as a function of advancing age. Late follicular levels are distinctly different; they seem to increase in women with older ovaries. Luteal phase levels of estrogen appear to decline with time. A potential explanation for these phenomena fits nicely with the histochemical, morphological, and ovarian secretion studies described earlier. The increased tendency toward atresia with advancing age and a reduced likelihood of antral follicular development could support the fact that the observed increase in follicle-stimulating hormone level[111] triggers more and more primordial follicles into the early maturational stages. Since the work of McNatty and others (described earlier) has shown that all follicles have the potential capacity to produce estrogens, it is possible that a large number of small follicles being stimulated by increasingly higher levels of FSH (observed with advancing years) would generate increasing levels of late follicular estrogen. Because the tendency with age is for a

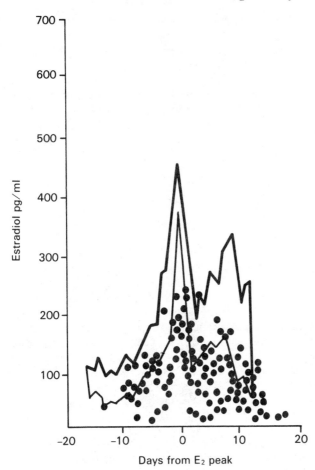

FIG. 1-6. Estrogen levels at different stages of the menstrual cycle: young cycling women vs. premenopausal women aged 45 to 50 (Sherman BM, West JH, and Korenman SG, 1976, J Clin Endocrinol Metab 42:629–636)

declining viability of the corpus luteum, the consistently observed decline in estrogen levels in the luteal phase is expected.

Once ovarian cyclicity ends, the situation changes. In almost every case of every study published, there is a clearly reduced (by about 80%) and noncycling estrogen level.[8,105,114] For example, in an elegantly designed study, Meldrum and colleagues presented data of 155 postmenopausal women aged 34 to 83 years.[105] They took the precaution of sampling plasma every 15 minutes for an hour and averaged those 4 samples for each woman. Estrogens remained constant throughout the menopause once ovarian failure had occurred. Estradiol levels ranged between 5 pg/ml and 27 pg/ml for all but 2 of the 155 women. The phenomenon held for both estradiol and estrone. Estrone levels averaged 40 pg/ml and did not vary with age across 50 years. Rare exceptions do occur. Estradiol levels that exceeded 25 pg/ml were noted in two postmenopausal 70-year-old women. A very strong relationship exists between the degree to which a woman is overweight and her circulating estrogen levels. Monroe and Menon (1977) compared age-matched postmenopausal women to ovariectomized women ranging from 51 to 65 years old.

Estradiol and estrone levels were not different in the two groups.[114] Thus, there is a large variation in estrogen production in aging women that should be appreciated.

The age at which ovarian failure occurs has not been resolved. The studies of Vermeulen showed that within the first four years after a loss of menstruation there was a significant reduction of estrogens. Figure 1–5 shows the pre- and postoophorectomy values in early postmenopause (Fig. 1–5A), *i.e.,* less than four years since last menstrual period, and in late postmenopause (Fig. 1–5B), more than four years after LMP.[169] In the early stage of menopause, estradiol levels are reduced by at least two-thirds after oophorectomy. By contrast, the late menopausal woman shows a relatively minor net loss of circulating estradiol levels after oophorectomy. Estrone levels show a similar trend but appear to be less influenced by oophorectomy at any age. Longcope has analyzed metabolic clearance and blood production rates of estrogen in postmenopausal women. He showed that the metabolic clearance rate is 25% lower in the postmenopausal woman.[91] Thus, even though older women could be suffering from decreased production as the metabolic rate slows down with aging, increased estrogen production in some older women is possible. The relative balance between clearance and production defines the circulating levels in weight-matched postmenopausal women. Age *per se* does not appear to influence production rates of estrogens; menopausal status and physical stature do.[93]

The presence of an adrenal secretion of estrogen has engendered controversy.[78] Estrogens that would be produced in the adrenals can be bound to sex hormone-binding globulin (SHBG) and then converted to estrone. The estrone source is more complex: 10% to 50% (depending on the time of the cycle in younger women) appears to be derived from androstenedione. After menopause, the estrone levels exceed levels of estradiol, with the average mean level of estrone being about 30 pg/ml, although in some women levels as high as 60 pg/ml are noted. These variations relate to the weight of the

FIG. 1-7. Estrogen levels as a function of time of menstrual cycle and age of the woman (*EF*=early follicular; *LF*=late follicular; *L*=luteal) (Reyes FI, Winter JSD, Faiman C, 1977, Am J Obstet Gynecol 129:557–564)

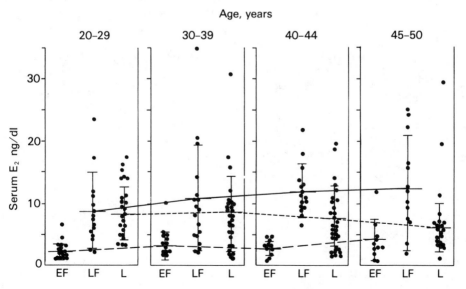

woman. Conversion from androstenedione into estrone increases in the fat cells of the body.[78,123] Although this general estrogen picture has been relatively consistently reported in the literature,[128] one study in 1976 noted that while estrone and estradiol levels were consistently low after the menopause, there was an "inexplicable increase" in some of the women some 10 years later.[20] Subsequent studies revealing the role of obesity in promoting estrogen levels provide a potential explanation.[93,105,123,169]

Androgens

Since the ovary loses its competence to produce estrogen, the remaining sources become critical. Certain key observations reveal that the principal source derives from conversion of androstenedione into estrone.

Androstenedione, the principal premenopausal ovarian androgen, is essentially noncyclic, except for a (15%) rise at mid cycle that apparently is due to ovarian contributions to secretion.[78] It is bound loosely to albumin and minimally to SHBG. Before menopause, the source of androstenedione is derived 50% each from ovaries and adrenal glands with a mean premenopausal level approximating 1800 pg/ml; after menopause is reached, the mean level is reported at a lower value, 831 pg/ml. This postmenopausal loss in androstenedione concentration has been attributed principally to a decrease in ovarian secretion.[78] With the loss of the ovarian cycle, the little monthly variation in androstenedione that did exist is lost.[77]

Androstenedione levels decline with age.[22,31,78,93,105,127] The postoophorectomy levels decline more severely in the early postmenopausal years than in the late ones, indicating some ovarian contribution to circulating androstenedione levels that diminishes with time. Figure 1–8 shows pre- and postmenopausal plasma levels of the following steroids: E2, E1, androstenedione, testosterone, dehydroepiandrosterone (DHEA) and cortisol.[176] The relationship between advancing age and androstenedione levels is well characterized in Figure 1–9.[105] Levels show a gradual decline from age 50 to 80. The characteristic drop in adrenal output of androstenedione that occurs in the early 50s is shown in Figure 1–10 presenting androstenedione level changes in oophorectomized women. One notes the decrement in mean levels of androstenedione with increasing age in these oophorectomized women. Support for this concept was provided more recently by data

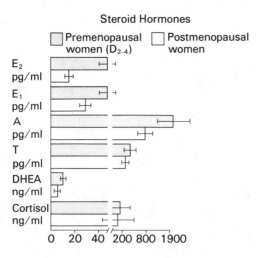

FIG. 1-8. Premenopausal vs. postmenopausal typical hormone levels: E2, E1, androstenedione, testosterone, DHEA, cortisol (Yen SSC, 1977, J Reprod Med 18:287–296)

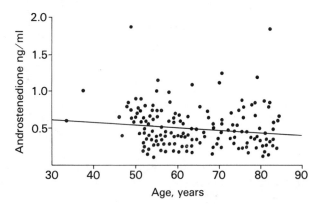

FIG. 1-9. Androstenedione levels in the menopause as a function of age (Meldrum DR, Davidson B, Tataryn I, Judd H, 1981, Obstet Gynecol 57: 624–628)

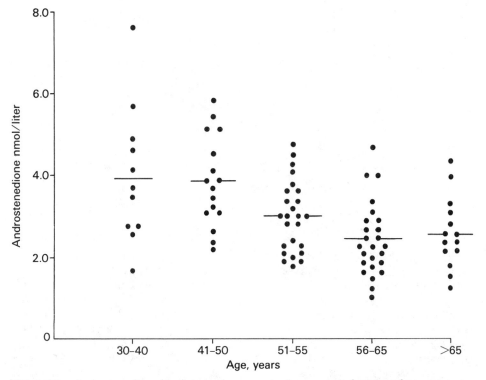

FIG. 1-10. Androstenedione levels in oophorectomized women as a function of age—stepwise drop noted (Crilly RG, Marshall DH, Nordin BE, 1979, Clin Endocrinol [Oxf] 10(2)199–201)

of Purifoy and co-workers.[127] They evaluated normal-weight, nonhirsute volunteers who were not taking any form of endocrine therapy. Each had intact ovaries, uterus, and adrenals. Consistent temporal sampling shows a phenomenon (Fig. 1–11) similar to the concept described by Crilly.

Studies of androstenedione production rate have also been described. Loncope and co-workers evaluated women aged 45 to 90 and concluded that age does not appear to

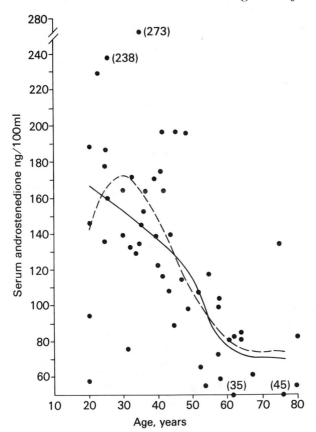

FIG. 1-11. Androstenedione levels as a function of age— sharp decline noted (Purifoy FE, Koopmans LH, Tatum RW, 1980, Hum Biol 52:181–191)

influence production rates for androstenedione but that the menopausal status and subject's weight do.[93] However, after age 62 or 63, there is a clear ceiling on the androstenedione production rate that is approximately 50% of former peak levels. There appears to be some inconsistency in the literature, however, for Hemsell states that there is an increased production rate of androstenedione at the menopause.[67] Regardless of a potential or loss of potential for androstenedione production with age, a weight-related increase in peripheral estrone levels probably accounts for much of the estrogen differences among different postmenopausal women. This estrone derives from the peripheral conversion of androstenedione.

Testosterone levels increase slightly in many women with the passage of years. Mean testosterone levels within the first 5 years post menopause were slightly lower than the mean testosterone levels taken more than 10 years after the menopause in the studies of Grattarola and colleagues.[55] Meldrum and coworkers (1981) also report a slight tendency for plasma testosterone levels to increase with age.[105] Purifoy shows free testosterone in plasma to increase with age.[127] There is some variation in the literature however. Judd and colleagues show a slight decline in small samples of premenopausal women who were compared with postmenopausal women.[76] Premenopausal average values for testosterone were approximately 325 pg/ml, postmenopausal averages approximated 230 pg/ml.[78]

If the production rate would decline somewhat in the face of slightly increased circulating levels of testosterone, there may be a decline in the metabolic clearance rate.

Other androgens in the metabolic pathway shown in Figure 1–3 have been studied; equivalent patterns have been noted.[78,105,110,169]

Androstenedione Conversion to Estrone

With advancing age there appears to be increased efficiency of the conversion of circulating androstenedione to estrone, even when the blood production rate of androstenedione does not increase.[66,67]

Summary of Plasma Steroid Change

A cohesive picture emerges that coincides with the behavioral and symptom alteration that is revealed through the years. Estrogen levels in the young cycling woman show two peaks per fertile cycle; the greater one occurs within a day of ovulation, the lesser peak coincides with the bloom of the corpus luteum approximately at the midpoint of the luteal phase. Beginning in the 20s and continuing until the menopause, the gradually increasing plasma estrogen in the late follicular phase of the menstrual cycle reflects the gradual increase in FSH through life and the gradual tendency toward increasingly larger follicular cohorts, often culminating in cystic ovaries as menopause dawns. In direct contrast, premenstrual estrogen levels move in the opposite direction throughout the reproductive years of the woman's life. The corpus luteum of the older woman shows less steroidogenic output. With age, postovulatory estrogen levels decline. Luteal progesterone secretion likewise diminishes with age. Thus, the highs get higher and the lows get lower as a woman's ovaries ripen.

THE ROLE OF OBESITY

Thin patients are disproportionately represented in populations with hip fractures. Moreover, hip fracture incidence reflects endocrine milieu (see Chap. 2). Balog reviewed charts of 100 postmenopausal women who were not taking hormone replacement therapy and who had been admitted to hospital because of fracture of the femoral neck. The average weight of the hip fracture group was significantly lower than the average weight of the nonfracture group. He suggested that heavier women may be less at risk for hip fractures.[7] The role of body fat in endocrine metabolism has been systematically evaluated. The findings follow a consistent pattern.

Plasma concentrations of estradiol and estrone tend to be higher in heavier women.[50,89,123,169,170] Figure 1–12 arrays the estradiol and estrone levels as a function of percent ideal weight in postmenopausal women with intact ovaries.[50] There is no relationship between height, age, or years postmenopause and estradiol or estrone levels. Likewise, there is no relationship between circulating levels of androstenedione or testosterone and any of these characteristics. Body weight appears to be an important influence on plasma levels of estrogen. Oophorectomized women more than 4 years after their surgery[89] also show plasma concentrations of estradiol that are positively correlated with body fat content.[89] Findings such as these led Vermeulen and co-workers to suggest a possible role of fat tissue in the aromatization of androgens.[170]

Production rates of estrone show no obvious relationship with age (Fig. 1–13A). A clear positive trend for increased weight to be associated with increased production rates of estrone is apparent (Fig. 1–13B). The picture for estradiol is similar though not as

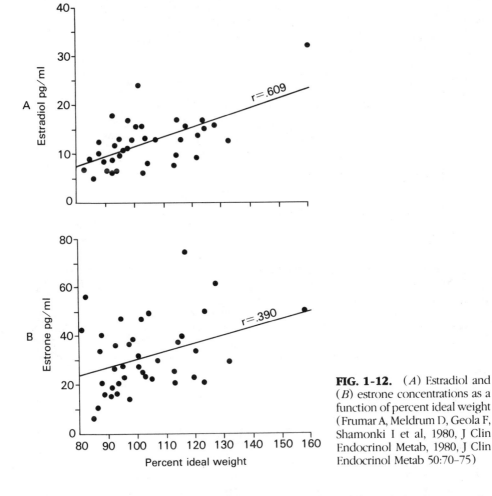

FIG. 1-12. (*A*) Estradiol and (*B*) estrone concentrations as a function of percent ideal weight (Frumar A, Meldrum D, Geola F, Shamonki I et al, 1980, J Clin Endocrinol Metab, 1980, J Clin Endocrinol Metab 50:70–75)

FIG. 1-13. Estrone production rates as a function of (*A*) age and (*B*) weight (Longcope C, Jafee W, Griffing G, 1981, Maturitas 3:215–223)

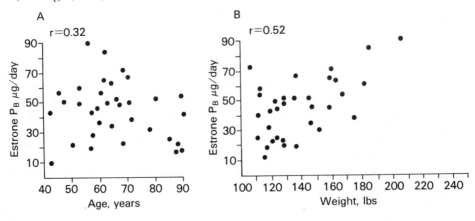

pronounced (Fig. 1-14).[93] A similar association of increased weight with increased androstenedione production rate exists.

The influence of obesity on the conversion of plasma androstenedione to estrone has been described.[43,78,95] Excessively heavy women (240-340 lbs.) showed an average conversion efficiency four times that of women of normal weight.[95] A direct correlation between the degree of obesity and the rate of conversion from androstenedione to estrone has been demonstrated by radiolabelled techniques *in vivo*.[43] The influence of dietary weight loss has also been reported.[122] The estrogen levels of obese women were similar to those of nonobese, age-matched postmenopausal women. Fasting reduced the estrogen level by 30%. When refeeding was resumed, estrogen levels rapidly returned to the nonfasting levels.[122] Testosterone levels were studied simultaneously, and no such effects occurred. Gonadotropin levels were also evaluated and found to change as a function of fasting and refeeding. Before fasting, obese women had significantly lower levels of gonadotropin than nonobese, age-matched women. Fasting induced an increase in both LH and FSH.

This general picture of the role of fat in metabolism of estrogens lends support to the earlier expression by Grodin and colleagues that the bulk of estradiol and estrone in postmenopausal women is produced by the peripheral conversion of androstenedione to estrone rather than by direct secretion of estrone by the ovary or adrenal.[60] The relative contribution of estrogens to the plasma pool derived from this conversion process remains to be elucidated but the overall trend is clear. Body fat serves as an efficient site for the metabolism of androstenedione into estrone, and estradiol levels in part reflect the levels of estrone.

HYPOTHALAMIC-PITUITARY AXIS

Although rapid oscillations of circulating gonadotropins have been noted in postmenopausal women,[103] clear developmental changes in average levels of the gonadotropins have been observed as well. Figure 1-15 shows the cyclic variation in levels of FSH with respect to the maturational process of women.[129] One notes the gradual and unmistakable increase in FSH levels as age increases. As the perimenopause approaches, excess FSH levels,[34,144] compared with levels of earlier years, are particularly pronounced. Figure 1-16 shows the FSH levels in cycling women aged 46 to 56. Individual dots reflect individual FSH values with respect to the day of the menstrual cycle. The younger female ranges of FSH levels are shown by the unbroken lines. FSH levels after the menopause continue to increase for the first few years, followed by a

FIG. 1-14. Estradiol production rates as a function of (*A*) age and (*B*) weight (Longcope C, Jafee W, Griffing G, 1981, Maturitas 3:215-223)

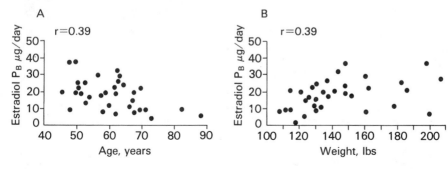

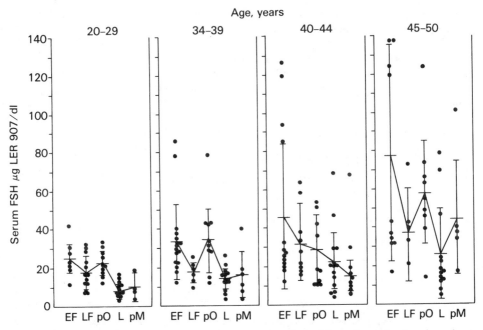

FIG. 1-15. Premenopausal FSH concentrations as a function of time of menstrual cycle and age (*EF*=early follicular; LF=late follicular; pO=periovulatory; *L*=luteal; pM=perimenstrual) (Reyes FI, Winter JSD, Faiman C, 1977, Am J Obstet Gynecol 129:557–564)

gradual decline in concentration that never reaches the premenopausal levels.[20] These phenomena are expressed in Figure 1–17. Support has been provided by other investigators as well, with a possibility that levels begin to increase again in the 80s and 90s.[139]

Changes in LH parallel changes in FSH with a much slower and more gentle increase with age. Figure 1–18 arrays the maturational changes in LH levels in different phases of the menstrual cycle.[129] One can see the clear and continuous trend for increased levels beginning in the 20s.

Yen has provided mean plasma level data of premenopausal and postmenopausal women for a variety of pituitary hormones, including FSH and LH (Fig. 1–19).[176] Pituitary secretion of gonadotropin is controlled in part by ovarian steroids and in part by hypothalamic secretions. Elements of the complex processes have been reviewed elsewhere.[25,32,82,174]

The gonadotropin response to luteinizing hormone releasing hormone (LH-RH) was earlier thought to be unchanged through time.[57] More recent studies have shown that the LH response to LH-RH is highest in the early postmenopausal years while estrogen levels are still relatively high.[52] The FSH response to LH-RH remains the same throughout menopause. These studies involved intravenous injection of a bolus of LH-RH.[52] LH-RH has been detected in the peripheral plasma of postmenopausal women when the plasma LH levels are relatively low.[42] The episodic LH release is apparently secreted in response to the episodic LH-RH release.

More recently, the studies of putative endogenous opiates (beta endorphins) in primates have indicated a critical role for these secretions in modulating the control of

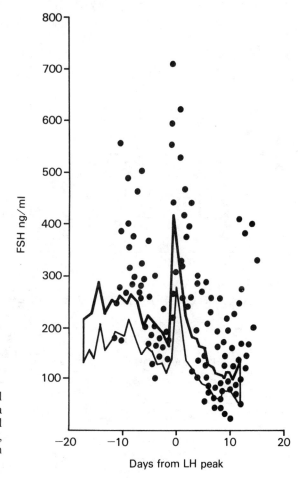

FIG. 1-16. Perimenopausal serum FSH concentrations as a function of time of menstrual cycle (Sherman BM, West JH, Korenman SG, 1976, J Clin Endocrinol Metab 42:629–636)

FIG. 1-17. Postmenopausal concentration of FSH as a function of years after the menopause (Chakravarti S, Collins WP, Forecast JD, Newton et al, 1976, Brit Med J 2:784–786)

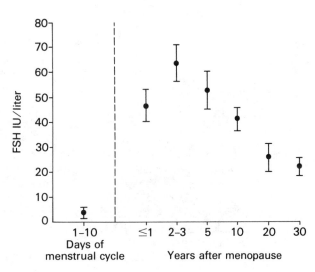

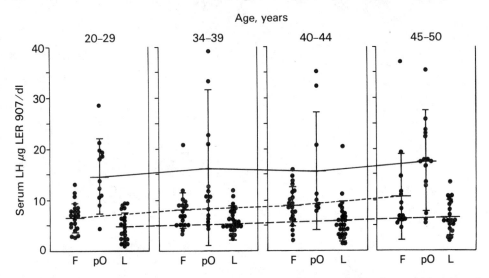

FIG. 1-18. Premenopausal serum LH concentrations as a function of time of menstrual cycle and age (Reyes FI, Winter JSD, Faiman C, 1977, Am J Obstet Gynecol 129:557–564)

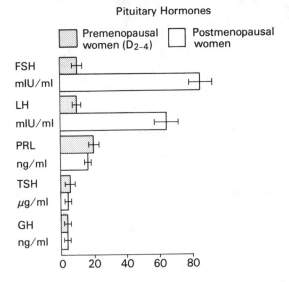

FIG. 1-19. Pre- and postmenopausal concentrations of pituitary hormones: FSH, LH, PRL, TSH, GH (Yen SSC, 1977, J Reprod Med 18:287–296)

the gonadotropins. Ovariectomized rhesus and pigtailed monkeys show startling deficits in pituitary stalk blood levels of endogenous opiates. When the animals are given injections of estrogen, portal blood levels remain in a deficient state. When 2 to 3 weeks of physiologic estradiol replacement therapy ensues, half of the animals exhibit a minor response. However, when estrogen and progestin replacement therapy is sufficient to provide physiologic replacement, the response is clear-cut. Pituitary stalk blood levels rise by more than 10 times the pretreatment level of beta endorphins.[172] Since morphine decreases the tonic gonadotropin secretion of ovariectomized monkeys, a potential role for the interaction between steroids and endogenous opiates in the control of gonadotropin secretions is implied but does not eliminate the involvement of neurotransmitters as well.

MENSTRUAL CHANGES IN THE PERIMENOPAUSE

AGE AT MENOPAUSE

A remarkable consistency in mean, median, and mode ages reported for menopause indicates that age 50 ± 1.5 years is the usual time for the occurrence of the last menstrual flow. Studies from midwestern United States, Scotland, Stockholm, Sweden, and Gothenburg, Sweden all show this pattern.[10,23,33,74,159,162,163,164,175] The meticulous reports of Treloar consist of prospectively collected menstrual cycle data of more than 25,000 woman years starting in the 1930s.[163] Analysis of the data for natural age at menopause without hormone replacement is depicted in Figure 1–20A. Data on menopause with estrogen replacement are shown in Figure 1–20B. One can observe the frequency of the onset of the menopause at various ages. Onset of the menopause in this sample occurred as early as age 41 and as late as age 59. The histogram also shows that the use of estrogen replacement therapy during the transition years was associated with a delayed onset of menopause. The mean menopausal age shifts by about 2 years.[163]

FIG. 1-20. (*A,B*) Age at menopause: frequency distribution (Treloar AE, 1981, Maturitas 3:249–264)

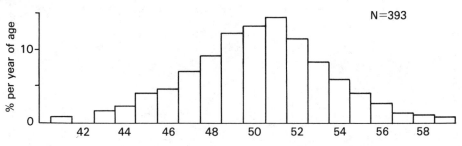

A. Menopause without hormonal replacement therapy

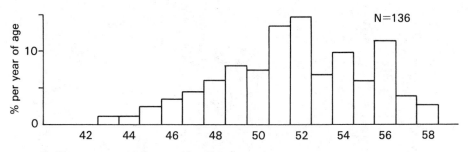

B. Menopause with hormonal replacement therapy

How To Determine Entry into the Menopausal Transition Years

During the transition years into the menopause, the observant woman will probably note a sudden change in the regularity of onset as well as quantity, quality, and duration of flow. If a record of the menstrual habit, recording the quality of each day of flow, is kept by the woman, this transition will be more apparent—reflecting the pattern of change from the ovulatory to the anovulatory decline in ovarian activity. These observations have been recorded in the biosocial as well as the clinical literature.[108,138,163] Figure 1–21 shows the classic array of menstrual cyclicity derived from the data collected by Treloar and presented according to gynecological and chronological age.[163] Even a brief glance will show the three very distinct phases of menstrual life. The reproductively fertile years are characterized by relative stability in cycle length and a relative trend toward a 29.5-day cycle. In contrast, the first 7 years and the last 7 years of menstrual cycle flow are characterized by a wide variation in the cycle length. Women are likely to have extremely long or extremely short cycles or some combination of the two. It is precisely this sudden

FIG. 1-21. Menstrual cycle length variation throughout life (Treloar AE, 1981, Maturitas 3:249–264)

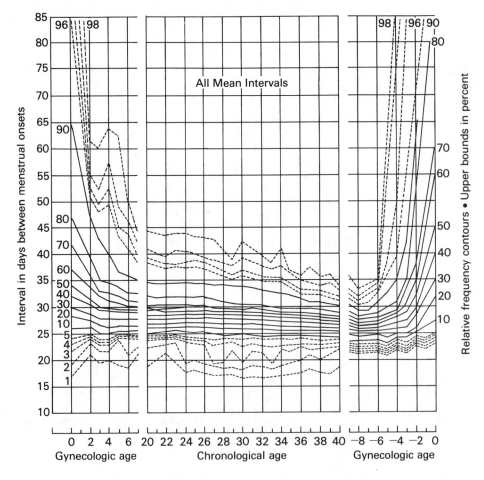

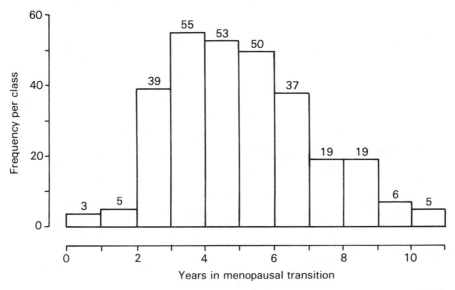

FIG. 1-22. Duration of menopausal transition (Treloar AE, 1981, Maturitas 3:249–264)

break in the stable pattern of cycling that serves to indicate that the menopausal transition has begun.

The duration of the transition has also been investigated. Figure 1–22 arrays the prospectively gathered data analyzed by Treloar to show how many years women can expect to be in the menopausal transition. One notes that, commonly, between 2 and 8 years pass in which widely variable menstrual cycles are experienced.[163] Bengtsson and co-workers have considered the question of amenorrhea at the perimenopausal time with respect to the likelihood that menopause has begun.[10] The likelihood of resuming menstruation after amenorrhea appears to be related both to the number of months of amenorrhea and the chronological age. If more than 6 months of amenorrhea occur, only 15% of women can be expected to menstruate again. Increasing length of amenorrhea portends a greater likelihood of menopausal state.

What the Menstrual Cycle Pattern Informs About Endocrine Milieu

It has long been appreciated that menstruation occurs in ovulatory as well as anovulatory cycles.[130] Clinically it is very difficult to distinguish between ovulatory and anovulatory uterine bleeding. The incidence of anovulatory cycles, evaluated by basal body temperature graphs, increases as a function of age.[26] More sophisticated efforts assessing either urinary pregnanediol or plasma progesterone to detect ovulation show that it is not the age but rather quality of flow and cycle length that signal the probable ovulation or anovulation.

Oligomenorrhea is a powerful predictor in the perimenopausal period. Oligomenorrhea is clearly associated with lower levels of urinary pregnanediol.[108] Oligomenorrhea is associated with relatively low levels of luteal phase plasma progesterone as well.[45]

The menstrual cycle length as well as recent change in cycle pattern offers the most important predictors of ovulatory status. Although ovulation occurs less often in women after 50, the potential for ovulation could be predicted by the length of the cycle (Table 1–1).[108] Saxena and co-workers showed that cycle length predicts ovulatory potential.[138] Thus, the patient presenting aberrant menstrual cycle length, especially if she is in her 40s, is very likely reflecting a normal transition-type menstrual pattern. Not all perimenopausal women have these irregular cycle patterns, but a significant number do.[1]

INFLUENCES ON AGE AT MENOPAUSE

A variety of potential influences have been studied with essentially unambiguous results. Smoking associates with an earlier spontaneous menopause, more cigarette consumption predicting earlier menopause than less smoking.[33,75,88] Mothers of twins entered menopause about a year sooner in one study of 3500 women.[175] Estrogen replacement therapy yielded menopause approximately 2 years later than menopause without hormonal support.[163] As is shown in Figure 1–20, estrogenic menopause shifts the histogram about 2 years later.

The age of menarche has been considered a potential predictor for the age at menopause. However, three studies found the two to be unrelated.[5,96,162] Marital status, parital status, and socioeconomic status were not found to associate with any particular age trends at menopause.[23] One study evaluating parity did report that women who had five or more children tended to enter menopause 1 year earlier than less parous women.[8]

PREMATURE MENOPAUSE

Reference is often made to the premature menopause. This reflects the onset of the menopause in the early 20s or 30s. Some use the label for a permanent amenorrhea before the age of 35.[9] No clear dichotomy between "normal" and "premature" exists. While some cite as causes of premature menopause hereditary factors that are not a sign of ill health but simply due to a genetic predilection, others reflect ovarian failure as being due to an autoimmune reaction secondary to rheumatoid arthritis or inflammatory reflections of mumps infections affecting the ovaries. Obviously, the surgical removal of both ovaries should be carefully guarded against unless it is absolutely indicated in the young woman. The premature menopause is differentiated from other causes of amenorrhea by highly elevated levels of the gonadotropins, plasma serum FSH, and LH. Since these individuals are chronologically young they must be viewed as special in regard to therapy. This will be reflected in discussions in Chapter 8.

One group of investigators report on four young amenorrheics (ages 23, 24, 36, 38) who were classified as exhibiting premature menopause. Hypergonadotropic and

TABLE 1-1. Ovulation potential in relation to cycle length

Cycle Pattern	No. of Women	Percent with Regular Ovulatory Cycles
No recent change	81	95%
Recent change	58	40%
21–35 Days	139	93%
<21 Days or >35 days	53	34%

Metcalf MG, 1979, J Biosoc Sci 11:39–48

hypoestrogenic stigmata were present. Subsequent to estrogen and progestogen therapy three of the four individuals treated became pregnant, suggesting a role of estrogen in initiating the sequence of events in re-initiating the ovulatory mechanisms.[154] The diagnosis of premature menopause is probably a semantic one. Ultrasound evaluation of follicular activity might also be useful.

TARGET ORGAN RESPONSES TO HORMONAL CHANGE

With the inevitable decline in steroid hormone concentration and the rise in gonadotropins, the target organs show a tendency to atrophy. Many studies have been published.

REPRODUCTIVE STRUCTURES

Vaginal Changes

With the menopause, the vagina becomes smaller with a diminution in the size of the upper vagina with increasing age. This conical tendency of the apex is also associated with a regression of the cervix and the vaginal epithelium becomes pale, thin, and dry; during this regression it can be easily traumatized and infected, resulting in a senile vaginitis. Similar atrophic changes occur in the vulva and in the vaginal orifice, which predisposes the person to dyspareunia. The epithelium of the labia minora and of the vestibule likewise gives a pale, dry appearance with a reduction in the fat content of the labia majora. Pubic hair becomes sparse and gray. The epithelium of the perivaginal and periurethral areas tends to develop erythematous areas that reflect local infection. The pelvic tissues and ligaments that support the uterus and the vagina lose their tone and predispose to prolapse.

Among oophorectomized women, pruritis vulva was associated with low estrogen plasma levels.[37] Symptomless oophorectomized women showed average E_2 concentrations of 114.2 ± 58.9 pmol/liter (n=36). In contrast, women with pruritis vulva showed average estrogen levels of 62.7 ± 31.0 pmol/liter.[37]

Vaginal Physiology

Vaginal change has been studied in two ways: by cytohormonal studies and by vaginal function studies. Cytohormonal studies employ the vaginal maturation index, which has varying usefulness in determining the current state of systemic estrogen activity on the vagina.[14]

The maturation index reflects the relative number of parabasal, intermediate, and superficial cells. Generally, a smear is best obtained from the upper lateral third of the vagina with a spatula. After staining, the ratio is achieved by counting some 300 intact squamous cells. Proliferation of the vaginal epithelium is estrogen dependent and is reflected in the vaginal smear by an increase in intermediate and superficial cells.

The "maturation value" is a function of the maturation index. Each cell type is given a score. Parabasal cells are assigned a score of 0, intermediate cells, 0.5, and superficial cells, 1. The total sum of the scores per 100 cells is defined as the maturation value.[173] This value tends to increase after estrogen stimulation. Vaginal cytohormonal evaluations show a progressive decrease in the vaginal maturation index after the menopause; 20% show complete vaginal atrophy, and 10% show high estrogenic activity.[104] Utian has described the estrogen influence on the parabasal cells. He reports that high oral doses of conjugated equine estrogen (5 mg/day) produce a significant decrease in the number of parabasal cells per field.[166] As just defined, this would tend to increase the vaginal maturation index. Clinically, Utian notes that atrophic vaginitis responds well to estrogen therapy in double-blind studies in which placebos were not effective.

Trauma to the genital tract is likely to cause profound changes in the resident microbial flora that may trigger proliferation of these organisms.[85] Because there is a tendency with age toward vaginal atrophy, sexual activity in estrogen-deficient women may yield such trauma and thereby increase the population of microorganisms. Pelvic infectious disease processes would ensue.[85]

Atrophic vaginal changes can and often do lead to increases in sexual discomfort. This is particularly noted in those women who have not given birth vaginally. Moreover, there are those with atrophic vaginitis who are sexually active during the menopausal transition and continue to be sexually active. These women may not have discomfort. However, among those who have a break in their behavioral continuity, many have severe problems that tend to occur promptly following the break in their sexual behavior and are noted particularly on the attempted resumption of such.[42] Postmenopausal women with regular coital activity, when compared to those of similar age without regular coital activity, had lesser degrees of vaginal atrophy in the face of equivalent plasma concentrations of estrogens in one sample not taking hormones.[86]

Semmens and Wagner noted a measurable decrease in vaginal secretions, their electrolyte content, an elevation of pH, and an approximately 50% increase in blood flow in response to estrogen therapy in postmenopausal women. Increases in vaginal blood flow were noted at 1 month and 3 months after the inception of hormone therapy. The levels of vaginal blood flow appeared to be heading back toward baseline after 6 months, but were still elevated well above the initial values. Vaginal fluid quantity showed a similar trend. Vaginal pH tended to become more acidic in harmony with the estrogen-dependent pattern of the vaginal fluid and vaginal blood flow changes. Likewise, transvaginal electropotential differences, measured in millivolts, also approached premenopausal condition at 3 months after the inception of estrogen therapy but seemed to head back toward basal levels at 6 months.[141] One of two doses (0.625 mg if uterus was intact, 1.25 mg if hysterectomized) was prescribed for 3 out of every 4 weeks. Both doses produced equivalent vaginal responses. The authors also noted that lubricative dysfunction occurred in 50% of their 50-year-olds and in 60% of their 60-year-olds. Cytological changes and the reversal of serum hormone levels were accompanied by the clinical improvement of atrophic vaginitis.

Vaginal relaxation and prolapses of the genital tract, including vaginal prolapse following hysterectomy, is often seen in the menopause. These vaginal relaxations are more a function of reproductive history than of estrogen levels. Although clear improvement in vaginal epithelium, blood flow, fluid quantity, pH, and electric potentials has been noted, pelvic floor tone is not improved by estrogen therapy and appears to be unrelated to plasma estrogen levels.[149]

Clitoral Changes

The term "clitoral index" has been defined as the product of sagittal and transverse diameters of the clitoris. Tagatz has described a characteristic enlargement in this index throughout the life span of a woman.[155] Huffman characterizes these "CI" changes (Fig. 1–23).[69] Women with excess androgen stimulation are said to have abnormally high clitoral index values. Clitoromegaly is clinically defined as an index that exceeds 35 mm

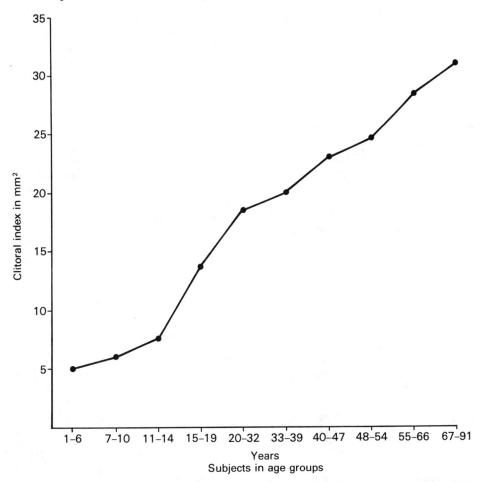

FIG. 1-23. Clitoral size as a function of age (Huffman JW, Dewhurst CJ, Capravio VJ, 1981, Anatomy and Physiology. in *The Gynecology of Childhood and Adolescence.* Philadelphia, WB Saunders Co)

squared and is a characteristic sign of excess androgen stimulation. As described earlier, many women show a tendency for testosterone increases with advancing age; this probably accounts for the clitoral enlargement tendency.

Cervical Innervation Changes with Age

The classic histochemical study of Rodin and Moghissi evaluating the intrinsic innervation of the human cervix noted two distinct changes with age.[132] Younger women had the greater sympathetic and parasympathetic innervation. Postmenopausal women had none.

Endometrium

Hysteroscopy reveals distinct changes in the appearance of postmenopausal uterine cavities.[59] The cavity was small and smooth. The endometrial tissue was sparse. No stalks were present. There were numerous small petechial hemorrhages. A white fibrotic band that stretches transversely across the fundus leading into the cornua and ending at the tubal ostia was apparent in the elder.

Myometrium

With the onset of the menopause, the myometrium and the endometrium atrophy, and the uterus diminishes in size. Fibroids, when present, also reduce in size; however, they do not disappear. They can and often do undergo hyaline and calcific degeneration.

Postmenopausal uteri likewise have alterations in their estrogen receptor binding. The postmenopausal estrogen receptor complex is unable to bind to the nuclear acceptor sites.[151] A threefold higher nuclear binding of estrogen in the premenopausal woman is observed over that of tissue of the myometrium obtained from surgical specimens obtained at surgery for benign conditions in postmenopausal women. This is felt to be the underlying cause or to reflect the mechanism leading to the age-related diminution in size of the uterus. It is thought that estrogen binding somehow stimulates myometrial growth, and, as the estrogen binding decreases, the concomitant decrease in uterine size follows.

Oviducts

In aging women distinct changes are noted in the oviduct, particularly the fimbrial portion. Little age-related change appears to occur in the isthmus or ampulla.[51] Likewise, there is a significant decline in the epithelium when compared to that of the premenopausal women. However, estrogen treatment for a year or longer maintains the tissues at levels comparable to those of younger women. A higher proportion of ciliated cells is seen in older women taking estrogen therapy. Here again, cytoplasmic nuclear estradiol receptors have been identified that vary as a function of estrogen level.[131]

Age Changes in Female Urethra

Urethral changes coincide with the vaginal cellular changes described earlier.[146] Both urethral and vaginal epithelium therefore appear to be estrogen-dependent tissues. The tendency is toward depletion and subsequent atrophy; the phenomenon is not inevitable. The maturation index may or may not reflect these deficiencies.

The urinary sediment has a reflective cytological characterization similar to that of the vaginal epithelium and has been used to detect ovulation. With the menopause, the urinary sediment reflects a reduction in the maturation index corresponding to that of the vaginal epithelium. Thus the increased frequency of urinary symptoms due to the cystitis, which is often correlative, responds to estrogen therapy. The frequency of cystitis is lower when the postmenopausal woman is on estrogen.

Breasts

With the gradual diminution of estrogen support, glandular breast tissue changes follow. There is a general loss of turgor, form, and fullness. Larger breasts are more susceptible to obvious change than are smaller ones.

BONES

The changes in bone physiology and anatomy are so profound and so critically important to menopausal management that an entire chapter is devoted to the subject. The reader is referred to Chapter 2 for a detailed discussion of topics on bone physiology and osteoporosis.

INTEGUMENT

Skin

Since 1966, studies of the microcirculation of the skin in old age have shown that the papillary capillaries disappear with age.[134,135] The papillary capillaries are the main source of a microcirculation that nourishes the surface epithelia of younger skin. Castration has profound influences on skin. Punnonen in 1972 reported that, when women were not replaced with estrogen, castration produced a continuously declining epidermal thickness that was proportional to the time since oophorectomy.[126] He compared the effect of different estrogen therapies on the epidermal thickness by taking samples of thigh tissue. Interestingly, a weak estrogen (estriol succinate, 2 mg for 24 hours) improved thickness and DNA synthesis; however, a strong estrogen (estradiol valerate, 2 mg for 24 hours) sometimes produced the opposite effect. Mechanisms for such a phenomenon are unclear, but one should be aware that weak estrogens appear to be optimal for skin physiology. Marks and Shahrad noted that trends with age that include dermal thinning, decrease in tensile strength of the skin, decrease in compressibility and mobility of the skin, general loss of turgor, slight decreases in total skin collagen, decreases in the quantity of melanocytes by 10% to 15% per decade, and decreases in sweat gland responses to emotional and thermal stimuli.[99] They also noted that estrogen therapies lead to a definite trend toward dermal thickening. Their reports evaluated estriol succinate, 4 mg per day. Although they disputed Punnonen's findings, saying that they were in the midst of work that did not support the earlier reports, one should recall the opposing effects that different strengths of estrogen had on skin in the work of Punnonen. Marks and co-workers used *in vitro* analytic methods rather than the *in vivo* methods of Punnonen. Marks used large concentrations of estrogens. Punnonen used smaller ones. In 1977, Punnonen and Rauramo reported further on the effects of long-term oral estriol succinate therapy on the skin of castrated women. After 3 years of estrogen therapy, they noted no significant decline in epidermal thickness in skin from the thigh. In contrast, there was a significant decline for skin biopsy planimetry values in age-matched, postoophorectomy untreated women.[126]

In 1980, the first characterization of estrogen receptors in human skin was published.[64] Estimates of the highest to the lowest levels of estrogen binding per mg of protein revealed the following relative E-binding levels: greatest was human uterine cytosol, followed by face skin, breast skin, thigh skin, lung cells, and adipose tissue.[64] The face skin evidenced much greater concentrations of receptor than thigh or breast skin and may account for the noticeable differences in women's facial skin texture after ingesting therapeutic estrogen.

Figure 1–24 shows the skin-fold thickness as a function of age.[30] Until the menopause there appears to be a steady state in skin-fold thickness. After approximately age 49 or 50, the regression line shows a clearly decreasing slope, indicating that with the passage of the years the skin-fold thickness decreases. Skin-fold thickness was further evaluated with respect to broad classifications of estrogen level. Figure 1–25 shows the skin-fold

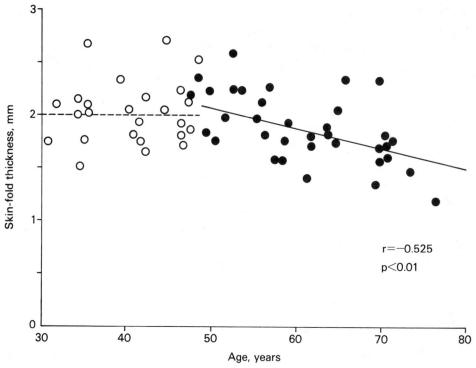

FIG. 1-24. Skin-fold thickness as a function of age in women (Crilly HR, Horsman A, Marshall DH, Nordin BEC, 1978, Front Horm Res 5:53–75, S. Karger AG, Basel)

thickness in women grouped according to whether they were postmenopausal osteoporotics or postmenopausal age-matched nonosteoporotics; a third group, those taking corticosteroids, were included. One notes that age-matched postmenopausal women show a difference in skin-fold thickness as a function of their endocrine condition. As detailed in Chapter 2, osteoporosis is associated with reduced levels of estrogen. It is therefore not surprising that osteoporotic women show, on average, a lower skin-fold thickness than normals. Corticosteroid therapy, as is discussed in Chapter 2, also further reduces plasma estrogen levels. Corticosteroid-dependent women show even lower levels of skin-fold thickness than osteoporotic women.[30]

Thus, while the details of skin physiology and its response to estrogen are currently unresolved, it does seem clear that profound influences of estrogen on skin do exist.

Hair

Developmental changes in the distribution of body hair have been noted in aging women. With the increased circulation of plasma androgens, a tendency toward an increased quantity of body hair and its distribution somewhat toward the male pattern is to be expected. For further discussion, see the section on hirsutism at the end of this chapter.

Buccal Mucosa

The buccal mucosa appears to be responsive to the estrogen level. In young women, gingival exudation carried out after two control cycles and followed by oral contraceptive use showed that ovulation time is the highest point of exudation in women not using oral contraceptives. Progestogen therapy (oral contraceptive) increased gingival exudation.[87] Other studies of young menstruating women showed the maturation index for the palate and buccal mucosa to vary cyclically as a function of time of cycle.[97] It was noted that one woman did not show a cyclic variation and coincidentally she was amenorrheic. The authors considered there was an ovulatory peak in the maturation index value.

More recently, Pisantry and co-workers have evaluated postmenopausal dental patients complaining of oral problems with dryness, viscosity of saliva, bad taste, and burning sensation, and compared these with postmenopausal noncomplainers and

FIG. 1-25.   Skin-fold thickness in normal, estrogen-deficient (osteoporotic) and corticosteroid-treated women (Crilly HR, Horsman A, Marshall DH, Nordin BEC, 1978, Front Horm Res 5:53–75, S. Karger A.G., Basel)

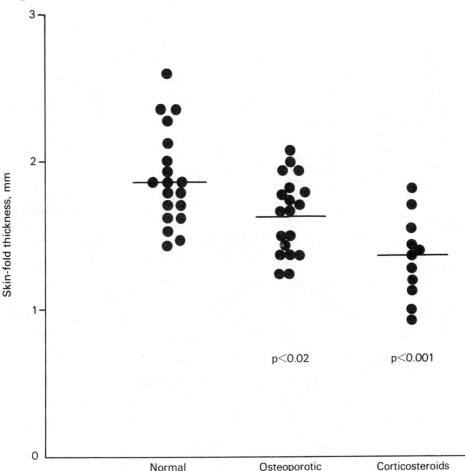

younger women still cycling who had no problems. Their results showed that the complainers had a thin atrophic epithelium and that any form of cream (estrogen, progestogen + estrogen, or placebo) when massaged into the gingiva three times a day always yielded a restoration of the mucosa, inducing proliferative changes in the buccal mucosa.[124] Concomitantly, they noted a significant increase in saliva. Thus it seems that vaginal epithelial changes characteristic of menopause are likely to be mirrored in buccal epithelial changes in the postmenopausal woman. The mechanical factors induced by massage undoubtedly play a confounding but significant role.

SYMPTOM FORMATION AND ENDOCRINE RELATIONSHIPS TO SYMPTOMS

As the average life expectancy for women age 50 is 27 additional years, the concerns of symptom formation at menopause are considerable. General trends toward symptomatology reveal that hot flushes (flashes) are the predominant symptom and that in general they are more relevant to the biological age than to the chronological age of women.[74] Symptoms found to be most severe before menses stop are fatigue, headaches, irritability, depression, and mental imbalance. In considering the different symptoms, hot flushes occur in 60% in early postmenopause (between 12 and 24 months after last menstrual period). Forty-five percent reported muscle aches and 20% tingling of extremities. The picture changes somewhat 5 to 10 years after the last menstrual period. At that time 45% still have hot flashes and 12% to 13% have tingling. In an attempt to categorize the various symptoms that commonly are reported, Greene presented a factor analytic study of climacteric symptoms.[58] Three factors emerged: psychological, somatic, and vasomotor.[58] The three factors are independent from each other; each is distributed normally; and a woman's presence in one category of problems has no bearing on whether she would be in the other two. Women who enter menarche later report fewer menopausal complaints than women who enter menarche earlier.[74] Likewise, nulliparity and unmarried status produce fewer complaints at menopause. A last pregnancy that occurs after age 40 is also protective against severity of menopausal complaints. One notes that all of these conditions are reflective of an endocrine milieu. Interestingly, higher income and education levels were each protective.[74] Most reports reveal no class differences in the reporting of menopausal symptoms.[98,101,167] Likewise, the influence of outside work does not necessarily improve the symptomatology of the menopausal woman.

Actual incidence of menopausal distress is very high. In different approaches to gathering these data, different statistics are gleaned. Notelovitz has stated that 25% to 30% of menopausal women complain of menopausal distress.[119] Crawford, in a grandparents clinic, showed that only 25% of the grandparents who came who were than checked for presence of symptoms at menopause reported they had escaped symptoms.[29] Stadell and Weiss, surveying King and Pierce counties in Washington, reported that 26% of menopausal women surveyed had "much trouble" with hot flushing at some point during the menopausal transition years.[148] They also noted that estrogen therapy users tended to be younger, more highly educated, and to have had a hysterectomy and a higher likelihood of hot flushes before taking the hormones.[148] Rutherford recorded that various unpleasant symptoms occur in about 50% of women.[133] He particularly noted menstrual habit changes and menorrhagia as well as hot flushes.[133] In contrast to this general picture of menopausal symptomatology sequence, Waldron has analyzed the causes of sex differences in mortality and morbidity.[171] She noted that women live longer than men, had lower death rates in most of the common causes of mortality, and had much higher rates of doctor visits and more frequent reports of complaints. She concluded that the situation probably reflects the greater sensitivity of women to symptoms of illness and that this very sensitivity leads to a focus on the illness and subsequent correction of the problem.[171]

Climacteric symptoms most often persist for more than 10 years after the menopause.[15] The incidence of hot flushes has been further assessed several different ways. In a large group undergoing a routine health screening, it was found that currently, 28% of the patients were experiencing hot flushes.[54] The distinction between current flushes and ever having flushes is an important one, however. An early report suggests that 62% of the women undergoing the menopause experience hot flushes[5] and only 16% of the women are free of all symptoms of distress as they pass through the menopause. Married women experience worse symptoms than single women, as in the other report.[5] Although previous general health is not related to menopausal distress, prior dysmenorrhea tends to associate with it. Specifically, 4 or 5 major categories of problems have been studied extensively. Vasomotor symptoms, their relationship to hormones, their relief by hormone replacement therapy, and their return when hormone therapy is stopped, have been well characterized. A relationship between endocrine milieu and potential for distressful menopausal experience has been noted.[5]

Osteoporosis, the gradual deterioration of bone because of a loss of bone mass, is continuous and progressive and has been extensively studied. This subject forms the content of Chapter 2. Emotional distress, depression, neurosis, and sleep disturbances have formed a cluster of complaints that have been studied both for their epidemiologic aspects and their relation to hormone therapies. Urinary problems, vaginal atrophy problems, and headaches have also been considered as they relate to the menopausal woman. Vasomotor symptoms with respect to menopause are probably the most clear-cut of the early disturbances and are considered in detail first.

THE VASOMOTOR SYMPTOMS

Physiological Aspects

Physiological reactions to hot flashes have been characterized. Molnar provided continuous data of a woman with respect to her skin and internal (rectal, vaginal, and tympanic) temperatures as well as onset and duration of a number of hot flashes.[112] The mean flash duration of this woman was 3.8 minutes, with a range of 2.4 to 4.7. Sweatprints showed that during the flash there was a profuse amount on the forehead and nose and moderate sweating on the sternum and adjacent areas without affecting the cheeks. Finger and toe temperatures always showed a sharp rise at the onset of the flash with a slower fall after it had peaked. Core temperatures dropped. The heart rate accelerated 13% at the onset of the flash but rapidly abated. There never was a premonitory sign of flash imminence (but other women have reported 30- to 45-second premonitions that the flashes were coming). Some studies of night sweats showed that women tended to waken some 45 seconds before the physiological evidence of the flash begins. Internal temperatures fell after each flash had begun at all three sites: rectal and vaginal and tympanic. Sturdee and co-workers, in trying to provoke a small sampling of hot flashes with the aid of electric blankets and water bottles, showed that simply warming a woman to create a very high skin surface temperature (that cannot be dissipated) is ineffective.[153] For those women who were experiencing flashes the data were in accord with the studies of Molnar just described. Each time a flash occurred there was an acute rise in hand, arm, and forehead temperature of about 1 degree centigrade on the skin surface. There was also a significant increase in heart rate at the onset of the flush (71 ± 3 beats/minute basal to 86 ± 4 beats/minute at onset of the flush). Electrocardiogram measures fluctuated widely from one woman to another. There was a fall in skin resistance. In this study, there were no significant changes in blood pressure. The temperature elevation persisted after the flush sensation had ceased and probably reflects the time it takes for the body to dissipate the heat it has just created.

Although one cannot liken a hot flash to simply warming a person, it does seem clear that ambient temperature influences the frequency and severity of hot flashes. Hotter days produce more flashes.[113] Thus, a woman who is suffering from hot flashes is more likely to experience more of them in the summertime than in the winter if she lives in a climate in which the summers are warm and the winters are cold.

Hormonal Control

Exactly what is triggering a flash has been a subject of some intricate investigations. Low levels of estrogen are clearly one of the associates of hot flashes because flashes commence as estrogen levels begin to decline precipitously in the perimenopausal transition. However, it is clear that estrogen levels by themselves cannot account for flashes unless other components of the endocrine system coordinate. Adolescents with low levels of estrogen do not report hot flashes. Men with testicular insufficiency have been reported to experience hot flashes.[47] Studies of 29 postabdominally hysterectomized subjects with bilateral salpingo-oophorectomy showed that no relationships could be clearly defined between the group that had hot flashes and the group that had no hot flashes with respect to E1 or E2 levels, nor could the vaginal maturation index be used to predict which of these women would or would not suffer hot flashes.[150] Nonetheless, there clearly are relationships between reduced estrogen level and potential for hot flashes. Hutton and co-workers, in their studies of postmenopausal women, showed that, of age- and weight-matched subjects, women with both superficial dyspareunia and hot flashes had significantly lower mean concentrations of plasma estradiol (but not of estrone) than symptomless women.[73] However, flushes alone were not related to plasma estrogen levels in that study. More recently, Hagen and colleagues reported lower levels of E2 in early post menopause among women with hot flashes than among those without flashes (131 ± 5 vs. 164 ± 10 pmol/1).[62] Women with hot flashes also had lower levels of androstenedione.[62]

Although basal levels of steroids do not permit one to predict the propensity for hot flashes, it does seem clear that estrogen withdrawal at that time of life when estrogen levels are rapidly dropping may be a critical steroid associate. Several studies have explored the minute to minute endocrine milieu during the hot-flash period. Gonadotropin pulses at first appeared to be a trigger. In 6 postmenopausal women, 55 flush episodes were studied among women who were quietly at rest without caffeine or cigarettes.[18] The menopausal flush episodes were invariably associated with the initiation of pulsatile pituitary release of luteinizing hormone. Flashes were not accompanied by significant change in circulating catecholamines or prolactin. The pulses of LH and FSH were not invariably predictive of flashes.[2,18] The authors expressed their belief that flashes were associated with withdrawal mechanisms since hypogonadal women never have flushes unless pretreated with estrogen and then taken off it. There is an implication of a central catecholamine role because adrenergic agonists decrease adrenergic activity centrally and provide symptomatic relief of flushes. Moreover, LH was positively correlated with skin temperature but FSH was not. These factors suggested to the authors that LH or factors associated with its pulsatile release are related to the flush mechanism.[156] Moreover, Meldrum and co-workers provided further data in their studies of postmenopausal women with flashes who had 8-hour continuous recordings of finger temperature with frequent serum serial measurements. Their results showed that the finger temperature elevation averaged $3.1 \pm 0.3°C$. The duration of the finger temperature elevation averaged 44 minutes. The time of the maximal rise after the onset of the flash was more than 7 minutes. The maximum LH elevation occurred approximately 5 to 10 minutes after the onset of the finger temperature rise. There were significant rises of DHEA, androstenedione, and cortisol with the maximum percentage changes of $56\% \pm 25\%$, $18\% \pm 7\%$, $45\% \pm 16\%$, respectively. They noted no acute changes of FSH, estrone, or $17\text{-}\beta$ estradiol with the pulses or with the flashes or with the temperature rises. These findings suggest that adrenal activity may occur *after* the hot flash.[107] Further indications of central peptide changes have been more recently provided.[84] Changes in thermoregulation, immunoreactive neurotensin, catecholamine, and LH during menopausal hot flashes have all been noted.[84]

Although the usual perimenopausal and postmenopausal circumstance of low steroids and elevated gonadotropins appear to suggest a gonadotropin cause for hot flashes, the situation appears more complicated. Two hypophysectomized patients (therefore with low gonadotropins) were found to have moderate flushing.[115] Two other young women with pituitary insufficiency were also shown to have hot flushes without pulsatile changes in LH.[106] Central catecholamines as well as catecholestrogens have been considered, but not yet proved, to influence the flashes.[18] It thus seems clear that the neuroendocrine link between various endocrine states and the propensity toward hot flashes is a complex one whose individual components will probably reveal a multifactorial etiology.

Answers to questions of mechanism continue to elude investigators. Although there are clear relationships between reduced estrogen levels and a propensity to flushes and between pulsatile LH release and actual onset of flushes, neither the estrogen nor the LH phenomenon can adequately explain the presence of flashes. Hot flashes were clearly shown not to be caused by gonadotropin pulses in several ways. The antigonadotropin danazol fails to relieve flushes. Clomiphene, an antiestrogenic drug, provokes hot flushes that disappear on cessation of drug use.[11] More recently, pituitary gonadotropin desensitization by a potent luteinizing hormone releasing factor agonist was administered. LH suppression did not alter flushes in the five flushing menopausal women given this gonadotropin agonist. The agonist produced lower and flat gonadotropin levels across the 4 hours of treatment. Thus, the authors concluded that the flushes cannot be caused by the LH pulses.[19]

Despite a failure to explain the mechanisms of the hot flash, symptomatic relief from flashes has proved obtainable. A variety of studies have evaluated multiple effects of hormones (estrogens, progesterones, testosterone), clonidine, propranolol, and other agents. The results are clear in showing the excellent therapeutic results obtained with estrogens. Progesterone appears to be active although somewhat less so than estrogen.[39] Placebos and antihypertensives as well as sedatives appear to produce a minor. transient, reduction in some cases.[2,24,27,136] However, they are not recommended.

Women who are experiencing hot flashes (1) are more likely to have lower estradiol levels than women who are not and (2) probably have elevated FSH levels.[21] These women are the ones who are most likely to respond to hormone therapies.

Regardless of the exact mechanism of a hot flash, it is clear that estrogen replacement therapy for perimenopausal or postmenopausal women offers the most effective way of relieving the symptoms. Although the exact dose that is most effective appears to vary from woman to woman and probably reflects her own degree of withdrawal as well as her basal level of estrogen, some data have been gleaned to suggest usual effective doses. For details of the studies, the reader is referred to Chapter 4 on hormone replacement therapy and to Chapter 7 on the dosages studied experimentally.

WELL-BEING AND MENTAL PERFORMANCE: THE RELATION TO HORMONES

The question of the affective symptoms—depression, insomnia, irritability, and loss of concentration—is elusive. Some investigators have shown an excellent response to hormone therapy in women who have affective symptoms. Others have not. There are many reasons for depression, and when the affective symptoms are related to an altered endocrine milieu, one can expect a positive response to hormone therapies. The question will be for the clinician to determine the causes and the relative components involved in the affective problems. Only time with the patient and patience and understanding are likely to bring out that information.

Depression in middle-aged women is a common phenomenon.[4,6,140] Schleyer-Saunders noted that depression occurs more commonly in three specific phases of a woman's life: after childbirth, at the menopause, and during the secretory phase of the menstrual cycle. Declines in endogenous estrogen occur coincidentally with these phases.[140]

Women commonly report that, as they approach the menopause, their premenstrual mood swings (tension, depression, irritability) are becoming increasingly more severe. If one looks at Figure 1–7 and considers the life and monthly cycle of change in estrogen level, a simple explanation emerges. With increasing age, the tendency is for increased *preovulatory* estrogen levels (perhaps due to higher gonadotropins, more cystic follicular content, and general incompetence of the ovulatory mechanism). At the same time, the *premenstrual* levels of estrogen show a trend toward lower levels than in earlier years. Thus, the swings from high (first part of cycle) to low (premenstrual) get wider with age. The fact that this swing in menstrual cycle levels of estrogen fluctuation coincides with the common affective experience of women probably reflects a strong influence of ovarian steroids on these mood swings. A sensitive clinician will be, at the very least, able to offer the patient the comfort of this information to show that this too will pass—or he or she may choose to treat it with premenstrual estrogen as the menopause approaches.

Gonadotropins have also been studied. Altman and co-workers showed that LH levels are significantly lower in depressed women than in age-matched controls.[3] Their findings provided additional support for the idea of diminished hypothalamic noradrenergic activity in depressive illness. Several investigators have evaluated the influence of estrogens or estrogens with progestins on the well-being and mental performance of perimenopausal and postmenopausal women.[38,46,53,116] One particularly complex study evaluated three groups of outpatients with climacteric complaints, all of whom were told (though not necessarily given) that they were getting estrogen treatment. Two forms of estrogen, both with progestins, were administered; a placebo was given to the third group. Assessments were made before treatment and then at 1, 3, and 6 months after treatment had begun.[46] Results were particularly reflective of changes in well-being in those on hormones that did not occur in those on placebos. Thyroid function was unchanged as were cholesterol and triglyceride levels. Plasma estrogen levels increased gradually throughout the period of the study, but not significantly until after 6 months had passed in those women who were taking estrogen. As expected, plasma estrogens did not increase in those women who were taking placebos. Behavior and emotional scales indicated that women who took hormones became less neurotic with passage of time, more extroverted, less depressed, and that their concentration improved. Estrogen was noted to have a positive effect in improving libido, sexual activity, satisfaction, fantasy, and capacity for orgasm. Postmenopausal women consistently showed pretreatment levels of libido that were lower than perimenopausal women's pretreatment levels of libido. Placebos were not helpful; hormone therapies were. As time passed, the placebo group deteriorated slightly on all scales of affect and sexual response that were measured. Because the study was double-blind and the groups given placebos were told they were taking hormones, the positive changes in those on hormone therapy are particularly noteworthy. Others have provided data suggesting similar positive responses to hormone therapies. Dennerstein and co-workers, in a double-blind study of 49 postoophorectomy patients, found that estrogen and progestogen had a pharmacological effect on mood, anxiety, irritability, and insomnia. All improved on ethinyl estradiol therapy (50 μg/day for 3 months). Progestins (levonorgesterol 250 μg/day) initially produce less favorable results, but initial problems with progestins diminished by the third therapy month and patients showed a trend toward improvement.[38] Other studies have confirmed this one.[53,116] For details of the research design and results, the reader is referred to Chapter 4.

Sleep disturbances are common during the menopausal transition as well; they often are coincident with night sweats.[44] These sweats at night are commonly associated with daytime hot flashes. Nocturnal hormone changes are revealing. The relationship between nocturnal plasma estrogen concentration and free plasma tryptophan in perimenopausal women has been established.[160] Estrogen fluctuations and free plasma tryptophan from three perimenopausal women showed positive correlation of 0.9995, suggesting that the two are directly related to each other. The author suggested that since both tryptophan and estrogen bind to albumins, the correlation is due to a direct action of estrogen on the tryptophan binding site of albumin. The same authors also studied the effect of estrogen on the sleep, mood, and anxiety of menopausal women.[161] In sleep laboratories, patients on estrogen therapies showed marked improvements in all parameters of sleep. Dream-stage sleep tended to increase in those on estrogen therapies, and sleep disruptions during the night tended to decrease. Because the psychological literature has occasionally indicated a relationship between the loss of dream sleep and psychological disturbances, it may be that one of the influences of estrogen on well-being is to increase the amount of time an individual can be dreaming and thereby, in some as yet undefined way, improve well-being during the daytime.

Dennerstein evaluated the effect of estrogen therapies on the tendency to have headaches in postoophorectomy patients.[36] These patients reported significantly more headaches in the estrogen-free period of the cyclic hormone regimen as well as when shifting (in double-blind crossover study) from estrogen to placebo.[36]

HIRSUTISM AND HORMONES

Hirsutism is a reflection of an androgen excess and can be caused by any one of a number of different alterations. In the menopause, hirsutism commonly does not reflect pathology, but rather the shifting in balance from an estrogen-dominated ovary to an androgen-dominated one. The consideration of categories of etiology of androgen excess is beyond the scope of this book, but the most common causes include the following:

Functional disorders of the adrenal
neoplastic disorders of the adrenal
functional disorders of the ovary
neoplastic disorders of the ovary
hypersensitivity of the target organs

These conditions are all variances from the normal and should be investigated. Treatment should be designed for the specific need.

It is useful to define the normal changes with age and consider their implications. The persistent release of androgens, particularly testosterone, by the postmenopausal ovary, probably explains in part some of the hirsutism and defeminization so common in older women.[22] Strickler and Warren have defined hirsutism as the growth of terminal coarse hair on the midline area of the lip, chin, chest, abdomen, and back, reflective of androgen overproduction.[152] They note that only the free hormone is biologically active, and 99% of testosterone is bound to SHBG, albumin, and transcortin. Potency in different androgens has been evaluated by a bioassay on seminal vesicles of male rat. If testosterone is given a scale of 100, the relative potency of dihydrotesterone is 200, that of androstenedione is 20, DHEA, 3, and DHEAS, also 3. One notes that androgens are metabolized in tissue. For example, there is biotransformation in the lung, the liver, the placenta, and the skin.[152] Lobo and co-workers recently showed that peripheral transformation accounts for a very large fraction of hirsutism.[90] Strickler notes that 95% of hirsute women have hypersecretion of testosterone from the ovary or peripheral biotransformation and that a pure adrenal source for hirsutism in adult women is rare.[152] The 17-ketosteroid concentration usually provides a poor index of hyperandrogenism, because testosterone is not associated with this condition. Serum testosterone is the single best monitor of the endocrine milieu of androgen excess and a free testosterone level above 45 pg/ml or a total testosterone level above 2 ng/ml correlates with severe hirsutism.[152]

Appropriate therapy for androgen excess depends upon the source of the problem. Ovarian suppression, adrenal suppression, cosmetic approaches, and other approaches are all potentially useful, and the interested clinician is referred to specialty papers on this subject.[63,65]

Thus the clinician should be alerted to the range of underlying conditions that may be reflective of the appearance of hirsutism in the menopausal woman. Having ruled out an underlying pathologic condition, the physician should consider the severity and, most often, treatment will not be necessary.

OSTEOARTHROSIS AND HORMONES

Dequeker and colleagues have evaluated the effect of long-term estrogen treatment on the development of osteoarthrosis of the small hand joints.[40] No significant difference in osteoarthrosis between treated and untreated women after 5 years of estrogen replacement therapy was observed. The development of osteoarthrosis was therefore assumed to be independent of endocrine status at menopause.

URINARY PROBLEMS AND HORMONE LEVELS

As described earlier, there are age changes in the female urethra that parallel estrogen decline. Urinary incontinence appears more commonly to reflect a muscle tone deficiency than a hormone deficiency. Postmenopausal urinary problems are similar to those of earlier years but some authors have suggested that they are accelerated with estrogen deficiencies.[13] The physiological aging process speeds up after menopause and there appears to be no clear hormonal cause for these problems. Nonetheless, effective physiological therapy for urinary stress incontinence has long been available in the form of the Kegel exercises.[80] According to Kegel, who quantified his terms, loss of function of the pubococcygeus muscles is present in all women with true urinary stress incontinence. In those with normal function, there is a 30- to 60-mm Hg reading (of transducer in vagina) on contraction. In those with urinary stress incontinence, the muscular function is poor or absent and readings of 0 to 5 mm Hg are common. Therapy consists of retraining the woman to tense the pubococcygeus muscles by teaching her to localize the contracting muscle surrounding a tampon or other agent in the vagina. Patients should be encouraged to continue with their efforts at contracting these pubococcygeus muscles, although their efforts may appear to be puny. In time these muscles do strengthen in response to repeated contractions.[80] Kegel has suggested 20 minutes, 3 times a day for a total of 300 contractions as a level to aim for. It appears not to matter whether the contractions be broken into 3 sessions a day or 20; it is the overall exercise to the muscles that is important. He reported complete relief in 6 to 8 weeks if the problem was of the simple type. Those with incapacitating urinary incontinence yielded an 84% complete relief in spite of prior failure to respond to surgery.[80] Kegel noted that he had gratifying responses in women even into their eighties. The tone and function of the muscles of the pelvic outlet can be restored through this muscle reeducation; and active exercise is desirable.

In contrast, Brown noted that although skeletal muscle is little affected by hormone deficiencies, connective tissue is; the latter condition alters the support of the pelvic organs, mainly the pelvic floor and transverse ligaments, therefore contributing to uterine prolapse.[13] In reviewing the literature, Brown noted that stress incontinence afflicts over 25% of women but is not an age-dependent phenomenon. Nocturnal frequency of micturition, though not associated with infection, is associated with central deterioration, which may be secondary to atherosclerosis or cerebral senescence. Sixty-one percent of the elderly (65+) experienced nocturnal frequency. Those under 65 had half the incidence. Obesity also was a contributing factor to urinary trouble, and its reversal could improve leakage problems. Estrogen cream (0.01 mg estradiol) vaginally applied (nightly) initially reversed those atrophic urogenital changes of a hormonal-dependent nature.[13]

It therefore seems that the estrogen-dependent tissue will respond to hormone therapy, although the muscle tone itself will respond most effectively to exercise of the pubococcygeus muscles.

CONCLUSIONS

There are major age-related changes in ovarian function that in turn produce menopausal changes characteristic of estrogen decline. The critical problem confronting the clinician is to differentiate pathology from ovarian atrophy. Those conditions caused by ovarian atrophy and reflective of drops in steroid production respond readily to estrogen replacement therapies.

Chapter 2 describes, in detail, the changes in bone physiology and their relationships to hormones. Following this, several chapters discuss hormone replacement therapy: benefits, indications, and contraindications; risks in relation to cancer; and the role of hormones in heart disease.

It is interesting to note that the great Eastern philosophies have a recurrent theme in their prescriptions for a well-lived existence. They state that a woman should not devote more than 20 years, or the middle stage of her life, to reproductive and child-care functions. Evidence gathered by anatomists and physiologists shows that the ovary may be a "pacemaker" for such a design.

REFERENCES

1. Abe T, Furuhashi N, Yamaya Y, Wada Y, Hoshiai A, Suzuki M (1977) Correlation between climacteric symptoms and serum levels of estradiol, progesterone, follicle stimulation hormone and luteinizing hormone. *Am J Obstet Gynecol* 129:1:65–67.
2. Albrecht BH, Schiff I, Tulchinsky D, Ryan K (1981) Objective evidence that placebo and oral medroxyprogesterone acetate therapy diminish menopausal vasomotor flushes. *Am J Obstet Gynecol* 139:631–635.
3. Altman N, Sachar EJ, Gruen PH, Halpern FS (1975) Reduced plasma LH concentration in postmenopausal depressed women. *Psychosomat Medicine* 37:3:274–276.
4. Ballinger CB (1975) Psychiatric morbidity and the menopause: screening of general population sample. *Br Med J* 3:5979:344–346.
5. Barret L, Cullis W, Fairfield L, Nicholson R, MacNaughton M, Williamson CF, Sanderson AE (1933) Investigation of menopause in 1000 women. Subcommittee of the Council of Medical Women's Federation of England. *Lancet* 1:106–108.
6. Bart, P (1971) Depression in middle-aged women. In: *Women in a Sexist Society.* Gornick V, Moran BK (eds). Spring Valley CA, Mentor.
7. Balog J (1980) Obesity and estrogen. *Am J Obstet Gynecol* January 15, 1980:242.
8. Barlow J, Emerson K, Saxena (1969) Estradiol production after ovariectomy for carcinoma of the breast. *N Engl J Med* 28:633–637.
9. Bates GW (1981) On the nature of the hot flash. *Clin Obstet Gynecol* 24:231–241.
10. Bengtsson C, Lindquist O, Redvall L (1979) Is the menopausal age rapidly changing? *Maturitas* 1:159–164.
11. Bohler C, Greenblatt RB (1974) The pathophysiology of the hot flush. In: *The Menopausal Syndrome.* Greenblatt RB, Mahesh VB, McDonough PG (eds). New York, Medcom Press.
12. Botella-Llusia J, Oriol-Bosch A, Sanchez-Garrido F, Tresquerres JAF (1980) Testosterone and 17 B oestradiol secretion of the human ovary. 11 normal postmenopausal women, postmenopausal women with endometrial hyperplasia and postmenopausal women with adenocarcinoma of the endometrium. *Maturitas* 2:7–12.
13. Brown ADG (1977) Postmenopausal urinary problems. *Clin Obstet Gynecol* 4:181–206.
14. Budoff PW, Sommers J (1979) Estrogen-progesterone therapy in postmenopausal women. *J Reprod Med* 22:5:241–247.
15. Bye PB (1978) Review of the status of oestrogen replacement therapy. *Postgrad Med J* 54:2:7–10.
16. Calkins E (1981) Aging of cells and people. *Clin Obstet Gynecol* 24:165–179.
17. Campbell S, Goswamy R, Goessens L, Whitehead M (1982) Real time ultrasonography for determination of ovarian morphology and volume. *Lancet* Fe 20 1982:425–426.
18. Casper RF, Yen SSC, Wilkes MM (1979) Menopausal flushes: a neuroendocrine link with pulsatile luteinizing hormone secretion. *Science* 205:823–825.
19. Casper RF, Yen SSC (1981) Menopausal flushes: effect of pituitary gonadotropin desensitization by a potent luteinizing hormone releasing factor agonist. *J Clin Endocrinol Metab* 53:1056–1058.
20. Chakravarti S, Collins WP, Forecast JD, Newton JR, Oran DH, Studd JWW (1976) Hormonal profiles after the menopause. *Br Med J* 2:784–786.
21. Chakravarti S, Collins WP, Thom MH, Studd JWW (1979) Relation between plasma hormone profiles, symptoms, and response to oestrogen treatment in women approaching the menopause. *Br Med J* 1:983–985.
22. Chang RJ, Judd HL (1981) The ovary after menopause. *Clin Obstet Gynecol* 24:181–191.
23. Christensson T (1976) Menopausal age of females with hypercalcaemia. A study including cases with primary hyperparathyroidism, detected in a health screening. *Acta Med Scand* 200:5:361–365.

24. Claydon JR, Bell JY, Pollard P (1974) Menopausal flushing: double blind trial of a non-hormonal medication. *Br Med J* 1:409–412.

25. Coble Y, Kohler P, Cargille CM, Ross GT (1969) Production rates and metabolic clearance rates of human follicle-stimulating hormone in premenopausal and postmenopausal women. *J Clin Invest* 48:359–363.

26. Collet ME, Wertenberger GE, Fiske VM (1954) The effect of age upon the pattern of the menstrual cycle. *Fertil Steril* 5:437.

27. Coope J, Williams S, Patterson JS (1978) A study of the effectiveness of propranolol in menopausal hot flushes. *Br J Obstet Gynaecol* 85:6:472–475.

28. Costoff A, Mahesh VB (1975) Primordial follicles with normal oocytes in the ovaries of postmenopausal women. *J Am Geriatr Soc* 23:5:193–196

29. Crawford MP, Hooper D (1973) Menopause, ageing and family. *Soc Sci Med* 7:469–482.

30. Crilly RG, Horsman A, Marshall DH, Nordin BEC (1978) Postmenopausal and corticosteroid induced osteoporosis. *Front Horm Res* 5:53–71.

31. Crilly RG, Marshall DH, Nordin BE (1979) Effect of age on plasma androstenedione concentration in oophorectomized women. *Clin Endocrinol (Oxf)* 10:2:199–201.

32. Cutler WB, Garcia CR (1980) The psychoneuroendocrinology of the ovulatory cycle of woman. *Psychoneuroendocrinology* 5:89–111.

33. Daniell HW (1976) Osteoporosis of the slender smoker. *Arch Intern Med* 136:298–304.

34. DeKretser DM, Burger HG, Dumpys R (1978) Patterns of serum LH and FSH in response to 4 hour infusions of luteinizing hormone releasing hormone in normal women during menstrual cycle, on oral contraceptives, and in postmenopausal state. *J Clin Endocrinol Metab* 46:227–235.

35. Dennefors B, Janson P, Knutson F, Hamberger L (1980) Steroid production and responsiveness to gonadotropin in isolated stromal tissue of human postmenopausal ovaries. *Am J Obstet Gynecol* 136:997–1002.

36. Dennerstein L, Laby B, Burrows G, Hyman G (1978) Headache and sex hormone therapy. *Headache* 18:146–153.

37. Dennerstein L, Wood C, Hudson B, Burrows G (1978) Clinical features and plasma hormone levels after surgical menopause. *Aust NZ J Obstet Gynaecol* 18:3:202–205.

38. Dennerstein L, Burrows G, Hyman G (1979) Hormone therapy and effect. *Maturitas* 1:247–259.

39. Dennerstein L, Burrow G, Hyman G (1978) Menopausal hot flushes: a double blind comparison of placebo ethinyl oestradiol and norgesterel. *Br J Obstet Gynaecol* 85:852–856.

40. Dequeker J, de Proft G, Ferin J (1978) The effect of long-term oestrogen treatment on the development of osteoarthrosis at the small hand joints. *Maturitas* 1:27–30.

41. Dor P, Muquardt C, L'Hermite M, Borkowski A (1978) Influence of corticotrophin and prolactin on the steroid sex hormones and their precursors in postmenopausal women. *J Endocrinol* 77:263–264.

42. Easley EB (1978) Sex problems after the menopause. *Clin Obstet Gynecol* 21:1:269–277.

43. Edman CD, MacDonald PC (1978) Effect of obesity on conversion of plasma androstenedione to estrone in ovulatory and anovulatory young women. *Am J Obstet Gynecol* 130:456–461.

44. Erlik Y, Tataryn IV, Meldrum DR, Lomax P, Bajorek JG, Judd HL (1981) Association of waking episodes with menopausal hot flushes. *JAMA* 245:1741–1744.

45. Erickson B (1979) Emotional, sexual and hormonal differences in women with long and short menses. *Eastern Conference on Reproductive Behavior,* Tulane University, June 1979.

46. Fedor-Freybergh, P (1977) The influence of estrogens on the well-being and mental performance in climacteric and postmenopausal women. *Acta Obstet Gynecol Scand* 64:1–66.

47. Feldman JM, Postlethwaite RW, Glenn JF (1976) Hot flashes and sweats in men with testicular insufficiency. *Arch Intern Med* 136:5:606–608.

48. Fienberg R, Cohen RB (1965) A comparative histochemical study of the ovarian stromal lipid band, stromal theca cell, and normal ovarian follicular apparatus. *Am J Obstet Gynecol* 92:958–969.

49. Finch CE (1976) The regulation of physiological changes during mammalian aging. *O Rev Biol* 51:49–83.

50. Frumar A, Meldrum D, Geola F, Shamonki I, Tataryn I, Deftos L, Judd H (1980) Relationship of fasting urinary calcium to circulating estrogen and body weight in postmenopausal women. *J Clin Endocrinol Metab* 50:70–75.

51. Gaddum-Rosse P, Rumery RE, Blandau RJ, Thiersch JB (1975) Studies on the mucosa of postmenopausal oviducts: surface appearance, ciliary activity, and the effect of estrogen treatment. *Fertil Steril* 26:10:951–969.

52. Geller S, Scholler R (1980) FSH and LH pituitary reserve and output in the postmenopause. *Maturitas* 2:45–52.

53. Gerdes LC, Sonnendecker EWW, Polakow ES (1982) Psychological changes effected by estrogen-progesterone and clonidine treatment in climacteric women. *Am J Obstet Gynecol* 42:98–104.

54. Goodman MJ, Stewart CJ, Gilbert F Jr. (1977) Patterns of menopause: a study of certain medical and physiological variables among caucasian and Japanese women living in Hawaii. *J Gerontol* 32:291–298.

55. Grattarola R, Secreto G, Recchione C (1975) Correlation between urinary testosterone or estrogen excretion levels and interstitial cell-stimulation hormone concentrations in normal postmenopausal women. *Am J Obstet Gynecol* 121:3:380–381.

56. Greenblatt RB (1974) Reprise. In: *The Menopausal Syndrome* Greenblatt RB, Mahesh VB, McDonough PG (eds). New York, Medcom Press.

57. Greenblatt RB, Natrajan PK, Tzingounis V (1979) Role of the hypothalamus in the aging woman. *J Am Geriatr Soc* 27:3:97–103.

58. Greene J-G (1976) A factor analytic study of climacteric symptoms. *J Psychosom Res* 20:5:425–430.

59. Gribb JJ (1960) Hysteroscopy as an aid in gynecologic diagnosis. *Obstet Gynecol* 15:593–601.

60. Grodin JM, Siiteri PK, Macdonald PC (1973) Source of estrogen production in postmenopausal women. *J Clin Endocrinol Metab* 36:207.

61. Guraya S (1976) Histochemical observations on the corpus luteum atreticum of the human postmenopausal ovary with reference to steroid hormone synthesis. *Arch Ital Anat Embriol* 56:189–202.

62. Hagen C, Christiansen C, Christensen MS, Transbol I (1982) Climacteric symptoms, fat mass, and plasma concentrations of LH, FSH, Prl, oestradiol 17B and androstenedione in the early postmenopausal period. *Acta Endocrinol* (Copenh) 100:4:486–491.

63. Hammond CB, Riddick DH, Wentz AC (1983) Gynecologic problems in gynecologic endocrinology. *Sixteenth Annual Postgraduate Course: The American Fertility Society.*

64. Hasselquist M, Goldberg N, Schroeter A, Spelsberg T (1980) Isolation and characterization of the estrogen receptor in human skin. *J Clin Endocrinol Metab* 50:76–82.

65. Hatch R, Rosenfield RL, Kim MH, Tredway D (1981) Hirsutism: implications, etiology and management. *Am J Obstet Gynecol* 140:815–830.

66. Hemsell DLI, Grodin JM, Brenner PF, Siiteri PK, MacDonald PC (1974) Plasma precursors of estrogen II Correlation of the extent of conversion of plasma androstenedione to estrone with age. *J Clin Endocrinol Metab* 38:476.

67. Hemsell DL, Siiteri PK, MacDonald PC (1972) Estrogen derived from plasma androstenedione. *Presentation to the Armed Forces District Meeting of the American College of Obstetricians and Gynecologists, Seattle,* October 1972.

68. Hertig AT (1944) The aging ovary, a preliminary note. *J Clin Endocrinol Metab* 4:581.

69. Huffman JW, Dewhurst CJ, Capravio VJ (1981) Anatomy and physiology. In: *The Gynecology of Childhood and Adolescence.* Huffman JW, Dewhurst CJ, Capravio VJ (eds). Philadelphia, WB Saunders Co.

70. Hunter J (1787) An experiment to determine the effect of extirpating one ovarium upon the number of young produced. *Philos Trans R Soc Lond (Biol) London* 77:233.

71. Hutton JD, Jacobs HS, James VHT, Murray MAF, Rippon AE (1977) Episodic secretion of steroid hormones in postmenopausal women. *J Endocrinol* 73:25.

72. Hutton JD, Jacobs HS, James VHT, Murray MAF, Rippon AE (1977) Acute effect of dexamethasone and adrenocorticotrophin on steroid hormone concentrations of postmenopausal and ovariectomized women. *J Endocrinol* 73:26.

73. Hutton JD, Jacobs HS, Murray MA, James VH (1978) Relation between plasma oestrone and oestradiol and climacteric symptoms. *Lancet* 1:8066:678–681.

74. Jaszmann LJB (1973) Epidemiology of climacteric and post climacteric complaints. *Front Horm Res* 2:22–34.

75. Jick H, Porter J, Morrison AS (1977) Relation between smoking and age of natural menopause: report from the Boston Collaborative Drug Surveillance Program, Boston University Medical Center. *Lancet* 1:8026:1354–1355.

76. Judd HL, Lucas WE, Yen SC (1974) Effect of oophorectomy on circulating testosterone and androstenedione levels in patients with endometrial cancer. *Am J Obstet Gynecol* 38:793–798.

77. Judd HL, Yen SSC (1973) Serum androstenedione and testosterone levels during the menstrual cycle. *J Clin Endocrinol Metab* 36:475–481.

78. Judd HL (1976) Hormonal dynamics associated with the menopause. *Clinical Obstet Gynecol* 19:775–788.
79. Judd HL, Judd GE, Lucas WE, Yen SSC (1974) Endocrine function of postmenopausal ovary: concentration of androgens and estrogens in ovarian and peripheral vein blood. *J Clin Endocrinol Metab* 39:1020.
80. Kegel AM (1951) Physiologic therapy for urinary stress incontinence. *JAMA* 146:915–917.
81. Kemeter P, Salzer H, Breitenecker G, Friedrich F (1975) Progesterone, oestradiol-17B and testosterone levels; in the follicular fluid of tertiary follicles and Graafian Follicles of human ovaries. *Acta Endocrinol* (Copenh) 80:686–704.
82. Kohler PO, Ross GT, Odell WD (1968) Metabolic clearance and production rates of human LH in pre- and postmenopausal women. *J Clin Invest* 47:38–47.
83. Korenman SG, Sherman BM, Korenman JC (1978) Reproductive hormone function: the perimenopausal period and beyond. *Clin Endocrinol Metab* 7:3:625–643.
84. Kronenberg F, Carraway R, Cote LJ, Linkie DM, Crawshaw LI, Downey JA (1981) *Proceedings of 62nd Annual Meeting of American Endocrine Society*, 141:abst. 236.
85. Larsen B, Galask R (1980) Vaginal microbial flora: practical and theoretic relevance. *Obstet Gynecol* 55:5 suppl. 100s–113s.
86. Leiblum S, Bachman G, Kemmann E, Colburn D, Swartzman L (1983) Vaginal atrophy in the postmenopausal woman: the importance of sexual activity and hormones. *JAMA* 249:2195–2198.
87. Lindhe J, Attstrom R, Bjorn AL (1969) The influence of progestogen on gingival exudation during menstrual cycles. *J Periodont Res* 4:97–102.
88. Lindquist O, Bengtsson C (1979) The effect of smoking on menopausal age. *Maturitas* 1:171–174.
89. Lindsay R, Coutts JR, Hart DM (1977) The effect of endogenous oestrogen on plasma and urinary calcium and phosphate in oophorectomized women. *Clin Endocrinol (Oxf)* 6:2:87–93.
90. Lobo R (1983) Presented at American Fertility Society Meeting, San Francisco.
91. Longcope C (1971) Metabolic clearance and blood production rates of estrogens in postmenopausal women. *Am J Obstet Gynecol* 111:778–781.
92. Longcope C, Hunter R, Franz C (1980) Steroid secretion by the postmenopausal ovary. *Am J Obstet Gynecol* 138:564–568.
93. Longcope C, Jatee W, Griffing G (1981) Production rates of androgens and oestrogens in postmenopausal women. *Maturitas* 3:215–223.
94. Longcope C, Pratt JH, Schneider SH, Fineberg SE (1978) Aromatization of androgens by muscle and adipose tissues in vivo. *J Clin Endocrinol Metab* 46:146–152.
95. MacDonald PC, Edman CD, Hemsell DL, Porter JC, Siiteri PK (1978) Effect of obesity on conversion of plasma androstenedione to estrone in postmenopausal women with and without endometrial cancer. *Am J Obstet Gynecol* 130:4:448–455.
96. MacMahon B, Worcester J (1966) National Center for Health Statistics, Age at Menopause, U.S. 1960–1962. Washington DC USPHS Publication 1000, Series 11, No. 19.
97. Main DMG, Ritchie GM (1967) Cyclic changes in oral smears from young menstruating women. *Br J Dermatol* 73:20–30.
98. Maoz B, Antonovsky A, Apter A, et al (1978) The effect of outside work on the menopausal woman. *Maturitas* 1:43.
99. Marks R, Shahrad P (1977) Skin changes at the time of the climacteric. *Clinics Obstet Gynaecol* 4:207–226.
100. Mattingly RF, Huang WY (1969) Steroidogenesis of the menopausal and postmenopausal ovary. *Am J Obstet Gynecol* 103:679–693.
101. McKinlay SM, Jeffreys M (1974) The menopausal syndrome. *Br J Prev Soc Med* 28:108–115.
102. McNatty KP, Makris A, DeGrazia C, Osathanondh R, Ryan KJ (1979) The production of progesterone, androgens, and estrogens by granulosa cells, thecal tissue and stromal tissue by human ovaries in vitro. *J Clin Endocrinol Metab* 49:687–699.
103. Medina M, Scaglia HE, Vazquez G, Alatorre S, Perez-Palacios G (1976) Rapid oscillation of circulating gonadotropins in postmenopausal women. *J Clin Endocrinol Metab* 43:5:1015–1019.
104. Meisels A (1966) The menopause: a cytohormonal study. *Acta Cytol* 10:49–55.
105. Meldrum DR, Davidson B, Tataryn I, Judd H (1981) Changes in circulating steroids with aging in postmenopausal women. *Obstet Gynecol* 57:624–628.

106. Meldrum DR, Erlik Y, Lu JK, Judd HL (1981) Objectively recorded hot flashes in patients with pituitary insufficiency. *J Clin Endocrinol Metab* 52:684–687.

107. Meldrum D, Tataryn I, Frumar A, Erlik J, Lu K, Judd H (1980) Gonadotropins, estrogens, and adrenal steroids during the menopausal hot flash. *J Clin Endocrinol Metab* 50:685–689.

108. Metcalf MG (1979) Incidence of ovulatory cycles in women approaching the menopause. *J Biosoc Sci* 11:39–48.

109. Mikhail G (1970) Hormone secretion by the human ovaries. *Gynecol Obstet Invest* 1:5–20.

110. Milewich L, Gomez-Sanchez C, Madden JD, Bradfield DJ, Parker PM, Smith SL, Carr BR, Edman CD, Macdonald PC (1978) Dehydroisoandrosterone sulfate in peripheral blood of premenopausal, pregnant, and postmenopausal women and men. *J Steroid Biochem* 9:12:1159–1164.

111. Mills TM, Mahesh VB (1977) Gonadotropin secretion in the menopause. *Clinics Obstet Gynaecol* 4:71–84.

112. Molnar GW (1975) Body temperatures during menopausal hot flashes. *J Appl Physiol* 38:3:499–503.

113. Molnar GW (1981) Menopausal hot flashes: their cycles and relation to air temperature. *Obstet Gynecol* 57:525–555.

114. Monroe SE, Menon KMJ (1977) Changes in reproductive hormone secretion during the climacteric and postmenopausal periods. *Clin Obstet Gynecol* 20:1:113–122.

115. Mulley G, Mitchell JRA, Tattersall RB (1977) Hot flushes after hypophysectomy. *Br Med J* 2:1062.

116. Navratil J, Novakova D, Pichner J (1975) The treatment of climacteric disorders with a combination of estradiol and testosterone—an outline of the pathogenesis of psychic symptoms in the climacterion. *Activ Nerv Supp (Praha)* 17:4:307–308.

117. Nelson JF, Felicio LS, Randall PK, Sims C, Finch C (1982) A longitudinal study of estrous cyclicity in aging C57BL/BJ mice: 1. cycle frequency, length and vaginal cytology. *Biol Reprod* 27:327–339.

118. Nicosia SV (1983) Morphological changes in the human ovary through life. In: *The Ovary.* Serra GB. New York, Raven Press. pp 57–81.

119. Notelovitz, M (1978) The menopause and its treatment. *J Fla Med Assoc* 65:341–344.

120. Novak ER (1970) Ovulation after fifty. *Obstet Gynecol* 36:903–910.

121. Novak ER, Goldberg B, Jones GS (1965) Enzyme histochemistry of the menopausal ovary associated with normal and abnormal endometrium. *Am J Obstet Gynecol* 93:669–673.

122. O'Dea JP, Wieland RG, Hallberg MC, Llerena LA, Zorn EM, Genuth SM (1979) Effect of dietary weight loss on sex steroid binding, sex steroids and gonadotropins in obese postmenopausal women. *J Lab Clin Med* 93:6:1007–1008.

123. O'Dea JP, Wieland RG, Hallberg MC, Llerena LA, Zorn EM, Genuth SM (1979) Effect of dietary weight loss on sex steroid binding, sex steroids, and gonadotropins in obese postmenopausal women. *J Lab Clin Med* 93:6:1004–1008.

124. Pisantry S, Rafaely B, Polishuk W (1975) The effect of steroid hormones on buccal mucosa of menopausal women. *Oral Surg* 40:3:346–353.

125. Punnonen R (1972) Effect of castration and peroral estrogen therapy on the skin. *Acta Obstet Gynecol Scand* (Suppl) 21:1–44.

126. Punnonen R, Rauramo L (1977) The effect of long-term oral oestriol succinate therapy on the skin of castrated women. *Ann Chir Gynaecol* 66:4:214–215.

127. Purifoy FE, Koopmans LH, Tatum RW (1980) Steroid hormones and aging: free testosterone, testosterone and androstenedione in normal females aged 20–87 years. *Hum Biol* 52:181–191.

128. Rader MD, Flickinger GL, deVilla GO, Mikuta JJ, Mikhail G (1973) Plasma estrogens in postmenopausal women. *Am J Obstet Gynecol* 116:1069–1073.

129. Reyes FI, Winter JSD, Faiman C (1977) Pituitary-ovarian relationships preceding the menopause. I. A cross-sectional study of serum follicle-stimulating hormone, prolactin, estradiol, and progesterone levels. *Am J Obstet Gynecol* 129:557–564.

130. Reynolds SRM (1949) *Physiology of the Uterus,* 2nd Edition. New York, Harper and Brothers.

131. Robertson DM, Landgren BM (1975) Oestradiol receptor levels in the human fallopian tube during the menstrual cycle and after menopause. *J Steroid Biochem* 6:3–4:511–513.

132. Rodin M, Moghissi KS (1973) Intrinsic innervation of the human cervix: a preliminary study. *The Biology of the Human Cervix.* Blandau RJ, Moghissi K (eds). Chicago, University of Chicago Press.

133. Rutherford AM (1978) The menopause. *NZ Med J* 87:251–253.

134. Ryan TJ (1966) The microcirculation of the skin in old age. *Geront Clin* 8:327–337.

135. Ryan TJ, Kurban AK (1970) New vessel growth in the adult skin. *Br J Dermatol* 82:5:92–98.

136. Salmi T, Punnonen R (1979) Clonidine in the treatment of menopausal symptoms. *Int J Gynaecol Obstet* 16:422–426.
137. Sanyal MK, Berger MJ, Thompson IE, Taymor ML, Horne HW (1974) Development of graafian follicles in adult human ovary. 1. Correlation of estrogen and progesterone concentration in antral fluid with growth of follicles. *J Clin Endocrinol Metab* 38:828–835.
138. Saxena BN, Poshyachinda V, Dusitin N (1976) A study of the use of intermittent serum luteinizing hormone, progesterone and oestradiol measurements for the detection of ovulation. *Br J Obstet Gynaecol* 83:660–664.
139. Scaglin H, Medina M, Pinto-Ferreira AL, Vazques G, Gual C, Perez-Palacios G (1976) Pituitary LH & FSH section and responsiveness in women of old age. *Acta Endocrinol (Copenh)* 81:673–679.
140. Schleyer-Saunders E (1974) Social and gerontological problems of the menopause: Hormonal implants. In: *The Menopausal Syndrome*. Greenblatt RB, Mahesh VB, McDonough PG (eds). New York, Medcom Press.
141. Semmens JP, Wagner G (1982) Estrogen deprivation and vaginal function in postmenopausal women. *JAMA* 248:445–448.
142. Seyler LE, Reichlin S (1973) Luteinizing hormone releasing factor (LRF) in plasma of postmenopausal women. *J Clin Endocrinol Metab* 37:197–203.
143. Sherman BM, Korenman SG (1975) Hormonal characteristics of the human menstrual cycle throughout reproductive life. *J Clin Invest* 55:699–706.
144. Sherman BM, West JH, Korenman SG (1976) The menopausal transition; analysis of LH, FSH, estradiol, and progesterone concentrations during menstrual cycles of older women. *J Clin Endocrinol Metab* 42:629–636.
145. Shettles LB (1973) Ovulation, normal and abnormal. In: *The Ovary*, p 128. Grady, Smith (eds). Baltimore, Williams & Wilkins.
146. Smith P (1972) Age changes in the female urethra. *Br J Urol* 44:667–676.
147. Somma M, Sandor T, Lanthier A (1969) Site of origin of androgenic and estrogenic steroids in the normal human ovary. *J Clin Endocrinol* 29:457–466.
148. Stadel BV, Weiss N (1975) Characteristics of menopausal women: a survey of King and Pierce Counties in Washington, 1973–1974. *Am J Epidemiol* 102:3:209–216.
149. Stark M, Adonia A, Milwidsky A, Gilon G, Palti Z (1978) Can estrogens be useful for treatment of vaginal relaxation in elderly women? *Am J Obstet Gynecol* 131:585–586.
150. Stone SC, Mickal A, Rye PH (1975) Postmenopausal symptomatology, maturation index, and plasma estrogen levels. *Obstet Gynecol* 45:6:625–627.
151. Strathy JH, Coulam CB, Spelsburg TC (1982) Comparison of estrogen receptors in human premenopausal and postmenopausal uteri: indication of biologically inactive receptor in postmenopausal uteri. *Am J Obstet Gynecol* 142:372–382.
152. Strickler RC, Warren JC (1979) Hirsutism: diagnosis and management. *J Clin Endocrinol Metab* 45:1039–1048.
153. Sturdee DW, Wilson KA, Pipili E, Crocker AD (1978) Physiological aspects of menopausal hot flush. *Br Med J* 2:6130:79–80.
154. Szlachter BN, Nachtigall LE, Epstein J, Young BK, Weiss G (1979) Premature menopause: a reversible entity? *Obstet Gynecol* 54:396–398.
155. Tagatz GE, Kopher RA, Nagel TC, Okagaki T (1979) The clitoral index: a bioassay of androgenic stimulation. *Obstet Gynecol* 54:562–564.
156. Tataryn I, Meldrum D, Lu K, Frumar A, Judd H (1979) LH, FSH and skin temperature during the menopausal hot flash. *J Clin Endocrinol Metab* 49:152–154.
157. Taylor, Howard, McAuley P, Engle E (1951) The morphologic basis of ovarian function. *Am J Obstet Gynecol* 61:5:1056–1064.
158. Tervila L (1958) The weight of the ovaries after stress ending in death. *Ann Chir Gynaecol* 47:232–244.
159. Thompson B, Hart SA, Durno D (1973) Menopausal age and symptomatology in a general practice. *J Biosoc Sci* 5:71–82.
160. Thomson J, Maddock J, Aylward M, Oswald I (1977) Relationship between nocturnal plasma oestrogen concentration and free plasma tryptophan in perimenopausal women. *J Endocrinol* 72:395–396.
161. Thomson J, Oswald I (1977) Effect of oestrogen on the sleep, mood and anxiety of menopausal women. *Br Med J* 2:6098:317–319.
162. Treloar AE (1974) Menarche, menopause and intervening fecundability. *Hum Biol* 16:89–107.

163. Treloar AE (1981) Menstrual cyclicity and the premenopause. *Maturitas* 3:249–264.

164. Treloar AE, Boynton RE, Behn DG, Brown BW (1967) Variation of the human menstrual cycle through reproduction life. *Int J Fertil* 12:77–126.

165. Tsang B, Moon Y, Simpson C, Armstrong D (1979) Androgen biosynthesis in human ovarian follicles: cellular source, gonadotropic control, and adenosine 3,5-monophosphate mediation. *J Clin Endocrinol Metab* 48:153–158.

166. Utian WH (1975) Definitive symptoms of postmenopause—incorporating use of vaginal parabasal cell index. *Front Horm Res* 3:74–93.

167. Van Keep PA, Kellerhals JM (1974) The impact of socio-cultural factors on symptom formation. Some results of a study of aging women in Switzerland. *Psychother Psychosom* 23:1–6:251–263.

168. Vermeulen A (1976) The hormonal activity of the postmenopausal ovary. *J Clin Endocrinol Metab* 42:2:247–253.

169. Vermeulen A (1980) Sex hormone status of the postmenopausal woman. *Maturitas* 2:81–89.

170. Vermeulen A, Verdonck L (1978) Sex hormone concentrations in postmenopausal women. Relation to obesity, fat mass, age and years post-menopause. *Clin Endocrinol* (Oxf) 9:59–66.

171. Waldron I (1982) An analysis of causes of sex differences in mortality and morbidity. In *The Fundamental Connection Between Nature and Nurture*. Gove WR, Carpenter GR (eds). Lexington, Massachusetts, Lexington Books.

172. Wardlaw SL, Wehrenberg WB, Ferin M, Antunes JL, Frantz AG (1982) Effect of sex steroids on beta endorphin in hypophyseal portal blood. *J Clin Endocrinol Metab* 55:877–881.

173. Wiegerinck M, Poortman J, Agema A, Thjissen J (1980) Estrogen receptors in human vaginal tissue. *Maturitas* 2:59–68.

174. Wise AJ, Gross MA, Schalch DA (1973) Quantitative relationships of the pituitary gonadal axis in post-menopausal women. *J Lab Clin Med* 81:28–36.

175. Wyshak G (1978) Menopause in mothers of multiple births and mothers of singletons only. *Soc Biol* 25:1:52–61.

176. Yen SSC (1977) The biology of menopause. *J Reprod Med* 18:287–296.

Osteoporosis

As more attention has been paid to the ever increasing proportion of our mature population, a greater awareness and interest has been focused on the problems of bone degeneration. Although it was well described years ago, osteoporosis has, more recently, been extensively investigated.[11] The term describes the increased porosity (rarefaction) of bone. Usually it is a disease of the axial skeleton with most of the loss accruing to trabecular bone with thinning of the cortex.[21,125] The definitive clinical signs are vertebral or hip fractures, but by the time these fractures have been discovered, the disease is generally well progressed. Even so, vigorous treatment can help halt a further loss of bone at whatever state the treatment begins. Recovery from the fracture itself is generally underway at three weeks. Guided exercise after fracture helps speed the recovery process, perhaps through the improved morale.[125]

Osteoporosis has been characterized statistically by the degree of bone that is lost. When the percent of cortical area (to bone cross-sectional area) has diminished to a level that corresponds to minus 1.64 standard deviations of the general population average, a stage of decay has been reached that exceeds the 95th percentile of the range of bone densities among normal individuals.[47] This is statistically defined as osteoporosis. The measurements of total bone width, medullary bone width, and cortical bone width are all interrelated. By using the percentage of cortical area as an index of measurement, Garn was able to quantify these terms.[47] Figure 2–1 illustrates these regions.

INCIDENCE OF OSTEOPOROSIS

Only recently has the scope of this disease begun to be appreciated.

MORBIDITY RATES

The incidence of bone fracture varies depending both upon location of the fracture and upon geographic region of the population studied. For hip fracture, a variety of statistics has been gathered. Table 2–1 shows the annual age-specific incidence of hip fractures in males and in females in five different areas of the world: Britain, Hong Kong, Singapore, Sweden, and among the South African Bantu.[21] A comparison of these incidence rates indicates that Scandinavia and England experience the highest rates, whereas China has intermediate rates and the South African Bantu seem to have the lowest. Whether these influences are caused by genetics, by the influence of sun on skin, or by patterns of exercise is currently unclear but all factors appear to play a role. In the United States it is estimated that about 113,000 women and 34,000 men per year sustain a proximal hip

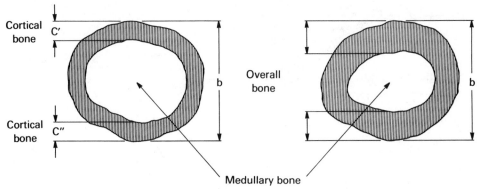

FIG. 2-1. Model of osteoporotic and normal bone cross section; cortical bone thickness C' + C" (Davis ME, Strandjord NM, Lanzl LH, 1966, JAMA 196:219–224)

TABLE 2-1. Annual age-specific incidence of hip fractures per 100,000 population in different countries

Age (Years)	Britain Male	Britain Female	Hong Kong Male	Hong Kong Female	Singapore Male	Singapore Female
35–44	6	1	3.3	1.6	6	1
45–54	13	10	11.2	13.2	14	3.2
55–64	29	30	33.6	33.4	43.7	25.6
65–74	78	159	111.7	102.7	100.5	68.6
75–84	302	633	377.8	351.8	344	129

Age (Years)	Sweden Male	Sweden Female	South African Bantu Male	South African Bantu Female
30–39	6	2	2.5	0.6
40–44	12	8	3	3
45–49	15	22	3	1
50–54	23	51	6	4
55–59	45	80	10	12
60–64	67	150	14	17
65–69	104	290	27	12
70–74	257	491	8	16
75–79	372	830	0	50
80+	560	577	116	80

Chalmers J, Ho KC, 1970, J Bone Joint Surgery 52b:667–675

fracture.[44,51] Approximately 32% of white American women can expect to have one or more hip fractures some time in their lives if the current inadequate methods of prevention and treatment are maintained.[51] The same appears to be true for Scandinavian and British women. In the United States, among Medicare enrollees, the incidence of hip fracture is currently about 1% per year. One should note that this is much higher than the rate of the combined death risks attributed to certain unopposed estrogen therapies.

The occurrence of spinal osteoporosis increases the likelihood by a factor of three that the individual will have other fractures elsewhere, for example, in the wrist. Spinal fracture predictably appears in a progressive series of three separate occasions, generally spaced about 5 years apart.[125] Figure 2-2 illustrates these three locations and ages. Note that these fracture points occur at the curve points on the spine, which comprise the areas of least resistance and therefore greatest susceptibility to mechanical stress. The disease is typically silent, although it can be accompanied by pain. One often becomes aware of it only after the fractures have occurred. As the osteoporotic process progresses, the bones that break and fuse produce a shortened and deformed posture and, in time, a severely weakened individual, walking with a bent-over, slow gait often accompanied by pain. However, it is not always painful.[51] With each vertebral compression, further loss of height of at least a centimeter occurs.

There is a relationship between spinal osteoporosis and hip fractures. The disease process, when present, occurs throughout the skeleton, regardless of where it first was revealed. For example, Hutchinson and co-workers (1979) reported that 33% of hip

FIG. 2-2. Spinal osteoporosis—location of bone fractures (Urist MR, Clinics Endocrinol Metab 2:159-176)

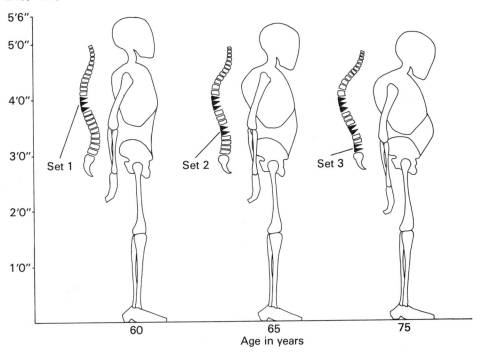

fracture cases in the Yale New Haven Hospital also showed osteoporosis on a chest plate.[63]

Current expectations of fractures for those white American women who do not take preventive measures are alarming. The same appears to be true for Scandinavian and British women. Crilly, in 1978, suggested that 30% of women reaching age 75 will have sustained at least one osteoporotic fracture.[28] By pooling data from many countries, Garn, in his extensive studies, was able to show that approximately half of all women in their sixth decade and beyond exhibited statistically defined osteoporosis.[47]

RISK FACTORS FOR OSTEOPOROSIS

Role of Gender

There are clear differences between men and women. Figures 2–3 and 2–4 illustrate the general age-related changes for both men and women. Throughout life the sexes behave differently with respect to bone loss and gain. During the growth stage, the male gains more subperiostally; the female gains more endosteally.[47] With advancing age, women demonstrate clinical osteoporosis about twice as frequently as men except for the oriental populations that have been studied.[7] Men, however, tend to show one larger drop in bone mass (of approximately 10%), which occurs typically at age 55. This age corresponds to the timing of the "adrenopause" that was described by Crilly and co-workers.[29] See Figure 1–10. At that age the adrenals show a marked decrease in output

FIG. 2-3. Changes in bone density with age—Men (Albanese AA, Edelson AH, Lorenze EJ Jr, Woodhull E, 1975, NY State J Med 75:326–336)

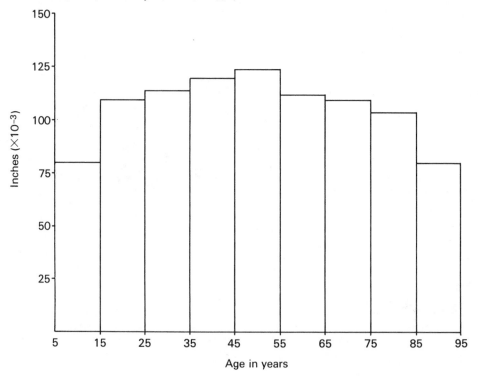

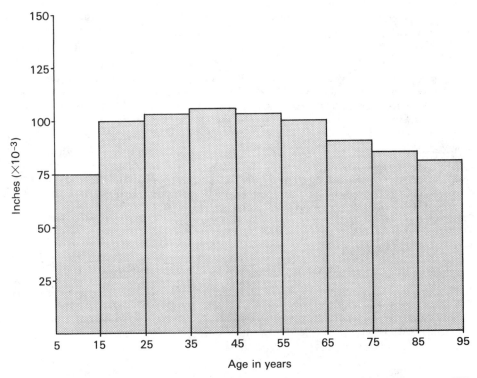

FIG. 2-4. Changes in bone density with age—Women (Albanese AA, Edelson AH, Lorenze EJ Jr, Woodhull E, 1975, NY State J Med 75:326–336)

of their steroid secretions. A review of the data of Longcope (1981) supports the concept of an adrenopause. Levels of androstenedione showed a clear upper limit after age 65 that was about half of that found before age 65.[74] Since androstenedione, as described earlier, appears to be the principal precursor to estrone and since estrone levels are sensitive indicators of possible concern for osteoporosis,[79] this connection between adrenal declines and the onset of obvious osteoporosis is likely to be directly related. Other comparisons of sex differences in hip fractures show that, by age 70, women experience two and one-half times the incidence of hip fracture experienced by men.[44] This sex difference seems to be a function of both age and country. Women in Hong Kong are at a slight advantage over men in hip fracture. In Singapore, they have about one and one-half times the fracture rate that men have after age 55.[21] In the United States four out of five of those afflicted with hip fractures are likely to be women. The reader might like to reappraise Table 2–1, which arrays these sex and age geographic region differences. The implications are grave and the probable explanations will unfold in the ensuing sections of this chapter.

Role of Age

A number of investigators have evaluated loss of bone mass by age. The overall age trend actually parallels the decline in ovarian and adrenal sex steroids.[29] These declines are nonlinear, the losses being greatest in the younger menopausal women at the onset of the loss.[113] Nonetheless, when Albanese recorded bone density data from 4000 normal subjects of widely varying ages, he showed that approximately 10% to 15% of individuals had shown significant bone density loss by the age of 25.[8] Albanese further showed, in cross-sectional data arrays, that from age 40 through age 90 there was a stepwise decline in the x-ray photodensitometry measurements of the 5-2 phalanx. By age 90 there was an unequivocal 30% loss compared to bone mass measurements at age 40.[7] Meunier and colleagues have provided similar data. They noted that, by age 90, women have lost an average of 43% of the trabecular bone they had at age 20.[88] These general age trends notwithstanding, the Meemas, in their studies of Caucasian women, measuring either cortical bone thickness or bone mineral mass in the proximal shaft, showed that regardless of the age of the woman the mass tended to be maintained until the menses stopped.[86,87] Once menopause ensues, whether surgically or naturally, a progressive loss ensued. Figure 2-5, showing the declines in bone mass, clarifies this relationship between bone mass and menopausal status.

Role of Skeletal Size

The size of the skeletal frame also appears to have some bearing on the likelihood of osteoporosis. Women with smaller frames are more susceptible. Alfram, studying the population of over 200,000 in the city of Malmo, Sweden (Scandinavia), evaluated all reported cases of fracture of the proximal end of the femur. Those with small frames were most at risk.[12] Likewise people with low initial bone mass lose relatively more with age than those with larger bones.[88]

FIG. 2-5. Declines in bone mass begin at menopause and continue (Meema HE, Bunker MI, Meema S, 1965, Obstet Gynecol 26:333–343)

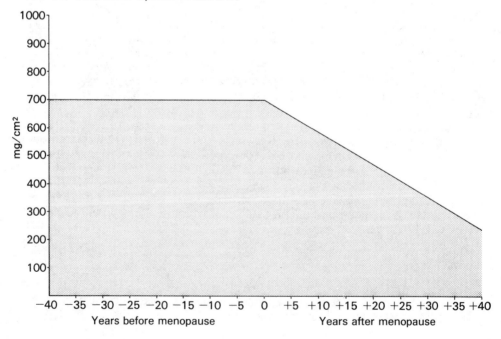

Role of Race

Race effects also have been suggested. Studies support the observation that black women rarely suffer the disorder.[7,134] American cross-sectional studies of healthy women showed that black women average 17% more finger bone mass than white women.

Role of Steroid Milieu

Osteoporosis has been associated with decreased estrone and androstenedione levels.[80] This association was noted when comparing the age-adjusted averages of estrone and androstenedione, but was not found for levels of estradiol and testosterone. It is also of note that when the replacement therapy has been used for longer than 5 years, a decreased risk of hip fracture has been observed.[96,129] Likewise when women were catagorized in terms of the rate of loss of their bone, it was noted that rapid bone-losers have lower estrogen levels as judged by the vaginal maturation index than slow losers.[95] Studies of castrated women provide, perhaps, the clearest data of all. When measuring loss of bone mass as a function of time since the operation, results form a consistent picture. Immediately after oophorectomy the bone loss is most rapid. Three or four years later bone loss continues but at a slower rate. The studies of Lindsay and co-workers indicate an initial 2.5% annual loss of bone mass (evidenced by cross-sectional studies); followed three or four years later by an approximate 0.75% annual rate of bone loss.[57,72] The time course after oophorectomy has been evaluated in a different way also. All women showed a decline in metacarpal mineral content in their first postoperative year; in the third postoperative year, 50%; and in the sixth postoperative year approximately 60% showed a continual loss of bone mass.[4] Studies consistently show that age *per se* is less relevant; time since ovarian loss is the key issue.[57,69,70,87]

Role of Exercise

While there appears to be a general impression that the degree of physical activity has some bearing on the amount of bone mass, the review of actual data indicate a subtly different effect.[32] It is true that some relationship exists between overall activity and bone mass, for the dominant hand tends to have 8% to 12% more bone density than the nondominant hand.[8] Likewise, amateur baseball players have shown a significant bone mineral hypertrophy of the dominant versus the nondominant humerus.[128] However, in a study in which cross-country runners were compared with office workers, there was little observable effect of exercise on the axial skeleton.[26,32,45] There was, however, some evidence for an effect on the axial stress areas. Among Olympic caliber athletes who were compared with healthy age-matched other young men and measured for bone density (by the photon absorption method in water), it was shown that (1) athletes had higher bone density in the distal end of the femur than nonathletes; (2) swimming was not effective but running was; and (3) control subjects who reported that they exercised regularly had a higher bone density than those who reported that they did not exercise.[92]

Lack of exercise, that is, complete immobilization, does appear to lead to an acute loss of bone mass that becomes progressively less marked with time as the formation and remodeling process stabilizes at a new lower total skeletal mass.[53]

There has been no convincing evidence that decreased levels of activity among normal populations are associated with any increase of bone loss. In one report, women who were more than one year post menopause and over 50 years of age were followed prospectively and compared with others evaluated in a cross-sectional array. In both groups the older women showed a significant reduction in the rate of mineral loss and concomitantly less activity than the younger women.[113] Although one cannot be sure that there is no phase lag effect of earlier activity promoting later bone mass retention, there is no evidence to suggest this.[113] There was some attempt to relate a program of physical activity (3 times/week, 30 min per session) to bone changes in a rest-home population of women over age 81 both with and without calcium therapy. Results of this study provided no clear support for a beneficial effect of exercise.[114,115]

One should note that although exercise has not been systematically shown to affect the bone mass of menopausal women, albeit it perhaps does in younger individuals, exercise clearly strengthens muscle. Women should, therefore, be encouraged to maintain a regular program of exercise so that, at the very least, the support structure surrounding the bone can be maintained at maximum strength. Moreover, improvement through exercising will enhance the stability and gait of the individual thus reducing the propensity of falls leading to fractures.

Role of Diet

Trends in osteoporosis do appear to be somewhat a function of dietary inadequacy although the influence is not a clear-cut one. Deficient calcium intake has been implicated in the osteoporotic process.[9] In fact, Albanese suggests that it is the calcium-deficient diet that is responsible for putting some women at risk for osteoporosis.[8,10]

The data do not appear strongly to support this position.[13] Garn, in his elegant cross-population studies, has suggested that calcium itself cannot be the answer because populations studied that were high in calcium intake lost bone in much the same fashion as elsewhere[47] (*e.g.,* United States).

Role of Smoking

Smoking appears to increase the risk of osteoporosis. The risk of hip fracture was elevated in smokers who were thin women but it was not elevated in smokers who were fat.[33,131] There is a positive correlation between body fat content and plasma estrogen concentration in oophorectomized women.[71] Presumably, women with increased fat content had estrone excess to protect them against whatever negative influence smoking had.

MORTALITY RATES

A good amount of data has accrued to provide information relative to the high rate of mortality after hip fracture. Although no demographic data are available to permit accurate statistics of total death rate after hip fracture, the sum of the evidence suggests that within four months of a hip fracture, on the average, 16% of those afflicted have died.[12,16,44,54,99] Figure 2–6 shows the survival rate 3, 6, and 12 months after cervical and intertrochanteric fracture as a function of age and sex, reported in 1964. These data were collected from a 1600-bed general hospital in Malmo, Sweden.[12] One notes that as age increases, postfracture survival rate declines. Figure 2–7 details the death rate as a function of time after hospital discharge from all hip fractures, reported in 1972. This study showed that the highest death rate occurred approximately two months after the hospital discharge.[16] Figure 2–8 further defines the cause of death of those postdischarged hip fracture cases. One sees that pneumonia, heart failure, myocardial infarction, and cerebral vascular accident each account for a significant fraction of the

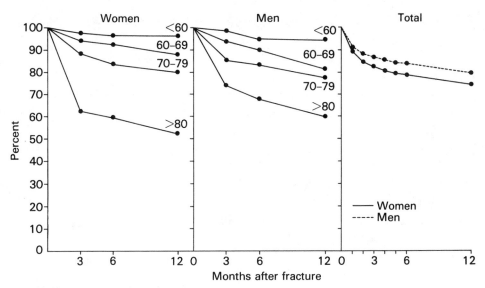

FIG. 2-6. Survival rates 3, 6, and 12 months after fracture as a function of age and sex (Alfram PA, 1964, Acta Orthop Scand [Suppl] 65:40–46)

FIG. 2-7. Death rate after hospital discharge following hip fracture (Beals RK, 1972, J Chron Dis 25:235–244)

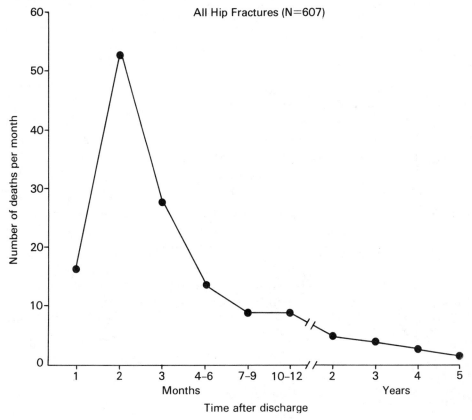

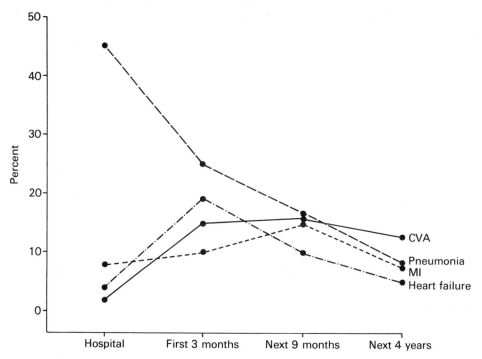

FIG. 2-8. Cause of death following discharge after hip fracture (Beals RK, 1972, J Chron Dis 25:235–244)

deaths after hip fracture.[16] Thus, a number of factors contribute to the death rate after a hip fracture; age appears to be the most significant predictor of survival after this trauma. Thus preventive measures are essential.

REGULATION OF BONE REMODELING

BONE STRUCTURE: DIFFERENTIAL VULNERABILITY

Bone structure can be broadly dichotomized under the headings of cortical and trabecular. About 80% of the skeleton is cortical, about 20%, trabecular.[94] Cortical bone loss during the osteoporotic process is relatively minor. Generally, in advanced stages of osteoporosis, only about 5% of the cortical bone mass is lost. In contrast, 50% of the trabecular bone has deteriorated.[94] That the rate of bone loss varies in different bones is graphically illustrated in Figure 2–9, which shows specific bones and distinguishes which of them is cortical and which is trabecular.[28] The osteoporotic bone loss is restricted to the endosteal bone envelope—that is, the marrow cavities—and to the trabeculae of cancelous or medullary bone.[54]

REGULATION OF BONE REMODELING

The bone remodeling process, that is, the continual cycling of resorption and formation, is under the control of a number of hormones and other factors that include mechanical stress, inorganic phosphate levels, and plasma calcium levels.[100] Table 2-2 shows the currently understood controlling factors in skeletal remodeling at the endosteal and haversian surfaces. Note that resorption and formation can each be increased or decreased by a variety of factors. Because bone remodeling is a dynamic process and because studies attempting to evaluate this process must select only a few of the factors at a time to study, the difference of opinion on the issue of control of the disease process that has pervaded the literature is not unexpected.

Calcium Requirements

Garn has pointed out that populations with diets that are deficient in calcium have no greater incidence of osteoporosis than those with rich calcium intakes, but others have shown an important role for calcium in the disease process.[47] Dietary requirements for calcium have been evaluated by balance studies as well as by absorption studies.

FIG. 2-9. Bone loss by type of bone and location in skeleton (Crilly RG, Horsman A, Marshall DH, and Nordin BEC, 1978, Front Horm Res 5:54, S. Karger AG, Basel)

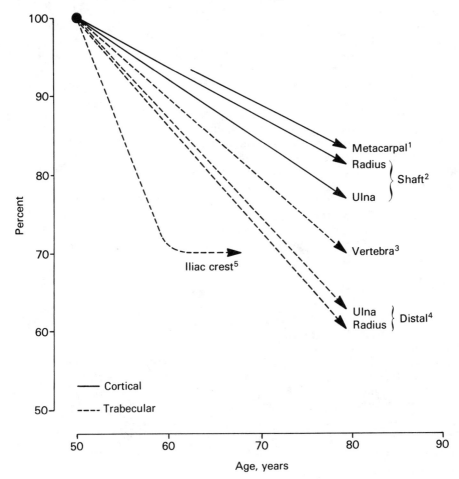

TABLE 2-2. Skeletal remodeling controls: endosteal and haversian surfaces

Resorption Rate (rate of conversion of osteoprogenitor cells to osteoclasts)		Bone Formation Rate (rate of conversion of osteoclasts to osteoblasts)
increased by	*decreased by*	*increased by**
parathyroid hormone	calcitonin	estrogen
1,25(OH)$_2$D$_3$	estrogen	calcitonin
calcium ion		growth hormone
		mechanical stress
		inorganic phosphate

*reductions in, for example, estrogen, cause the cells to stay longer in the resorptive stage

Calcium balance was studied in nuns initially ranging in age from 35 to 45 who returned each five years for hospital stays to allow testing of their calcium balances. On dietary averages of 660 mg of calcium per day, absorption averages of 33%, or 195 mg of calcium, were noted. At this level of absorption, negative calcium balance ensued. Between 40 mg and 50 mg of calcium a day was lost in the feces and urine. Within this group the individual balance scores were dependent upon the individual dietary intake levels.[55] Elsewhere, among normal postmenopausal women on a mean calcium intake of 778 mg a day, a 50-mg net loss of calcium was also noted.[94] Thus, at this dietary level, women are losing bone. The loss was attributed to a high obligatory calcium loss rather than to an absorption problem.

In addition to an obligatory loss of calcium each day, calcium absorption has been shown to decrease with age. In one study of men and women ranging from 30 to 90 years, a clear age-related decline in absorption rate was noted. A decline in circulating levels of vitamin 1,25(OH)$_2$D$_3$ appeared responsible because this vitamin is the absorbing metabolite.[46] However, other studies of circulating levels of vitamin 1,25(OH)$_2$D$_3$ cast doubt on such a conclusion.[41,83] Diets lower in calcium produce higher calcium absorption rates. In studies of the same individuals after 200- or 300-mg calcium diets, these compensatory effects were clear.[64] In addition, age effects were pronounced: Older people absorbed less well at all levels, and older subjects had somewhat higher urinary calcium in spite of lower absorption of calcium. There were no sex differences.[64]

Calcitonin

Calcitonin, a 32-amino acid peptide, varies from species to species.[75] Moreover, there is immunologic heterogeneity in plasma calcitonin;[49] specifically this applies to thyroidal and nonthyroidal fractions, which are different.[38] The various species of sequences that have been isolated form three main groups: (1) the primate/rodent group, which consists of five forms; (2) the teleost group (*e.g.,* eel and salmon); and (3) the antidactyl group (*e.g.,* ox and sheep).[75] The biological activity varies by species; rats have the least (2) amino acid substitutions and therefore are most like the human.[117] In contrast, salmon calcitonin contains 16 amino acid substitutions.[117] Biological activity varies by species: Salmon calcitonin is most active on bone, GI, and kidney.[117]

In the human, the hormone is secreted at peak levels at midday with a circadian variation of peaks and troughs.[119] This information is pertinent when evaluating a patient's calcitonin level.

The actions vary. At the kidney, calcitonin enhances the secretion of electrolytes (Na, K, phosphate, Ca, and Mg) and enhances the renal production of $1,25(OH)_2D_3$, the active form of vitamin D.[117] Although the relative sensitivity of various parts of the skeleton probably do vary, experiments at the cat tibia have shown that isolated perfusions of skeletal bone with porcine calcitonin caused a retention of calcium in bone. Arteriovenous differences of 5% resulted after one pass.[76] The major action of calcitonin in the human, as shown by both *in vivo* and *in vitro* experiments, appears to be the direct inhibition of bone resorption.[111,119]

The principal site of calcitonin production is the C cell of the human thyroid.[110] Figure 2–10 illustrates plasma calcitonin levels in normal men and women as well as in pregnant and lactating women. One notes that during pregnancy the levels are elevated fourfold.[110] Figure 2–10 shows sex differences: The man's level is more than four times greater than that of the woman.[56,58] Moreover, the response of calcitonin to calcium infusion is also sex dependent. Men show a rapid and much higher level of calcitonin than women in response to the calcium infusion.[56] Likewise, after pentagastrin administration, men show a surge in calcitonin; women show a gentle elevation.[56]

The role of steroids in controlling calcitonin levels has been examined by several different studies. Oral contraceptive users have on average five times the plasma level of calcitonin that normal women have.[58] Figure 2–11 shows the plasma calcitonin increases in response to estrogen replacement therapy—either percutaneous estradiol or ethinyl estradiol. More recently, calcitonin response to either of two estrogens, oestrogel or

FIG. 2-10. Plasma calcitonin levels in normal men and women and during pregnancy and lactation (MacIntyre I, Evans IMA, Hobitz HHG, Joplin GF et al, 1980, Arthritis and Rheumatism 23:1139–1147)

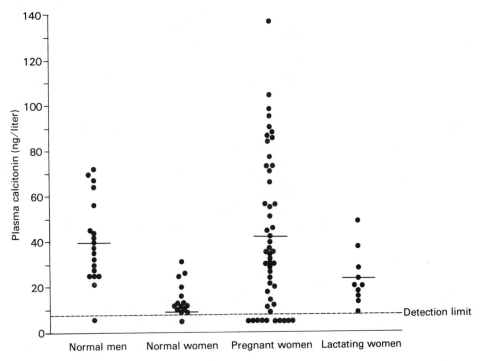

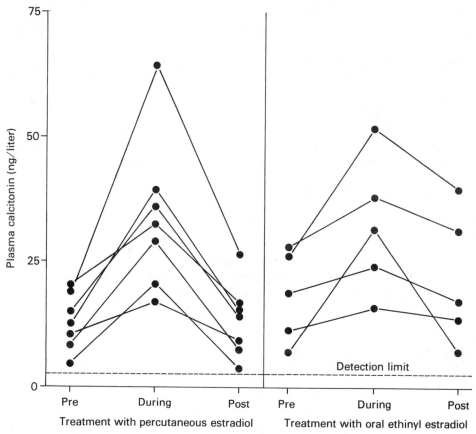

FIG. 2-11. Plasma calcitonin levels in postmenopausal women before, during, and after 12 weeks of treatment with either percutaneous estradiol or ethinyl estradiol (MacIntyre I, Evans IMA, Hobitz HHG, Joplin GF et al, 1980, Arthritis and Rheumatism 23:1139–1147)

ethinyl estradiol, was shown to follow a circadian pattern: It is demonstrable in the midday sample but not in the night and 9:00 a.m. sample.[118]

The influence of calcium on basal calcitonin levels has also been investigated after 10-minute infusions in men and women ranging in age from 20 to 79. Figure 2–12 delineates these age and sex differences in response to a 10-minute infusion of calcium. One notes that the male response in calcitonin level is higher than the female response and that the calcitonin response occurs rapidly, within 10 minutes. Furthermore, as people age, the response diminishes.

Parathyroid Hormone

The role of parathyroid hormone in the bone remodeling process has been characterized by several studies. This hormone initiates bone remodeling,[54] principally by stimulating the resorption phase. It is opposed by calcitonin. Estrogen loss limits the calcitonin level, thus throwing the balance toward an increased ratio of parathyroid hormome to calcitonin. A study of individuals with hyperparathyroidism showed that the menopausal women had significantly lower bone density. The premenopausal women and men with elevated parathyroid levels did not show lower bone density than normal.[97] It would therefore seem that high parathyroid hormone in combination with lower calcitonin and/or reduced estrogen levels, which produce reduced calcitonin levels, combine to shift the remodeling process in favor of resorption. Sex and age differences of

FIG. 2-12. Responses of plasma calcitonin and serum calcium to a 10-minute infusion of calcium in 58 normal men (solid circles) and 83 normal women (open circles). Stippled bars denote infusion of calcium (as the chloride salt) at a dosage of 3 mg per kg of body weight. Values represent mean ± SE for each determination. Indicated at the top are the numbers of male and female subjects in each decade. Plasma calcitonin is greater in men than in women (P<0.05 to 0.001), and there is a progressive decrease with age in both sexes. To convert calcium values to millimoles per liter, multiply by 0.25. (Deftos L, Weisman MH, 1980, N Engl J Med 302:1351–1353; reprinted by permission of the New England Journal of Medicine)

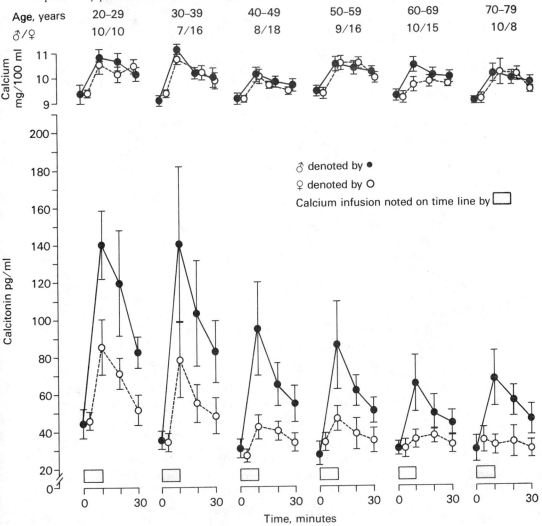

parathyroid hormone levels support such a view. One study of men and women aged 20 to 89 showed that women under age 40 had about double the level of parathyroid hormone as men (466 pg/ml vs. 226 pg/ml). After age 69 the female average was again much higher than the male's and even higher than in the younger population (728 pg/ml vs. 466 pg/ml).[132]

Thus it would seem that the role of parathyroid hormone is clearly a resorptive one whose action is facilitated both by reduced estrogen levels and reduced calcitonin levels.

Estrogens

Estrogens have been suggested to inhibit the bone resorbing action of parathyroid hormone as shown by studies in tissue culture.[43] The previously described studies add clarity to this perspective. Estrogens decrease parathyroid hormone, thus inhibiting resorption; estrogens stimulate calcitonin secretion, thus stimulating bone formation.

Vitamin D

The role of vitamin D in bone resorption, its cutaneous photosynthesis from steroids, its distribution and storage, its regulation and metabolism, and the influence on regulation and metabolism of sun, season, pregnancy and lactation, and age, and finally the clinical uses of vitamin D measurements are all relevant [35,65,98,109]—the specific role is presented herein.

Bone resorption appears to be one major influence of excess levels of vitamin D.[23,94,103] Two metabolites (25 OH D_3 and 1,25(OH)$_2$ D_3) are potent stimulators of bone resorption, but vitamin D_3 itself is inactive. The 1,25 form is 100 times more potent than the 25 form. The 1,25 form acts at doses low enough to indicate that it may be very important in the normal turnover of bone.

The cutaneous photosynthesis of previtamin D_3 has been studied.[59] Figure 2-13 illustrates and outlines the events involved in the cutaneous previtamin D_3 conversion by sun from the 7-dehydrocholesterol already residing in the skin. This conversion is limited by three forces: photochemical regulation (10%–15% maximum), pigmentation (darker skins take longer to reach maximum conversion of 7-DHC, that is the previtamin D), and latitude (the closer to the equator, the faster the conversion process) as well as a seasonal dependency.[59,120] Vitamin D_3 conversion to 25 OH D_3 occurs in the liver and the 25 OH D_3 conversion to 1,25 (OH)$_2$ D_3 occurs in the kidney.[59] The main circulating form that is biologically active is the 1,25 form.

Studies of the distribution and storage of vitamin D and its metabolites in human tissues show that adipose tissue and voluntary muscle are principal regions of storage.[83]

Ultraviolet radiation effects on vitamin D synthesis have also been studied.[1,38]

A seasonal variation in vitamin D metabolites exists in Great Britain where foods are not fortified with the vitamin.[65,70,116] The peak levels occur in July and the troughs in late winter and early spring. Older men and women (ages 75–86) always show lower levels than younger men and women.[116] Women show higher levels in summer than men, presumably due to the large area of skin exposed by their summer dresses. In Wisconsin and Ohio, similar studies indicated an absence in seasonal variation of 1,25 OH form despite a rise of the 25 OH form in the summer in healthy young people.[22] The fortification of milk with vitamin D would seem to account for these differences between the United States and Great Britain.

The clinical implications of measurements of circulating vitamin D metabolites are somewhat ambiguous. The time course of metabolic response to a single injection of

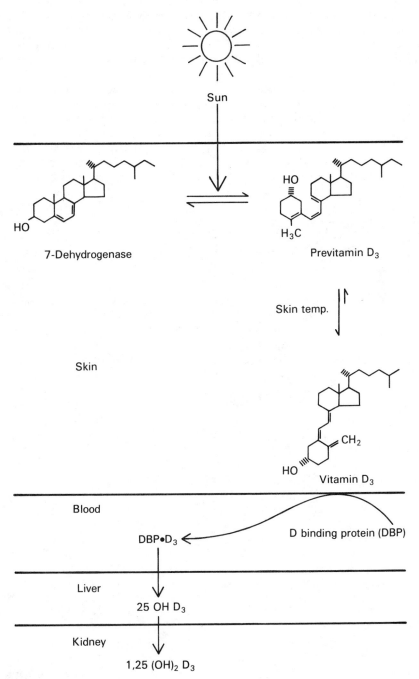

FIG. 2-13. Cutaneous previtamin D conversion process from skin and sunlight through kidney (modified from Holick MF, J Invest Dermatol 76:51–58)

vitamin D_3 is different in normal vs. D-deficient individuals.[86] A single assay of D and its metabolites is not too useful because of the dynamic changes in time course of metabolism.[83] Figure 2–14 shows that plasma levels of $1,25(OH)_2D_3$ in normals and others.[18] Note that levels are elevated during pregnancy, acromegaly, and primary hyperparathyroidism.

The regulation of the metabolism of vitamin D, although a very complex and somewhat well-defined phenomenon, appears not to be a critical factor in the osteoporotic process. The literature reveals that vitamin D metabolic deficiencies are not likely to be the critical problem in postmenopausal osteoporosis. Promotion of calcium absorption by vitamin D is clinically useful principally in vitamin D- or calcium-deficient states.[41] However, it is not recommended to achieve high increases in vitamin D levels since these will simultaneously effect both calcium absorption and bone resorption.[10,94,103]

One should be cautioned that excess levels of vitamin D have been implicated in increasing the resorption phase of the bone remodeling process. Likewise, deficient levels are implicated in a failure of intestinal resorption of calcium. A variety of studies have indicated that a proper daily dose is somewhere in the range of 400 IU.

FIG. 2-14. Plasma $1,25(OH)_2D_3$ (ng/liter) concentrations in all subjects studied. Bars indicate mean + SE of mean values. (Brown DJ, Spanos E, Macintyre I, 1980, Br Med J 1:277–278)

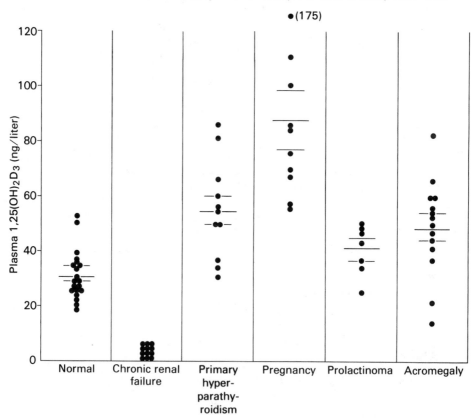

CHANGES AT MENOPAUSE

Nordin and co-workers (1979) believed that postmenopausal bone loss is due to increased sensitivity of bone to the resorbing action of parathyroid hormone and/or the bone resorbing action of $1,25(OH)_2D_3$. A possible impairment of the conversion of vitamin 25 OH D to the $1,25(OH)_2D_3$ form after age 65 has been reported.[46] This might account for the impaired absorption of calcium in older men and women. The intestinal absorption of calcium declines with age in both sexes, a process evident after age 69 in which the absorption seems to decrease by about 50%.[19] The initial cause of these changes at menopause may well be the declining levels in estrogen.

ASSESSMENT OF OSTEOPOROSIS

In order for the physician to assess osteoporosis, he or she can proceed along three lines of evaluation:

- The clinical details retrieved from the subject's medical history and physical examination
- The evaluation of bone density that can be carried out by several methods
- Clinical laboratory assessments, *e.g.,* calcium/creatinine (Ca/cr) levels, certain steroid levels, or calcitonin levels

These may be quite revealing of a state of osteoporosis.

CLINICAL DETAILS FROM MEDICAL HISTORY AND PHYSICAL EXAMINATION

The presence of pain in a postmenopausal woman, particularly a pain emanating from the lower spine area that is not radiating, should be a clear warning of potential osteoporosis. Albanese, after studying 4000 individuals, concluded that a persistent pain that does not radiate, originating in the lower spine, is often the first symptom of osteoporosis.[5] Gallagher and colleagues also noted that among their postmenopausal patients with one or more vertebral compression fractures all had backaches.[42] These women ranged in age from 45 to 82.

The presence of fractures, especially without a major trauma to have initiated them, should serve as a clear signal for the investigation of potential osteoporosis. Studies evaluating the association between fractures in one region of the skeleton with bone mass loss in other areas of the skeleton have confirmed the ubiquitous degeneration process of the skeleton once osteoporosis is extant. Among patients with cervical and hip fractures subsequent evaluation of their records indicated that 26% had had a previous x-ray film showing vertebral fractures.[44]

The overall appearance of the patient can also serve an alert physician as a signal of incipient osteoporosis. A progressive alteration in posture with the development of a fat pad forms the characteristic hump known as "the Dowager's Hump" (Fig. 2–15). The presence of Dowager's Hump should be understood as one of the end results of osteoporosis.[6] Often overlooked is the etiology of this deformity. A general decline in height is another predictive signal for osteoporosis. Figures 2–3 and 2–4 also show these related changes in bone density with age for women and for men.

The timing of the osteoporotic process has been resolved. By the time conventional x-ray films show osteoporosis the condition is very far advanced.

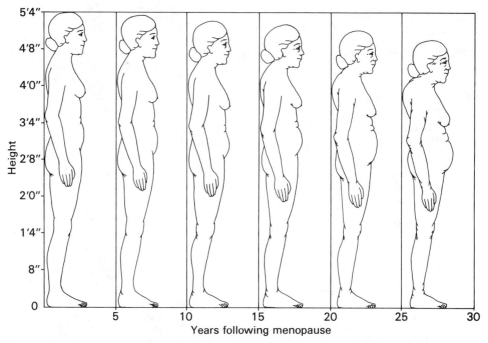

FIG. 2-15. Dowager's Hump (Albanese AA, 1978, Postgrad Med J 63:3:167–172)

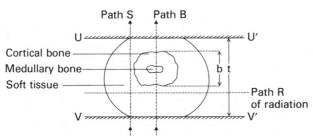

FIG. 2-16. Model of bone in cross section as revealed in photodensitometry (Davis ME, Strandjord NM, Lanzl LH, 1966, JAMA 196:219–224)

EVALUATING BONE DENSITY

The cortical bone as illustrated in Figure 2–1 surrounds the medullary bone; it is this cortical bone that tends to thin out with the passage of time. A bone with less cortical thickness or less cortical density is shown adjacent to a normal one. One sees that while the overall diameter of the bone may be the same, the medullary region expands. Scanners have been applied to cross-sections of cortical bone. The soft tissue is least resistant to the beam; the path of radiation is illustrated Figure 2–16. One sees that the radiation path has varying resistance relative to what lies in its way. Cortical bone will absorb less of the photons than soft tissue; medullary bone will tend to absorb more than cortical bone; and through complex mathematical functions and the aid of a computerized densitometer, replicable measurements can be achieved. One such common unit of measurement is the linear absorption coefficient. The lower the linear absorption coefficient, the lower is the amount of bone mineral content in the path of the measuring radiation beam.[36]

A number of different bone scanners have been developed, many after the Cameron and Sorenson bone scanners.[36] As early as 1966 clear data had been collected from these scanners to show that estrogen therapies (doses not reported) yielded higher bone density readings than absence of therapy in age-matched women.

The simplest method of early assessment is the measurement of cortical thickness using a conventional standardized photon absorptiometry method that is directed at the metacarpal or radius. Unfortunately, the machines available to do this are expensive, in the $25,000 to $40,000 range. An isotope source beams photons through the bone with the density of bone obstructing the passage of the beam. Computerized programs for evaluating the readings are built into this equipment.

Bone mineral content in normal and osteoporotic women has been estimated using a variety of methods. One comparability trial of 4 methods and 7 bone sites[50] showed that all the methods worked but some were simpler. The methods included: I-absorption scan, spinal x-ray, finger x-ray, and forearm x-ray. Elbows and heels are less sensitive for screening purposes although they can effectively show advanced stages of osteoporosis.[50] Bone mineral content can be estimated through studies of bone mass and through bone biopsy. Neutron activation analysis for whole-body calcium is not generally useful.[25]

Iliac crest biopsy analysis reveals a reduction of 8 to 19% of normal bone mass in women, aged 45 to 82, with vertebral crush fractures.[42] In other studies, iliac crest biopsy was also evaluated to show that there is a significant fall in bone formation with age in both men and women.[93] Bone resorption increased by 30% in women, with no change for men. These results could reflect the calcitonin sex differences described earlier. In 1982, White and co-workers reported data of iliac crest biopsy in untreated women aged 50 to 83 who did have osteoporosis. The results of the biopsies did not permit one consistently to distinguish the disease. About one-third had no evidence of active bone formation but about 70% did. The author suggested that since the chemistry of numerous parameters did not distinguish those with from those without histologic deficits, the condition we call osteoporosis might well be a heterogeneous class of disorders.[130] These data appear in Table 2–3. An alternate perspective might be that sampling variation in the tiny bone portions evaluated might be inadvertently selecting for tissue that is currently in one or another stage of the disease. The iliac crest biopsy, although probably the most accurate and refined method of scientific analysis, is an intensely painful procedure, both in its process and aftermath. It does not lend itself to routine studies.

Bone mass has also been successfully measured by phalanx bone density in the work of Albanese. In 1969 he established x-ray photodensitometry of the 5-2 (fifth digit, second plalanx) using an aluminum step-wedge equilibration system. In that report he established the validity of such measures by studying chicken bones and subsequently ashing the bone to measure its calcium content.[7] Although Garn objects to the use of the 5-2 phalanx because of the large individual variation he has seen in that finger,[47] Albanese, through this 5-2 phalanx technique, has been successful in distinguishing those at risk and those who are helped by various therapies.[7] In his patients, a close correlation between fracture incidence (hip, vertebral, and long-limb) and subnormal coefficient of bone density of the 5-2 phalanx was clearly demonstrated.[8] The phenomenon was especially strong for women over age 45.

Metacarpal cortical width has been more generally accepted as a valid site for measurement. Age-matched, pre- vs. postmenopausal women show clear differences in radiologic metacarpal cortical width. Premenopausal women show no decline regardless of how old they are while they are still menstruating; however, in one report of women

TABLE 2-3. Histomorphometric assessment of trabecular bone from 26 women with untreated postmenopausal osteoporosis

Parameter	Patient Mean ± SE	Control* Mean ± SE	Patient Range	Control Range
Total bone volume (%)	12.0±1.3	21.3±2.6	3.7–30	4.6–33
Relative osteoid volume (%)	2.9±0.4	1.9±0.8	0–7.8	0–8.9
Total osteoid surface (%)	17.0±2.0	12.0±5.0	1–35	0–56
Osteoblastic osteoid surface (%)	2.2±0.5	1.3±0.5	0–8.8	0–5.5
Mean osteoid seam width (μm)	7.8±0.6	9.8±8.3	0–15	0–32
Osteoclasts/mm² bone medullary space	0.13±0.03	0.11±0.04	0–0.34	0–0.39
Osteoclasts/mm trabecular perimeter	0.06±0.01	0.03±0.01	0–0.25	0–0.08
Total resorptive surface (%)	3.04±0.35	2.18±0.38	0.58–6.92	0.48–4.22
Osteoclastic resorptive surface (%)	0.25±0.06	0.13±0.06	0–1.1	0–0.6
Fibrotic surface (%)	0.19±0.16	0	0–4.0	0
Cellular rate of mineralization (μm/day)	0.55±0.09	0.64±0.02	0–1.3	—

*From 12 Caucasian women, ages 20 to 80 (mean 49 years) without history of bone disease
From Whyte M, Bergfeld MA, Murphy WA, Avioli LV et al, 1982, Am J Med 72:198–202

ranging in ages from 20–80, postmenopausal women always showed a decline.[93] In that study, medullary width showed a steep rise from 0.3 to 0.5 cm at the most advanced ages. This hollowing out of the medullary region of the bone is characteristic of the osteoporotic process.

Routine monitoring of the spinal regions most susceptible to osteoporosis or of the femoral neck would seem to be a logical choice for evaluating bone density. However, problems associated with alterations in red and yellow marrow composition as well as the loss of precision at the higher energies necessary for penetrating the regions have led some to conclude that computed tomography quantification of trabecular bone is not the monitoring method of choice.[84] Single photon densitometry does appear to be useful for monitoring the trabecular bone in the distal forearm (2 cm from ulna styloid) as well as the cortical bone more proximally measured on the radius.[52,112]

The controversy regarding the safety and accuracy of the various methods of bone monitoring continues. The single photon densitometry method still appears to be safe and, from a clinical point of view, useful in monitoring bone loss.[3,15,85]

Vaginal Maturation

Vaginal atrophy is significantly more frequent in compression fracture cases than in controls.[93] However, the vaginal maturation index is not useful as a diagnostic tool because there is a large variation in the vaginal maturation index that appears to progress independently of the osteoporotic process.

ASSAYING PLASMA CONSTITUENTS

Urinary hydroxyproline is a widely accepted measure as an indirect reflection of bone resorption. The hydroxyproline to creatine (OH Pr/Cr) ratio increases dramatically with hysterectomy.[93] However, Rasmussen[100] states that the hydroxyproline level is not necessarily a reflection of resorption. For example, when bone is formed, the metabolic by-products of the formation can also yield an increased quantity of urinary hydroxyproline. In general this represents a minor contribution in adults, but it can be quite large in growing adolescents. Thus, one would conclude that in an aged population measures of urinary hydroxyproline would reflect measures of bone resorption but such might not be the case in younger patients. The Ca/Cr in osteoporotic patients ranged between 0.037 and 0.318 vs. a normal range of 0.01 to 0.15.[130]

According to Gilbert Gordan, a definitive test for osteoporosis would be to find that serum calcium increases are present that are not related to hyperthyroidism and that serum phosphate levels are simultaneously rising. He states that tubular reabsorption of phosphate is normal in postmenopause but low in hyperthyroidism. One should recall that hyperparathyroidism stimulates the resorption process. Plasma calcitonin levels that fall below 30 pg/ml are strongly indicative of an osteoporotic condition, according to Whyte and colleagues,[130] and parathyroid hormone levels tend to be higher than normal in some osteoporotic patients.

It has been recently suggested by Stevenson and Whitehead[121] that the capacity of estrogen to minimize osteoporosis could well be mediated through calcitonin. Therefore, low calcitonin levels may herald a risk factor for the disease. Such a perspective is logical and a potentially fruitful area for research. Unfortunately, this issue has not yet been fully investigated.

Plasma steroid measurements do offer some predictive information about the likelihood of osteoporosis. Estrone and androstenedione deficiencies, relative to age-matched normals, are highly predictive.[30] Two other studies support such an influence.[34,42] In one, vertebral fractures among women 45 to 82 disclosed significantly lower urinary estrogen (24-hour collection) than control age-matched normals. The parathyroid hormone levels matched the normals.[42] Among crush fracture patients in one group all showed reduced androstenedione and estrone levels. However, plasma cortisol levels were not different in patients with hip fractures compared with age-matched subjects without hip fractures.[34]

MANAGEMENT OF OSTEOPOROSIS

GENERAL CONSIDERATIONS

Conservative estimates support that by age 75, 30% of women will have sustained at least one osteoporotic type fracture.[28] Hip fracture usually requires surgery and the average in-patient stay is about 24 days. The current annual cost in the United States exceeds one billion dollars.[44]

With the disease so ubiquitous in the aging female population and so expensive to the general population, it becomes imperative that an aggressive approach to the treatment and, hopefully, the prevention of the disease be universally accepted. Unfortunately, at this writing, the best available evidence suggests a current paucity of adequate medical care for the treatment and prevention of osteoporosis. In a 1981 survey, only 42% among 1000 specialists who direct their efforts to either bone diseases or menopausal women used hormone replacement therapy for postmenopausal osteoporosis.[17] Only half of these who did use hormone replacement therapy supplement estrogen with progestin, as is currently recommended for estrogen therapies. Clearly a more sophisticated approach is required.

PREVENTION

Despite an earlier difference of opinion about the potential for bone replacement after the osteoporotic process has begun, there is a unanimity of opinion that the disease can be prevented with an early application of estrogen replacement therapy. The Meemas showed, in their 8-year Premarin study (0.625 or 1.25 mg), that not only did the hormone therapy prevent bone loss, but an actual gain in bone mass was demonstrated after 8 years of therapy.[87] When estrogen replacement therapy (2.5 mg Premarin) was started within 3 years of the last menstrual period of menopause, among disease matched women, there was actually more bone mass after 10 years of therapy than prior to treatment.[91] If the treatment was initiated later than 3 years after the last menstrual period in this study, no new bone was formed; nonetheless, almost no bone was lost after 10 years on this therapy when compared to the initial values. By contrast, the placebo group lost bone and, among the 48 women on placebos, 7 fractures occurred in the span of those 10 years.[91] More recently, Christiansen and co-workers have shown a full gamut of the profound beneficial dose-related influences on bone remodeling. Early postmenopausal treatment with estrogen/progestin regimens is especially valuable.[26] Such beneficial changes, when comparing steroid to placebo treatment among 50-year-old women, disclosed the following:

Urinary hydroxyproline (decreases)
Urinary Ca/Cr (decreases)
Bone mineral content (increases)
Serum phosphate (decreases)
Serum alkaline phosphatases (decreases)

In contrast, according to Gallagher and Nordin, no therapy that they tested, among a combination and variety of them, could apparently replace bone already lost.[45] Nevertheless, these contrasting conclusions appear to be a function of dose dependency.[61] A 2.5-mg dose of Premarin did produce some bone accretion; however, Gallagher and Nordin used a Premarin dose of either 0.6 or 1.25, an estrone sulfate dose of 1 mg or of 2 mg, and estradiol dosage of 0.025 mg or 0.05 mg daily.[45] These lower doses did not associate with deposition. Progestogens did not prevent loss of bone mass in one study;[48] however, at higher doses, they were effective.[40,45,61,73]

According to Gordan, 0.625 mg conjugated equine estrogens or the equivalent of 0.01 mg ethinyl estradiol will prevent the development of osteoporosis in an individual who does not have it at the start of this therapy.[51] It seems reasonable to conclude that estrogen therapies are effective in preventing the progression of the osteoporotic process and that, in sufficiently high doses, they may even produce small amounts of bone deposition.

The issue of calcium deficiencies is a critical one for the practitioner who is considering estrogen therapy for the prevention of osteoporosis. It should be emphasized that if calcium intake is inadequate, steroid treatment may not help.

TREATMENT MODALITIES

Calcium

Calcium deficiencies limit the effectiveness of any estrogen therapy. Moreover, calcium treatment may reduce the estrogen dosage needed.[94] A necessary minimum must be maintained for the hormones to be effective and this minimum appears to vary from woman to woman. The recommended dosage of calcium ranges between 1000 mg a day and 1500 mg a day.[23,24,42,67,68]

Whether calcium alone, or calcium plus calcitonin, offers sufficient therapy has been debated in the literature. Albanese has concluded that calcium alone in sufficiently high dosage may be adequate to prevent or reverse osteoporosis. According to his conclusions it takes between 6 and 9 months to see bone density improvements (5-2 phalanx) when the calcium is supplemented with vitamin D.[8] However, high calcium intake (1.5 mg of dissolved powder) did not change skeletal deposition or absorption rate in osteoporotic patients followed for 2 years,[67] nor did calcium infusions to postmenopausal osteoporotic women.[127] Apparently one needs to distinguish the preventive from the degenerative process. Chestnut compared 1200 mg a day of $CaCO_3$ and 400 IUs of vitamin D_2, with and without calcitonin. He showed a decrease in bone mass after 18 months of 2.15% on the calcium. For the same time interval on the calcium supplemented with calcitonin, an increase of 0.24% in bone mass was seen. He used 100 MRC units of synthetic salmon calcitonin daily.[24] One should recall that with increasing age calcium absorption capacity of the intestine shows a clear decline and that large doses of oral calcium yield low indices of absorption. In 1981, Lee and co-workers reported on calcium deficiency in elderly osteoporotic females that could be corrected with 1000 mg a day of calcium.[68] After 6 months of this therapy, the researchers noted increases in bone density in 58%, no change in bone density in 16%, and a further loss in 32%. A conservative conclusion with respect to the calcium issue leads one to (1) supplement a calcium-deficient individual; (2) probably assume that older women are not ingesting enough calcium and; (3) recommend a minimum of 1200 mg a day be ingested. Table 2-4, shown on page 84, lists calorie and calcium values of foods.

Steroid Hormones

Estrogens.   As early as 1959, Wallach and Henneman reported that cyclic estrogens were effective in treating and preventing osteoporosis and that these steroids consistently eliminated low-back pain.[126] Recently, Horsman and co-workers have demonstrated a dose–response relationship between estrogen therapy (ethynil estradiol) and postmenopausal bone loss.[61] Furthermore, it is becoming clear that the estrogen benefit is limited by calcium malabsorption and that some low level of vitamin D, about 400 IU, should therefore be given in conjunction with estrogen.[78]

The issue of estrogen and osteoporosis has been investigated in a number of ways. Bone loss has been measured as a function of absence of treatment or administration of placebos and of different dosages of estrogen, calcium, and calcitonin. The previous description—that calcitonin levels increased after estrogen therapies (Fig. 2–11)—should be borne in mind. Bone loss as a function of different therapies forms a clear picture. Some dosage of estrogen, with sufficient calcium, combines to optimize the state of bone health in an aging female population. For example, in prospective trials of postmenopausal women, particular attention to oophorectomized women showed that the bone loss in the calcium-treated group was somewhere intermediate between the estrogen-treated group and the placebo group.[60,62] The investigators also noted that the loss is different in different locations. The ulna, the radius, and the metacarpals were compared (Fig. 2–17). One notes the influence of estrogen across 3 years in increasing bone mass and the fact that calcium therapy alone could not totally halt the decline in bone mass but was clearly better than no therapy. Moreover, estrogen and calcium offered no greater effectiveness than estrogen alone in this particular subset of women studied.[62]

Bone densitometry of the patient population of Purvis Martin showed a higher bone density, at each age, among women taking estrogens than among those not on such therapy.[81] Figure 2-18 also evaluates the patient population shown in Figure 2-17. Three therapies and placebo are compared for all the patients, and the mean change in cortical width is measured across the summation of time.[62] One notes that ethinyl estradiol with calcium was the most effective of the therapies; ethinyl estradiol without calcium was also effective although less so than with calcium added to the estrogen. More recently, the same group established a dose–response schedule among 120 postmenopausal women. They showed that at the lowest doses (<15 μg/day) a net loss of bone ensued; at intermediate levels (15–25 μg/day), bone mass was not increased or decreased; and at high doses (>25 μg/day), bone deposition outpaced bone loss.[61] Calcium alone was not adequate to halt the loss of cortical width across time. Placebos yielded the greatest loss of cortical width across the time studied.

Other investigators also have provided support for the general conclusions (1) that estrogen replacement therapy reduces the bone density loss per month most effectively; (2) that calcium carbonate is effective but less so and that controls continue losing bone with the passage of time.[102,107] Radiogrammetry and photon absorptiometry were both

FIG. 2-17.   A comparison of the loss of bone from the ulna (bone mineral content), radius (bone mineral content), and metacarpal (cortical width) in controls (dotted) and in groups of women treated with estrogen, calcium, and combined therapy (Horsman A, Nordin BEC, Gallagher JC, Kirby PA et al, 1977, Calcif Tissue Res (suppl) 22:217–224)

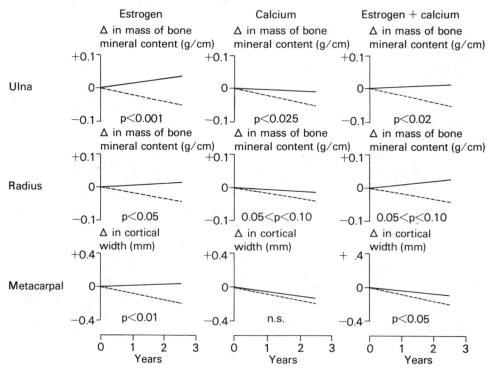

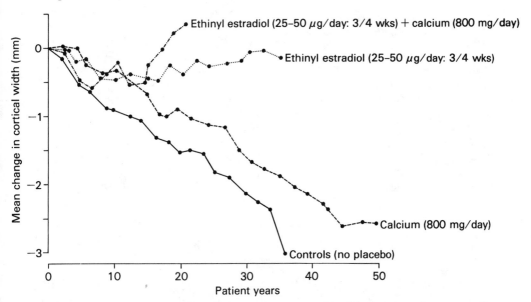

FIG. 2-18. Cumulative sequential changes in the mean width of the metacarpal cortices in the control and three treated groups (Horsman A, Nordin BEC, Gallagher JC, Kirby PA et al, 1977, Calcif Tissue Res (suppl) 22:217–224)

recorded in postmenopausal women given either estrogens alone, calcium carbonate alone, or no therapies. Radiogrammetry yielded slightly different percentage figures than did photon absorptiometry, but both showed the same general trends. The controls lost from 1.18% (radiogrammetry) to 1.82% (photon absorptiometry) of their bone mass per year; hormones reduce this loss to 0.15% or 0.73%. Calcium supplements without estrogen additions were somewhat intermediate; from 0.22% to 1.89% of bone was lost per year.[102]

Ethinyl estradiol (0.1–1.5 mg/day) reduced resorption, and temporarily, up to 15 months, increased formation in osteoporotic patients who were followed with exhaustive calcium-47 kinetic studies, nitrogen balance, and so forth.[67]

In addition to the foregoing studies of measurements of bone loss, plasma changes have been measured across time in response to different therapies. They confirmed that estrogens halted the outflow of calcium into plasma in postmenopausal women with vertebral compression fractures.[42] Comparisons were made between a series of hormones:

Ethinyl estradiol 0.025 mg/day or 0.05 mg/day
Oestriol hemisuccinate (Synapause) 2, 4, 6, or 8 mg a day
Estrone sulfate (Harmogen) 1 or 2 mg/day
Conjugated equine estrogen (Premarin) 0.625 or 1.25 mg/day

These estrogens were evaluated for their influence on plasma calcium, fasting urine Ca/Cr, urinary hydroxyproline/Cr, and calcium balance. The results showed that equivalent doses of hormone at 1 month of therapy were as follows:

6 mg oestriol succinate or
0.025 mg ethinyl estradiol or

1 mg estrone sulfate or
0.625 mg conjugated equine estrogens

The authors noted that plasma calcium levels did not change on most of the treatments.[45] Elsewhere, 3 mg a day percutaneous oestrogel as well as 20 μg a day of oral ethinyl estradiol was evaluated during 12 weeks of therapy. The urinary hydroxyproline to creatinine ratio dropped on both treatments and the two therapies appeared to provide equivalent responses.[118]

The influence of duration of treatment as well as the response to alternations in treatment, *i.e.,* stopping and then resuming treatment, has provided a somewhat consistent picture. It appears that as long as the treatment levels of estrogens and calcium are adequate, bone loss is halted; as soon as these levels fall below minimal requirements, osteoporotic processes resume. It further appears that at any time the therapy is initiated further loss of bone mass is prevented.

It therefore becomes clear that, for the individual at risk of osteoporosis, optimal treatment will be a lifelong event rather than a temporary palliative measure.[26] In 1977, Riggs and co-workers compared 4 months of treatment to 24 months, evaluating the percent of resorbing surface to estimate bone resorption. The effects of the 2.5-mg dose of conjugated equine estrogens were clear. Bone resorption decreased from approximately 16% of the surface to approximately 8% of the surface after 4 months of the treatment and further decreased to approximately 4% of the surface by 24 months of continuous treatment.[106] Other long-term studies have confirmed the beneficial effects of continuing treatment.[27,28] In the elegant studies of Christiansen (1981), particular interest was focused on bone mass after hormone replacement therapy was stopped, then changed to placebos, and then resumed in healthy postmenopausal women. Calcium (0.5 g/day) was included with the following hormone regimen: day 1–day 12: 4 mg 17,B estradiol plus 2 mg oestriol; day 13–day 20: same plus 1 mg norethisterone acetate; day 23–day 28: 1 mg estradiol plus 5 mg oestriol. Figure 2-19 clearly shows the beneficial effects of the estrogen therapies, both initially and even 2 years after taking a placebo. One notes that individuals on placebos show a continual loss of bone mineral content and that individuals on estrogen replacement therapy show a gradual deposition of bone through time.[27] There appears to be a value in estrogen therapy on the osteoporotic reduction at any of these times. Moreover, the early postmenopausal application of estrogens has the statistically greatest benefit because this is the time of most severe annual bone loss and estrogens prevent this loss.[26]

To date, the studies in the literature evaluating the effects of hormone therapies on the osteoporotic process have tended to study the oral therapeutic approach. However, with the recent focus on vaginal estrogen to avoid liver effects of high oral doses, investigators are beginning to suggest that vaginal doses are a preferred route.[48] Particularly critical was the finding that in cases of vaginal atrophy such high doses of oral estrogens were required to overcome these effects that the liver was subject to such excesses in SHBG and CBG as well as renin substrate that oral dosages were the dispreferred route.[48] For these details, see Chapter 7. Unfortunately, no clear studies of the influence of vaginal therapies on the bone processes have yet been reported. The demonstration that plasma estrone and plasma androstenedione are the critical plasma hormones that determine the likelihood of osteoporosis makes it likely that vaginal estrogens may be perfectly adequate for the osteoporotic treatment processes. One should be alert to future studies on these issues however.

Androgens. Androgens administered (at 6 mg a day) do halt osteoporosis.[23] They were shown to significantly decrease parathyroid hormone and to increase bone formation, in

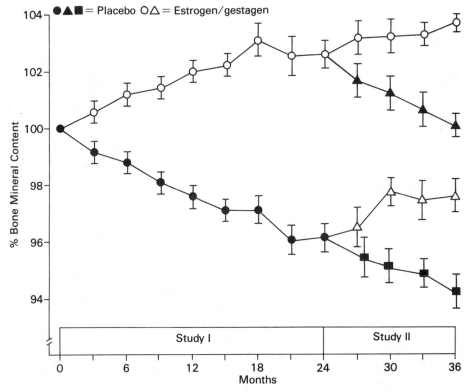

FIG. 2-19. Bone mineral content as a function of time and treatment in 94 (study I) and 77 (study II) women soon after menopause (Christiansen C, Christensen MS, 1981, Lancet Feb 28, 459–461)

the iliac crest biopsy evaluations. The androgens were effective in reducing resorption in osteoporotics; however, they were able to increase bone formation only temporarily, *i.e.,* up to 15 months.[67]

Although the androgens do have beneficial effects on bone deposition and on minimizing bone resorption they are not recommended due to the masculinization effects that they inevitably produce.

Progestogens. A potential beneficial influence of progestogens on bone mineral status has also been reported. In typical postmenopausal dosage ranges, progestins do not reduce bone resorption but were considered potentially able to stimulate bone formation.[70] Several Italian articles suggest, in individual cases, that medroxyprogesterone acetate limited the urinary loss of calcium in one subject;[89] that intravenous administration of medroxyprogesterone acetate for a "long period of time" had beneficial effects in "old" osteoporotics;[111] and that "ancient osteoporotic patients" showed increased intestinal calcium absorption rates in response to medroxyprogesterone acetate (dosage not stated) after 50 daily treatments.[123] Norethisterone (5 mg/day) showed effects on calcium metabolism similar to those of several regimens of estrogens.[45] Clear declines in urinary calcium loss within one month of treatment were demonstrated. Megestrol acetate also lowered the urinary calcium loss, particularly at high doses (80 mg/day) in a small sample but not to levels commensurate with premenopausal controls.[40] Likewise statistically significant but small reductions in hydroxyproline/creatinine ratios were shown at all doses (20, 40, 80 mg). Lindsay and co-workers reported that either a 40-μg/day oral dose of mestranol or a 200-mg injection of gestranol (19 or 17 beta hydroxyprogesterone) at monthly and then 3-month intervals was effective in reducing calcium excretion and retarding the loss of bone density in postmenopausal women.[73] Although the samples were small (10 women per treatment) the magnitude and the statistical significance of the effect, in comparison with placebo controls, was clear.

At this time progestins cannot be recommended as a treatment for osteoporosis because high doses appear necessary and these doses are potentially dangerous for lipid metabolism. Chapter 6 reviews the lipid/hormone studies.

Estrogens with Progestins.   One recent study of 79 postmenopausal women given 1 mg norethisterone acetate (10 days/cycle) opposed to 3 different estrogen strengths (17 beta estradiol and estriol: 4/2, 2/1, or 1/5) clearly showed a dose–response effect in which increased doses of estrogen had positive effects on several parameters of healthy bone metabolism.[26]

As new studies explore these relationships, it is likely that a beneficial role for the combinations of estrogen and progestin will become firmly established. The trend of findings is certainly headed in such direction.

Calcitonin

The role of calcitonin in the bone remodeling process was described earlier. Figure 2–11 showed that estrogen therapy increased plasma calcitonin levels.[75,118] Calcitonin was also shown to be increased within 10 minutes after a calcium infusion (see Fig. 2–12), and this response was less powerful with the passage of the years, so that by the time of menopause the response is less than half of what it is in a younger person.[39] Calcitonin acts on the remodeling process by decreasing bone resorption.[23]

It should be noted that calcitonin was not increased after a calcium challenge in a group of osteoporotic women, but it was increased in age-matched controls.[122] Although the authors of that study suggested that the osteoporotic group had a calcitonin deficiency and that this condition might be involved in the etiology of the disease, they did not consider that an estrogen deficiency may have been responsible. Since a known characteristic of osteoporosis is an estrogen deficiency, it seems as likely that the calcitonin influences on the bone remodeling process require some minimum level of estrone. Such studies have not yet been reported.

In one short-term, 6-month, double-blind study of postmenopausal osteoporotic women who were seeking an alternative to estrogen replacement therapy, placebos were compared with placebo plus calcitonin injection or with oral phosphate and calcitonin injections.[101] The results were supportive of a role for calcitonin in the process. There was new bone formation in response to the combined therapy by several different measures: There was a 37% increase in absolute bone volume, an 85% increase in active bone formation surface in all patients, and a 64% increase in the osteoid surface in 78%. The group receiving calcitonin only showed an increase in the osteoclasts. In this study there was no post-treatment hormone value assay presented, but pretreatment groups were presumed to have had equivalent values based on the fact that all of the women had osteoporosis and were randomly assigned to either one of the treatment groups.

Gordan[51] as well as Chestnut[23] considers calcitonin useful only as a last resort because it has a short half-life, requires frequent injection, has a cumbersome treatment regimen requirement, and has the additional problem of antibody formation to the commonly available porcine and salmon strains.[23,51]

Vitamin D

As described earlier, vitamin D has a homeostatic effect on plasma calcium levels. Vitamin D not only increases calcium absorption from the intestine, in excess doses it promotes bone resorption. It is currently recommended that vitamin D be given in conjunction with estrogen and calcium but not more than 400 IU per day. Higher doses increase the risk of a compression fracture.[23]

When doses of 1-hydroxy vitamin D_3 were increased from 1 to 2 μg per day resorption clearly increased if no hormone replacement therapy was given.[78] Estrogen therapies abolished this resorptive effect of the high dose of vitamin D.[78] It is now known that 40,000 international units daily (which was necessary to correct some malabsorption problems) led to increased bone resorption.[94] In Figure 2–20, one can see how vitamin D with and without calcium produced great losses in height as years of treatment increased.[94] This malabsorption problem exists in 50% of the crush fracture cases and therefore complicates the treatment for such individuals. The cause of the malabsorption is not assessed but the calcium malabsorption is generally present in spinal osteoporosis.[93]

Although large doses of vitamin D can usually correct the calcium malabsorption problems (10,000–20,000 IU per day), these are now known to be incompatable dosages because they also promote bone resorption.[23] Nordin (personal communication, 1983)

FIG. 2-20. Changes in height of menopausal women in response to different treatments (Nordin BEC, Hopman A, Marshall DH, Simpson M et al, 1979 Clin Orthop Related Res 140:216–239)

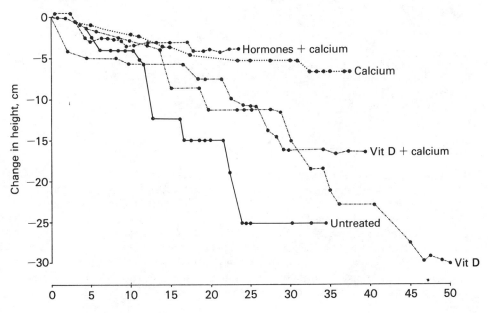

has suggested that when calcium malabsorption exists, very high dosages of calcium supplementation, that is, 1200 to 1500 mg a day, may be indicated. He describes that there is minimal or no risk of renal stone formation in such cases because the malabsorption limits the calcium to be absorbed to levels below that which would stimulate renal stones. Practitioners should be alert to the vagaries of the culture in which they practice medicine. In the United States, for example, milk is supplemented with vitamin D, but in Great Britain it is not. Being sensitive to the dietary habits of the patient with respect to the food processing patterns of the country will help to guide vitamin D ingestion levels. If the diet or pattern of exposure to sunshine provides adequate vitamin D, then supplements are contraindicated.

Sodium Fluoride

Although sodium fluoride appeared to increase bone formation, the bone that was formed was shown to be brittle.[23] Sodium fluoride was significantly better in reducing the fracture rate in 60% of those postmenopausal osteoporotic women receiving it, but it was not helpful for the rest.[108] Moreover, sodium fluoride has been shown to have adverse side effects in close to half of the patients given it; rheumatic symptoms (joint pain or swelling) or gastrointestinal symptoms of severe nausea and vomiting are common in persons receiving sodium fluoride treatments. Moreover, long-term fluoride treatment increased the bone fracture rate in one 6-year study of patients with primary osteoporosis given 40 to 65 mg.[105] In that study, daily calcium intakes ranged between 1 and 1.5 g; vitamin D to the majority included 50,000 IU twice a week. This combination of treatment yielded synovitis, painful plantar fascial syndrome, recurrent vomiting and anemia in 42% of the patients, and 0.3 new vertebral fractures per 10 years of observation.

Because sodium fluoride, as so far evaluated, has so many adverse effects, the current use of such a therapy would be ill advised.

Thiazides

Although it had appeared that thiazides, in the first 6 months, seem to influence some (urinary calcium excretion rate is reduced) but not other (bone mineral content) parameters of bone function, it is now established that the effect is transient.[124] The mechanism through which thiazide works is not understood. It appears to act by improving renal calcium conservation and also, initially, by increasing the intestinal calcium absorption.

NEED TO CONTINUE TREATMENT

Inadequate treatment is better than no treatment, as shown in Figure 2–19. Although there has been some suggestion that after 6 years have passed since an oophorectomy subsequent inception of treatment was ineffective,[4] the time course of that study only showed that within the first 2 years of estrogen replacement therapy in contrast with placebo, the two groups were not different in metacarpal mineral content. In light of the more recent studies showing beneficial effects of estrogen therapies with and without calcium, a more conservative conclusion would be that at any point a practitioner is faced with a patient undergoing a bone degenerative process, estrogen therapy should be beneficial. It may require time, perhaps 3 years of treatment, before benefits are apparent.

SPECIAL PROBLEMS WITH TREATMENTS

Practitioners should be alerted that calcium ingestion is often resisted in aging women.[9] Complaints of gastrointestinal disturbance on high-calcium diets as well as the reluctance to take large pills combine to inhibit patient acceptance. It becomes very important that enough time and energy be spent with the patient to explain the tremendous importance of calcium ingestion in preventing or limiting osteoporotic degeneration. A recently published guide, *Menopause: A Guide for Women and the Men Who Love Them,* coauthored by the authors of this text, was developed to explain, in accurate but simple terms, the importance of such health care practices.[31]

The question of calcium stones or the likelihood of stone formation on diets or supplementation so high in calcium should also be considered. In those patients who do have osteoporosis this appears not to be a problem because osteoporosis carries with it a reduced absorption. Moreover, with increased age, calcium absorption diminishes greatly. Nordin, in his 30 years of using high-dose calcium supplements, reports that he has never seen it produce renal stones. Women with renal stones may have a different calcium metabolism. Studies in these peri- and postmenopausal women are needed. The issue of calcium-induced gallstones remains unexplored.

SPECIAL TREATMENT CONSIDERATIONS

Treatment for Oophorectomized Women

Oophorectomized women appear to be at much greater risk for a rapid onset of osteoporosis than women whose menopause occurs naturally. They also show the greatest reduction in hip fracture risk-ratio when they take estrogens.[96] This is probably due to the menopausal ovarian output of androstenedione and its subsequent conversion to estrone.

In a double-blind placebo vs. mestranol (20 μg/day) study, healthy oophorectomized women in whom therapy was begun either 2 months postoperatively or 3 or 6 years postoperatively, showed both an effect of therapy and an effect of time since surgery on the effectiveness of therapy. Metacarpal mineral changes were prevented when treatment began within 2 months of the operation. Treatment within 3 years postsurgery produced less bone loss annually than was noted if 6 years had passed before therapy began. Treatment was always more effective than placebo if it began within 3 years after oophorectomy. For the group that waited 6 years after surgery to begin taking estrogen, no difference in metacarpal loss could be observed between the estrogen group and the placebo group. Calcium excretion was reduced by mestranol at all times taken. Hepatic function was not different for placebo vs. treatment using clinical evidence of this hepatic function as the criterion. Three women—one from the hormone group and two from the placebo group—had "biochemical evidence suggestive of hepatic dysfunction and in all instances these changes were transitory." Side effects of treatment included cramps in calves and feet at night in bed.[4] A more extended time course showed that after 5 years, on either placebo or 20 μg mestranol a day, there was a gradual increase in metacarpal mineral content in those who took mestranol while the controls gradually lost bone. Serum calcium did not change on any treatment regimen and serum phosphate decreased on mestranol after 1 year.

It thus appears that oophorectomized women form a special subset for whom preventive therapy should ideally begin immediately after surgery, but for whom treatment should be offered at any point at which it is possible to begin helping them.

Treatment for Arthritic and Asthmatic Women

Prolonged medication with corticosteroids has profound influences on estrone levels and increases the likelihood of subsequently developing osteoporosis.[2,14,37,52,90,104,112] In 1969, results of one study showed that prolonged prednisone medication yielded large calcium loss to urine that could be somewhat corrected with the androgen oxandralone ("AX-10"). This therapy produced a positive nitrogen balance and a decreased urinary calcium output. Confirmation of the negative influence of corticosteroid therapies on plasma estrone levels was provided in 1978.[80] Low plasma estrone in corticosteroid-treated postmenopause is considered a factor in the genesis of corticosteroid-induced osteoporosis. In 1978, Crilly and co-workers reported treatment with dehydroepiandrosterone, a precursor of androstenedione and thus of estrone. In four cases of corticosteroid-treated women it was effective in reducing the corticosteroid-induced changes in estrone and testosterone deficits. Elsewhere, Kimberg and colleagues showed that corticosterone reduces calcium absorption in their studies of everted gut sacks from the proximal 4 to 5 centimeters of rat duodenum.[66]

Hypercortisolism and hyperthyroidism are "well identified causes of osteoporosis."[133] In contrast, excesses of growth hormone produce the excess periosteal new bone growth that is characteristic of acromegaly. Figure 2–21 shows plasma estrone levels in three

FIG. 2-21.   Plasma estrone levels in normal, osteoporotic, and corticosteroid-treated patients. (Crilly RG, Horsman A, Marshall DH, and Nordin BEC, 1978, Front Horm Res 5:57, S. Karger AG, Basel)

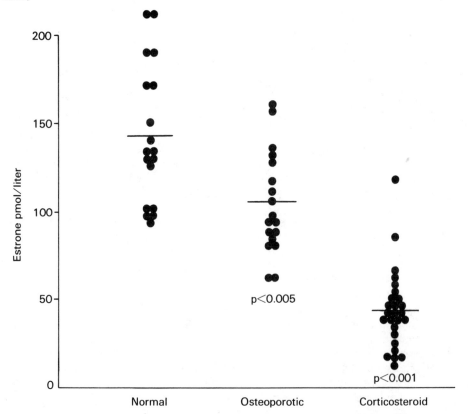

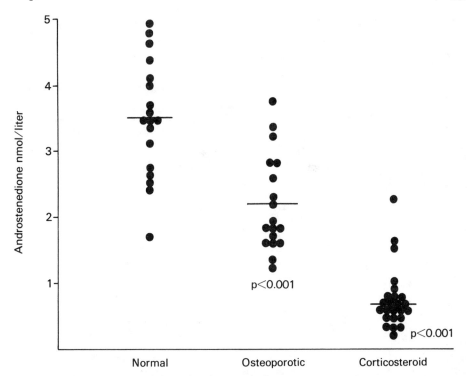

FIG. 2-22. Plasma androstenedione levels in normal, osteoporotic, and corticosteroid-treated patients (Crilly RG, Horsman A, Marshall DH, and Nordin BEC, 1978, Front Horm Res 5:57, S. Karger AG, Basel)

groups of women: normal, osteoporotic, and corticosteroid-treated. One notes that osteoporotic women have lower estrone levels than normal women,[77] but that corticosteroid-treated women have even lower levels than the typical osteoporotics.[28] Figure 2–22 details plasma androstenedione levels for normal, osteoporotic, and corticosteroid-treated women. It is interesting to note in this respect the results from the study by Manolagas,[77] who showed that after 10 years following oophorectomy without hormone replacement therapy, women who were fast losers of bone tended to have excessively high levels of urinary free cortisol compared to women who were slow losers of bone or who were estrogen-treated. It may well be that the fast loser mimics the steroid condition of the corticosteroid-treated woman. Figure 2–23 shows the testosterone levels of normal women, osteoporotic women, and corticosteroid-treated women.[28] Again it is noted that corticosteroid-treated women have characteristically reduced levels of steroids in contrast to the other two groups.

Because of these profound influences of corticosteroids on the relevant plasma steroids that control the bone remodeling process, it becomes particularly critical for the alert practitioner to be aware of whether his patients are on corticosteroids and if so to consider some form of therapy to protect the bony structures. The potential use of dehydroepiandrosterone or a precursor to counteract the suppressive effects of corticosteroids on estrone and androstenedione should be considered. For such patients, regular (every 3 months) plasma estrone or androstenedione level monitoring is probably a protective measure.

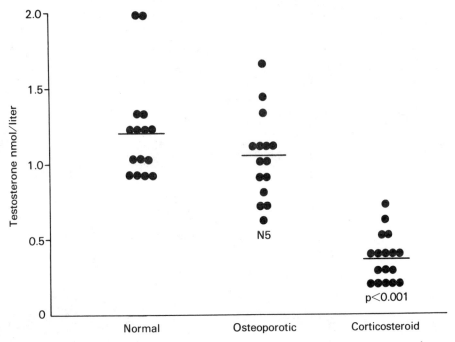

FIG. 2-23. Plasma testosterone levels in normal, osteoporotic, and corticosteroid-treated patients (Crilly RG, Horsman A, Marshall DH, and Nordin BEC, 1978, Front Horm Res 5:58, S. Karger AG, Basel)

CONCLUSIONS

We are thus faced with a major concern for fair-skinned women—osteoporosis. Because 60% of the female population is potentially at risk when no extraordinary measures are taken, osteoporosis constitutes a major concern for the health care of maturing women.

Prevention of the disease can be achieved, in most cases, by developing a plan for continued health care assuring the following:

1. Adequate vitamin D (400 IU a day or 15 minutes sun exposure).
2. Sufficient dietary calcium (about 800 mg in the early 40s, gradually increasing to 1500 mg by age 65).
3. Adequate estrogen levels (with hormone replacement regimens where the body produces insufficient steroid).
4. A regular program of exercise that assures maintenance of muscle tone. Table 2–4 provides calcium and calorie values of common food sources and is taken from *Menopause: A Guide for Women and the Men Who Love Them,* an easy-to-read version of the conclusions of this text.[31]

Treatment of osteoporosis should begin as soon as the clinician, screening for the disease, suspects its presence. The controversy regarding the safety and accuracy of the various methods of bone monitoring continues. The single photon densitometry method still appears to be safe and, from a clinical point of view, useful, in the monitoring of bone loss.[3,15,85] It is never too late to halt the severity of the degenerative process.

TABLE 2-4. The calcium values of common food sources

Food	Calcium Rich Foods		
	Portion	Calories	mg Calcium
Breads & Cereals			
Cream of Wheat, Instant	1 cup, cooked	130	185
Pabulum Cereal			
Barley or Rice	3/4 cup, cooked	108	188
Oatmeal or Mixed	3/4 cup, cooked	110	188
Thomas Protein Bread	1 slice	45	78
Dairy Products			
Cheese			
American	1 oz.	107	195
Cheddar	1 oz.	112	211
Cottage, Creamed	1 cup	239	211
Edam	1 oz.	87	225
Swiss	1 oz.	104	259
Ice Cream (Chocolate)	1/6 quart	174	131
Ice Milk (Vanilla)	1/6 quart	136	189
Milk			
Buttermilk, from Skim	1 cup	88	296
Skim	1 cup	89	303
Whole, Fat 3.5%	1 cup	159	288
Vanilla Pudding	1/2 cup	139	146
Yogurt from Skim with			
Nonfat Milk Solids	1 cup	127	452
Goat Milk	1 cup	163	315
Eggs			
Scrambled, Milk & Fat	1 medium	112	52
Fish & Shellfish			
Flounder	3 oz.	61	55
Mackerel, Canned	3 1/2 oz.	192	194
Oysters, Raw	5–8 medium	66	94
Sardines, Canned	8 medium	311	354
Scallops, Cooked	3 1/2 oz.	112	115
Shrimp, Raw	3 1/2 oz.	91	63
Fruits & Seeds			
Figs, Dried	5 medium	274	126
Orange	1 medium	73	62
Sunflower Seeds	3 1/2 oz.	560	120
Syrups & Sweets			
Blackstrap Molasses	1 tbsp.	43	116
Maple Sugar	4 pieces (2x1x1/2 in.)	348	180
Chocolate Candy	1 bar (2 oz.)	296	52
Vegetables			
Artichoke	edible portion (base and	44	51
Beans	soft end of leaves)		
Lima, Green, Cooked	6 tbsp.	111	47
Snap, Green, Cooked	1 cup	31	62
Wax, Yellow, Cooked	1 cup	22	50
Beet Greens, Cooked	1/2 cup	18	99

TABLE 2-4.   The calcium values of common food sources *(continued)*

Food	Calcium Rich Foods		
	Portion	Calories	mg Calcium
Vegetables			
(continued)			
Broccoli			
Raw	1 stalk (5 in. long)	32	103
Cooked	2/3 cup	26	88
Cabbage, Savoy, Raw	2 cups shredded	24	67
Chard, Cooked	3/5 cup	18	73
Chicory	30–40 inner leaves	20	86
Collards, Cooked	1/2 cup	29	152
Endive	20 long leaves	20	81
Escarole	4 large leaves	20	81
Fennel, Raw	3 1/2 oz.	28	100
Leeks	3–4 (5 in. long)	52	52
Lettuce, Romaine	3 1/2 oz.	18	68
Mustard Greens, Cooked	1/2 cup	23	138
Parsley, Raw	3 1/2 oz.	44	203
Parsnips, Raw	1/2 large	76	50
Rutabagas, Cooked	1/2 cup	35	59
Spinach, Raw	3 1/2 oz.	26	93
Cooked	1/2 cup	21	83
Sweet Potatoes, Baked	1 large	254	72
Watercress, Raw	3 1/2 oz.	19	151

Cutler WB, Garcia CR, Edwards DA, 1983, *Menopause: A Guide for Women and the Men Who Love Them,* New York, W.W. Norton Co., New York, adapted from Pennington J, Church HN 1980, Bowes & Church's Food Values of Portions Commonly Used, 13th ed. JB Lippincott, Philadelphia.

Hormone replacement therapy regimens that include both estrogen and progestins appear, on the basis of preliminary evidence, to offer the optimal hormone treatment approach. Although estrogens inhibit the resorption phase of the bone remodeling process, progestin opposition appears potentially able to increase the active bone formation rates.

REFERENCES

1. Adams JS, Clemens TL, Parrish JA, Holick MF (1982) Vitamin D synthesis and metabolism after ultraviolet irradiation of normal and vitamin D deficient subjects. *New Engl J Med* 306:722–725.

2. Adinoff A, Hollister JR (1983) Steroid-induced fractures and bone loss in patients with asthma. *N Engl J Med* 309:265–268.

3. Adinoff AD, Hollister JR (1984) reply in correspondence to Dr. Mazess. In: *N Engl J Med* 310:321.

4. Aitken JM, Hart DM and Lindsay R (1973) Oestrogen replacement therapy for prevention of osteoporosis after oophorectomy. *Br Med J* 3:515–518.

5. Albanese AA (1977) Osteoporosis *J Am Pharm Assoc* 17:252–253.

6. Albanese AA (1978) Calcium nutrition in the elderly. *Postgrad Med J* 63:3:167–172.

7. Albanese AA, Edelson AH, Lorenze EJ, et al (1969) Quantitative radiographic survey technique for the detection of bone loss. *J Am Geriatr Soc* 17:142–154.

8. Albanese AA, Edelson AH, Lorenze EJ Jr., Woodhull E (1975) Problems of bone health in the elderly: a ten year study. *NY State J Med* 75:326–336.

9. Albanese AA, Lorenze EJ, Edelson AH, Wein EH, Carroll L (1981) Effects of calcium supplements and estrogen replacement therapy on bone loss of postmenopausal women. *Nutrition Reports International* 24:2:403–414.

10. Albanese AA, Lorenze EJ, Wein EH (1978) Osteoporosis: effects of calcium. AFP (Privately printed) 18:160–167.

11. Albright F, Smith PH, Richardson AM (1941) Postmenopausal osteoporosis, its clinical features. *JAMA* 116:2465–2474.

12. Alfram PA (1964) An epidemiologic study of cervical and trochanteric fractures of the femur in an urban population. *Acta Orthop Scand* 65 (Suppl) 1:9–102.

13. Alhava EM, Puittinen J (1973) Fractures of the upper end of the femur as an index of senile osteoporis in Finland. *Ann Clin Res* 5:398–403.

14. Baylink DJ (1983) Glucocorticoid-induced osteoporosis. *N Engl J Med* 309:306–308.

15. Baylink DJ (1984) reply in correspondence to Dr. Mazess In: *N Engl J Med* 310:321–322.

16. Beals RK (1972) Survival following hip fracture: long term followup of 607 patients. *J Chronic Dis* 25:235–244.

17. Boyle IT (1981) Treatment for postmenopausal osteoporosis. *Lancet* June 20, p 1376.

18. Brown DJ, Spanos E, MacIntyre I (1980) Role of pituitary hormones in regulating renal vitamin D metabolism in man. *Br Med J* 1:277–278.

19. Bullamore JR, Gallagher JC, Wilkinson R (1970) Effect of age on calcium absorption. *Lancet* 2:535–537.

20. Cann CE, Genant HK, Ettinger B, Gordan GS (1980) Spinal mineral loss by quantitative computed tomography in oophorectomized women. *JAMA* 244:2056–2059.

21. Chalmers J, Ho KC (1970) Geographical variations in senile osteoporosis: the association with physical activity. *J Bone Joint Surg* 52b:667–675.

22. Chesney RW, Rosen JF, Hamstra AJ, Smith C, Mahaffey K, DeLuca HF (1981) Absence of seasonal variation in serum concentrations of 1,25-dihydroxyvitamin-D despite a rise in 25-hydroxyvitamin-D in summer. *J Clin Endocrinol Metab* 53:139–142.

23. Chestnut CH (1981) Treatment of postmenopausal osteoporosis: some current concepts. *Scott Med J* 26:72–81.

24. Chestnut CH, Baylink DJ, Nelp WB (1979) Calcitonin therapy in postmenopausal osteoporosis: preliminary results. *Clin Res* 27:85A Abstract.

25. Chestnut CH, Nelp WB, Lewellen TK (1981) Neutron activation analysis for whole body calcium measurement. In: *Osteoporosis: Recent Advances in Pathogenesis and Treatment,* pp 19–23. DeLuca HF, Frost HM, Jee WSS, Johnston CC (eds). University Park Press, Baltimore.

26. Christiansen C, Christensen MS, Larsen NE, Transbol IB (1982) Pathophysiological mechanisms of estrogen effect on bone metabolism. *J Clin Endocrinol Metab* 55:1124–1130.

27. Christianssen C, Christensen MS (1981) Bone mass in postmenopausal women after withdrawal of oestrogen/gestagen replacement therapy. *Lancet* Feb 28, 459–461.

28. Crilly RG, Horsman A, Marshall DH, Nordin BEC (1978) Post menopausal and corticosteroid induced osteoporosis. *Front Horm Res* 5:53–75.

29. Crilly RG, Marshall DH, Nordin BE (1979) Effect of age on plasma androstenedione concentration in oophorectomized women. *Clin Endocrinol (Oxf)* 10.2:199–201.

30. Crilly R, Horsman A, Marshall DH, Nordin BEC (1979) Prevalence, pathogenesis and treatment of post-menopausal osteoporosis. *Aust N Z J Med* 9.1:24–30.

31. Cutler WB, Garcia CR, Edwards DA (1983) *Menopause: A Guide for Women and the Men Who Love Them.* New York, WW Norton Co.

32. Dalen N & Olsson KE (1974) Bone mineral content and physical activity. *Acta Orthop Scand* 45:170–174.

33. Daniell HW (1976) Osteoporosis of the slender smoker. *Arch Intern Med* 136:298–304.

34. Davidson BJ, Riggs BL, Wahner WH, Judd HL (1983) Endogenous cortisol and sex steroids in patients with osteoporotic spinal fractures. *Obstet Gynecol* 61:275–278.

35. Davie M, Lawson DEM (1980) Assessment of plasma 25-hydroxyvitamin D response to ultraviolet irradiation over a controlled area in young and elderly subjects. *Clin Sci* 58:235–242.

36. Davis ME, Strandjord NM and Lanzl LH (1966) Estrogens and the aging process. *JAMA* 196:219–224.

37. Deding A, Tougaard L, Jensen MK, Rodbro P (1977) Bone changes during prednisone treatment. *Acta Med Scand* 202:253–255.

38. Deftos LJ, Roos BA, Bronzert D, Parthemore JG (1975) Immunochemical heterogeneity of calcitonin in plamsa. *Clin Endocrinol Metab* 40:409–412.

39. Deftos LJ, Weisman MH (1980) Influence of age and sex on plasma calcitonin in human beings. *N Engl J Med* 302:1351–1353.

40. Erlik Y, Meldrum DR, Lagasse LD, Judd HL (1981) Effect of megestrol acetate on fushing and bone metabolism in postmenopausal women. *Maturitas* 3:167–171.

41. Fraser DR (1980) Regulation of the metabolism of vitamin D. *Physiol Rev* 60:551–613.

42. Gallagher JC, Aaron J, Horsman A, Marshall DH, Wilkinson R, and Nordin BEC (1973) The crush fracture syndrome in postmenopausal women. *Clin Endocrinol Metab* 2:293–315.

43. Gallagher JC, Horsman A, Nordin BEC (1974) Osteoporosis in the menopause. In: *The Menopausal Syndrome*. Greenblatt RB, Mahesh VB, McDonough PG (eds). New York, Medcom Press.

44. Gallagher JC, Melton LJ, Riggs BL, Bergstrath E (1980) Epidemiology of fractures of the proximal femur in Rochester, Minnesota, U S A. *Clin Orthop* 150:163–171.

45. Gallagher J and Nordin BEC (1975) Effects of oestrogen and progestogen therapy on calcium metabolism in post-menopausal women. *Front Hor Res* 3:150–176.

46. Gallagher JC, Riggs BL, DeLuca HF (1978) Effect of age on calcium absorption and serum 1,25 OH2D3 *Clin Res* 26:680A.

47. Garn SM (1970) *The Earlier Gain and the Later Loss of Cortical Bone in Nutritional Perspective*, pp 69–137. Springfield, Illinois, Charles C. Thomas.

48. Geola F, Frumar A, Tataryn I, Lu K, Hershman J, Eggena P, Sambhi M, Judd H (1980) Biological effects of various doses of conjugated equine estrogens in postmenopausal women. *J Clin Endocrinol Metab* 51:620–625.

49. Girgis SI, Hillyard CJ, MacIntyre I, Szelke M (1977) An immunological comparison of normal circulating calcitonin with calcitonin from medullary carcinoma. *Mol Endocrinol* 175–178.

50. Goldsmith NF (1971) Bone-mineral estimation in normal and osteoporotic women: a comparability trial of four methods and seven bone sites. *J Bone Joint Surg* (Am) 53A:83–100.

51. Gordan GS (1981) Early detection of osteoporosis and prevention of hip fractures in elderly women. *Med Times* special section following page 104. pp 1s–17s. April

52. Hahn TJ, Boisseau VC, Avioli LV (1974) Effect of chronic corticosteroid administration on diaphyseal and metaphyseal bone mass. *J Clin Endocrinol Metab* 39:274–282.

53. Heaney RP (1962) Radiocalcium metabolism in disuse osteoporosis in man *Am J Med* 33:188–200.

54. Heaney RP (1974) Pathophysiology of osteoporosis: implication for treatment. *Tex Med* 70:37–45.

55. Heaney RP, Recker RR, Saville PD (1977) Calcium balance and calcium requirements in middle aged women. *Am J Clin Nutr* 30:1603–1611.

56. Heath H, Sizemore G (1977) Plasma calcitonin in normal man. *J Clin Invest* 60:1135–1140.

57. Hempel Von E, Kriester A, Freesmeyer E, Walter W (1979) Prospecktive studie zur osteoporose nach bilater ovarektomie mit und ohne postoperative ostrogenprophylaxe. *Zentralblatt fur Gynakologie* 101:309–319.

58. Hillyard CJ, Stevenson JC. MacIntyre I, (1978) Relative deficiency of plasma-calcitonin in normal women. *Lancet* 1:961–962.

59. Holick FM (1981) The cutaneous photosynthesis of previtamin D3; a unique photoendocrine system. *J Invest Dermatol* 76:51–58.

60. Horsman A, Gallagher JC, Simpson M & Nordin BEC (1977) Prospective trial of oestrogen and calcium in postmenopausal women. *Br Med J* 2:789–792.

61. Horsman A, Jones M, Francis R, Nordin C (1983) The effect of estrogen dose on postmenopausal bone loss. *New Engl J Med* 309:1405–1407.

62. Horsman A, Nordin BEC, Gallagher JC, Kirby PA, Milner RM & Simpson M (1977) Observations of sequential changes in bone mass in post-menopausal women: a controlled trial of oestrogen and calcium therapy. *Calcif. Tissue Res* (suppl) 22:217–224.

63. Hutchinson TA, Polansy SM, Feinstein AR (1979) Postmenopausal estrogens protect against fractures of hip and distal radius, a case-control study. *Lancet* 2:705–709.

64. Ireland P, Fordtran JS (1973) Effect of dietary calcium on age on jejunal calcium absorption in humans studied by intestinal perfusion. *J Clin Invest* 52:2672–2681.

65. Juttmann JR, Visser TJ, Buurman C, deKam E, Birkenhager JC (1981) Seasonal fluctuations in serum concentrations of vitamin D metabolites in normal subects. *Br Med J* 282:1349–1352.

66. Kimberg DV, Baerg RD, Dusius RT (1971) Effect of cortisone treatment on the active transport of calcium by the small intestine. *J Clin Invest* 50:1309–1321.

67. Lafferty FW, Spencer GE, Pearson OH (1964) Effects of androgens, estrogens and high calcium intakes on bone formation and resorption in osteoporosis. *Am J Med* 36:514–528.

68. Lee CJ, Lawler GS, and Johnson GH (1981) Effects of supplementation of the diets with calcium and calcium-rich foods on bone density of elderly females with osteoporosis. *Am J Clin Nutr* 34:819–823.

69. Lindsay R, Aitken JM, Anderson JB (1976) Long term prevention of postmenopausal osteoporosis by estrogen *Lancet* 1:1038–1040.

70. Lindsay R, Aitken JM, Hart DM, Purdie D (1978) The effect of ovarian sex steroids on bone mineral status in the oophorectomized rat and in the human. *Postgrad Med J* 54:2:50–58.

71. Lindsay R, Coutts JR, Hart DM (1977) The effect of endogenous estrogen on plasma and urinary calcium and phosphate in oophorectomized women. *Clin Endocrinol (Oxf)* 6:2:87–93.

72. Lindsay R, Hart DM, MacLean A, Clark AC, Kraszewski A, Garwood J (1978) Bone response to termination of oestrogen treatment. *Lancet* 1:8078:1325–1327.

73. Lindsay R, Hart DM, Purdie D (1978) Comparative effects of oestrogen and progestogen on bone loss in postmenopause women. *Clin Sci Mol Med* 54:193–195.

74. Longcope C, Jafee W, Griffing G (1981) Production rates of androgens and oestrogens in postmenopausal women. *Maturitas* 3:215–223.

75. MacIntrye I, Evans IMA, Hobitz HHG, Joplin GF, Stevenson JC (1980) Chemistry, physiology, and therapeutic applications of calcitonin. *Arthritis Rheum* 23:1139–1147.

76. MacIntrye I, Parsons JA (1967) The effect of thyrocalcitonin on blood bone calcium equilibrium in the perfused tibia of the cat. *J Physiol (Lond)* 191:393–405.

77. Manolagas SC, Anderson DC (1978) Detection of high affinity glucocorticoid binding in rat bone. *J Endocrinol* 76:379–380.

78. Marshall DH, Nordin BE (1977) The effect of 1-alpha-hydroxyvitamin D3 with and without oestrogens on calcium balance in postmenopausal women. *Clin Endocrinol (Oxf)* 7(suppl):159s–168s.

79. Marshall DH, Crilly RG, Nordin BE (1977) Plasma androstenedione and oestrone levels in normal and osteoporotic postmenopausal women. *Br Med J* 2:6098:1177–1179.

80. Marshall DH, Crilly R, Nordin BE (1978) The relation between plasma androstrenedione and oestrone levels in untreated and corticosteroid treated post-menopausal women. *Clin Endocrinol* (Oxf) 9:5:407–412.

81. Martin, P (1982) Unpublished data . . . kindly supplied and on file.

82. Mawer EB (1980) Clinical implications of measurements of circulating vitamin D metabolites. *J Clin Endocrinol Metab* 9:63–79.

83. Mawer EB, Backhouse J, Holman CA, Lumb GA, Stanbury SW (1972) The distribution and storage of vitamin D and its metabolites in human tissues. *Clin Sci* 43:413–431.

84. Mazess RB (1983) Errors in measuring trabecular bone by computed tomography due to marrow and bone composition. *Calcif Tissue Int* 35:148–152.

85. Mazess RB (1984) Steroid induced bone loss. (letter) *N Engl J Med* 310:321.

86. Meema HE, Bunker MI, Meema S (1965) Loss of compact bone due to menopause. *Obstet Gynecol* 26:333–343.

87. Meema S & Meema HE (1976) Menopausal bone loss and estrogen replacement. *Isr J Med Sci* 12:601–606.

88. Meunier P, Courpron P, Edourd C, Bernard J, Bringuier J, and Vignon F (1973) Physiological senile involution and pathological rarefaction of bone. *Clin Endocrinol Metab* 2:239–256.

89. Molinas G, Bompani R, Scali G, et al. (1970) Modifications induced by treatment with medroxyprogesterone acetate in the urinary excretion of the calcium after oral and intravenous load in old subjects. *Giornale de Gerontologia* 18:361–372.

90. Mueller MN (1976) Effects of corticosteroids on bone mineral in rheumatoid arthritis and asthma. *AJR* 126:1300, abstract.

91. Nachtigall LE, Nachtigall RH, Nachtigall RD, Beckman EM (1979) Estrogen replacement therapy 1:A 10 year prospective study in the relationship to osteoporosis. *Obstet Gynecol* 53:277–281.

92. Nilson BE and Westlin NE (1971) Bone density in athletes. *Clin Orthop* 77:179–182.

93. Nordin BEC, Gallagher JC, Aaron JE, Horsman H (1975) Postmenopausal osteopenia and osteoporosis. In Estrogens in the Postmenopause. *Front Hormone Res* Karger, Basel 3:133–149.

94. Nordin BEC, Horsman A, Marshall DH, Simpson M, Waterhouse GM (1979) Calcium requirement and calcium therapy. *Clin Orthop* 140:216–239.

95. Nordin BEC, Horsman A, Brook R, Williams DA (1976) The relationship between oestrogen status and bone loss in post-menopausal women. *Clin Endocrinol* 5 Supp 1353–361.

96. Paganini-Hill A, Ross RD, Gerkins VR (1981) A case-control study of menopausal estrogen therapy and hip fractures. *Ann Intern Med* 95:28–31.

97. Pak CYC, Stewart A, Kaplan R, Bone H, Notz C, Browne R (1975) Photon absorptiometric analysis of bone density in primary hyperparathroidism. *Lancet* 2:7–8.

98. Papapoulos SE, Clemens TL, Fraher LJ, Gleed J, O'Riordan JLH (1980) Metabolites of vitamin D in human vitamin-D deficiency: effect of vitamin D2 or 1,25-dihydroxycholecalciferol. *Lancet* September 20:612–615.

99. Pollner F (1979) When is estrogen replacement therapy justified? *Obstet Gynecol News* July 1, 1979, 1–16.

100. Rasmussen H & Bordier P (1974) *The Physiological Basis of Metabolic Bone Disease.* Baltimore, Williams & Wilkins.

101. Rasmussen H, Bordier P, Marie P, Auguier L, Eisinger JB, Kuntz D, Caulin F, Argemi B, Gueris J, & Julien A (1980) Effect of combined therapy with phosphate and calcitonin on bone volume in osteoporosis. *Metab Bone Dis Relat Res* 2:107–111.

102. Recker RR, Saville PC, Heaney RP (1977) Effect of estrogens and calcium carbonate on bone loss in postmenopausal women. *Ann Intern Med* 87.6:649–655.

103. Reynolds JJ, Holick MF, DeLuca HF (1973) The role of vitamin D metabolites in bone resorption. *Calcif Tissue Res* (suppl) 12:295–301.

104. Rickers H, Deding A, Christiansen C, Rodbro P, Naestoft J (1982) Corticosteroid-induced osteopenia and vitamin D metabolism: effect of vitamin D2 calcium phosphate and sodium fluoride administration. *Clin Endocrinol* (Oxf) 16:409–415.

105. Riggs BL, Hodgson SF, Hoffman DL, Kelly PJ, Johnson KA and Taves D (1980) Treatment of primary osteoporosis with fluoride and calcium. *JAMA* 243:446–449.

106. Riggs BL, Jowsey J, Goldsmith RS, Kelly PJ, Hoffman DL, and Arnaud CD (1972) Short and long-term effects of estrogen and synthetic anabolic hormone in postmenopausal osteoporosis. *J Clin Invest* 51:1659–1663.

107. Riggs BL, Jowsey J, Kelly PJ, Jones JD & Maher FT (1969) Effect of sex hormones on bone in primary osteoporosis. *J Clin Invest* 48:1065–1072.

108. Riggs BL, Seeman E, Hodgson SF, Taves DR & O'Fallon WM (1982) Effect of the fluoride/calcium regimen on vertebral fracture occurrence in postmenopausal osteoporosis. *New Engl J Med* 306:446–450.

109. Rushton C (1978) Vitamin D hydroxylation in youth and old age. *Age Aging* 7:91–95.

110. Samaan N, Anderson GD (1975) Immunoreactive calcitonin in the mother, neonate, child and adult. *Am J Obstet Gynecol* 121:622–625.

111. Scali G, Cosselli C, Palmari V, et al (1970) Modifications induced by the calcitonin load on the curve of disappearance of Ca++ from the serum in patients with osteoporosis treated with medroxyprogesterone acetate. *Gional di Gerontologia* 18:382–388.

112. Schlenker RA (1976) Percentages of cortical and trabecular bone mineral mass in the radius and ulna. *AJR* 126:1309–1312, abstract.

113. Smith DM, Khairi MRA, Norton J, Johnston OC Jr (1976) Age and activity effects on rate of bone mineral loss. *J Clin Invest* 568:716–721.

114. Smith EL, Reddan W, and Smith PE (1981) Physical activity and calcium modalities of bone mineral increase in aged women. *Med Sci Sports Exer* 13:60–64.

115. Smith EL, Reddan W (1976) Physical activity—a modality for bone accretion in the aged. Conference on Bone Mineral Measurement. *Am J Roentgenology* 126:1297.

116. Stamp TCB, Round JM (1974) Seasonal changes in human plasma levels of 25-hydroxyvitamin D. *Nature* 247:563–565.

117. Stevenson JC (1980) The structure and function of calcitonin. *Investigations and Cell Path* 3:187–193.

118. Stevenson JC, Hillyard CJ, Abeyasekara G, Phang KG, MacIntyre I, Campbell S, Young O, Townsend PT, Whitehead MI (1981) Calcitonin and the calcium-regulating hormones in postmenopausal women: effect of estrogens. *Lancet* 693–695.

119. Stevenson JC, Hillyard CJ, MacIntyre I (1979) A physiological role for calcitonin protection of the maternal skeleton. *Lancet* 2:769–770.

120. Styrd RP, Gilbertson TJ, Brunden MN (1979) A seasonal variation study oif 25 hydroxyvitamin D3 serum levels in normal humans. *J Clin Endocrinol Metab* 48:771–775.

121. Stevenson JC and Whitehead MI (1982) Calcitonin secretion and postmenopausal osteoporosis. *Lancet* April 3:804.

122. Taggart H, Ivey JL, Sison K, Chestnut CH III, Baylink DJ, Huber MB, and Roos BA (1982) Deficient calcitonin response to calcium stimulation in postmenopausal osteoporosis. *Lancet* Feb 27. 475–478.

123. Tonelli M, Cucinotta D, Gundi A et al (1970) Intestinal absorption of radioactive calcium in old patients with osteoporosis treated with medroxyprogesterone acetate. *Giornale di Gerontologia* 18:420–425.

124. Transbol I, Christensen MS, Jensen GF, Christiansen C, McNair P (1982) Thiazide for the postponement of postmenopausal bone loss. *Metabolism* 31:4:383–386.

125. Urist MR (1973) Orthopedic management of postmenopausal osteoporosis. *Clin Endocrinol Metab* 2:159–176.

126. Wallach S & Henneman PH (1959) Prolonged estrogen therapy in postmenopausal women. *JAMA* 171:1637.

127. Walton J, Dominguez M, Bartler FC (1975) Effects of calcium infusions in patients with postmenopausal osteoporosis. *Metabolism* 24:7:849–854.

128. Watson RC (1973) Bone growth and physical activity. *International Conference on Bone Mineral Measurements* 380–385.

129. Weiss NS, Ure CL, Ballard J (1980) Decreased rise of fractures of the hip and forearm with postmenopausal use of estrogen. *New Engl J Med* 303:1195.

130. Whyte MP, Bergfeld MA, Murphy WA, Avioli LV, Teitelbaum SL (1982) Postmenopausal osteoporosis: a heterogeneous disorder as assessed by histomorphometric analysis of iliac crest bone from untreated patients. *Am J Med* 72:193–202.

131. Williams AR, Weiss NS, Ure CL, Ballard J, Daling Jr (1982) Effect of weight, smoking and estrogen use on the risk of hip and forearm fractures in postmenopausal women. *Obstet Gynecol* 160:659–699.

132. Wiske PS, Epstein NH, Bell NH, Queener SF, Edmondson J & Johnston CC (1979) Increases in immunoreactive parathyroid hormone with age. *N Engl J Med* 300:1419–1421.

133. Worley RJ (1981) Age, estrogen, and bone density. *Clin Obstet Gynecol* 24:203–218.

134. Wylie, CM (1977) Hospitalization for fractures and bone loss in adults. *Public Health Rep* 92:33–38.

3

Sexuality and Hormones

SEXUALITY: GENERAL CONSIDERATIONS FOR STUDY

Professionals will frequently be called upon to give guidance and information to menopausal women about the many changes that are happening in their own and their partner's sexual lives. Not everyone may be prepared to respond to this important need. Some information is available for heterosexual couples; virtually no scientific studies have been published to guide those who express other sexual preferences. For this reason, discussions are limited to heterosexual dynamics although we acknowledge the needs of others.

Studies of human sexuality are necessarily incomplete in the information they can provide. Because sexual function is a dynamic process between two individuals—one that is intimately entwined in emotion—conclusions that can be drawn from individual studies often are distorted. Nonetheless, from the studies that are available, one can combine the facts that may be particularly useful in guiding a clinician's understanding and ability to advise and counsel the patient.

It is deplorable that much of the sexuality data is viewed in a priggish way by many immature sensationalists as well as uninformed moralists.[71] Moreover, in a rapidly changing moral climate such as has been witnessed over the last several decades, the message of society is clear: Times have changed. Many women have become more aware of and vocal in their demands for a sexually satisfying life-style. It is interesting to note that by 1973 an increasing convergence in sexual response to erotic films had been noted in both men and women.

The general harmony that affirms to both the man and the woman the complementary nature of their own roles, that is, their respective masculinity and femininity, can be called sexuality. Individual studies provide segments of the picture. A composite of the various studies offers a more cohesive and integrated view. It would appear, from the various studies, that the male endocrine system and sexual behavior are influenced by the female counterparts and *vice versa*. One elegant study by Persky and co-workers demonstrated a delicate phase-locking between the cyclic variation in a woman's sex drive and her partner's change in sexual behavior that correlated with rises in his testosterone levels.[96,97] A mathematical harmonic could be described for most of the couples; the man's behavior and his testosterone peaks were predicted by the woman's changing hormone secretions.

Nonetheless, disparities between the sexes have also been observed. There is a steady decline in the incidence and frequencies of marital coitus with advancing age.[28,45,46] In the 1950s Kinsey and Pomeroy, in observing this trend, considered it to be the result of the aging processes in the male.[60] They saw that the decline in sexual capacities of the female appeared much later in her life than her physical decline. Husbands and wives have long been known to report somewhat opposite trends in life-phase preferences for frequency of sexual intercourse. Sexual desire of the males when they were younger was greater, and this general pattern reversed as the couple matured.[60] More recently, Pfeiffer and co-workers collected data from men and women, ages 45 to 69. They reported that the women's sexual activity was primarily a reflection of the availability of a "socially sanctioned" sexual relationship.[98] They further concluded that, when there was a decline in the activity of a couple, the tendency was for both the man and woman to attribute the reduction to a decline in the *male's* function rather than to the female's responsiveness. A clear decline in each five-year increment for both frequency of sexual intercourse and desire for sexual activity was apparent.[98] Lief also concluded that the chief sexual problem after age 50 rests with the male—specifically his inability to maintain an erection.[73] Others comment on the decreasing availability of male sex partners with advancing years.[59] Because the clinician will need to be sensitive to a woman's situation (which perforce reflects what is happening with her partner), this chapter reviews studies of aging male sexual physiology as well as studies in the female.

THE SEXUAL RESPONSE IN AGING WOMEN

Measurements of sexual arousal in women were pioneered by several investigators. The reports of Masters and Johnson are widely known. In addition, the use of a vaginal photometry tool was reported in the 1960s.[124] It was further refined in the 1970s.[41,49,53] Vaginal photometry today generally uses an indirectly lighted photo cell probe that can reflect vaginal blood volume.[32,36,48,112] The tool has been useful in showing that the vaginal blood volume reaches a peak just before orgasm and this peak level is followed by a rapid decline in pooled volume.[36] After this decline there is often a rebound with postorgasmic blood volumes that are higher than the original base levels, which lasts for about 10 minutes. However, the phenomenon does not occur in all women. This measuring technique allows the subject to insert the probe in the privacy of a lab and, thereby, participate in the sex experiments without being directly viewed by anyone. Such methods allow a more natural kind of sexual response than the earlier directly viewed sexual activity studies pioneered by Masters and Johnson.[76-78] However, these direct measurements of genital response to arousal came into disfavor because, more recently, discoveries that the zephiran chloride (a sterilizing solution) that is applied to the probe between patients was reported to be ineffective against viruses such as herpes.[35,48] The vaginal and pelvic responses to sexual stimulation have been well characterized. Beginning with the classic work of Masters and Johnson and continuing to the more recent issues of a "G spot"* and uterine/cervical response to sexual stimulation, our developing understanding of female sexual response shows the potential for a very complex hierarchical orgasmic response, one that may show a clitorovulval orgasm that, if adequate, repeated massage of the G spot is supplied in a vaginally stimulable site, can effect more powerful vaginal contractions at orgasm.[38,94] More recently, the potential for a cervicouterine orgasmic response to deep coital thrusting has been described.[18,59a,125] Studies using intrauterine transducers to record uterine contractions during orgasm are currently underway in the laboratory of Dr. Julian Davidson at Stanford; oxytocin release

---

*Grafenberg described the site of maximal muscle reaction to vaginal stimulation on the superior–anterior region of the vagina.

at orgasm is under study as well. At this writing, positive results in both were obtained in a small sample.

In evaluating the age-related hormonally induced changes in sexual response, it is necessary to distinguish measurements of sexual arousal from measurements of orgasmic response. With the diminution of steroid levels characteristic of the menopause, a number of changes in both dimensions occur.[77,78] Masters and Johnson have described in great detail the characteristics of these changes. A senile involution of target organs (breasts, labia, vagina, and uterus) predictably follows the steroid declines of the menopause. An alteration in the timing of sexual arousal responses follows.

The breast continues to respond to sexual arousal with advancing age. Although nipple erection is unchanged, the vasocongestive response is diminished and breast swelling during arousal is less pronounced. Rectal contractions during orgasm are absent as aging advances. Clitoral responses to sexual excitement are less likely to occur: tumescence is less pronounced, the elevation of the clitoris during the plateau phase is unchanged, and the de-tumescence is more rapid at resolution. The labial responses tend to be lost with advancing age because the fatty deposits that facilitate flattening, separation, and elevation during arousal are diminished. The responses of the labia minora also show changes. The youthful vasocongestive thickening is reduced as the woman ages and there is an obvious loss in the consistency of the minor labial sex skin reaction. The vagina also changes with age, shortening from an average of 7 to 8 cm (during the 20s to 40s) to a smaller 4.5 to 6 cm in length. The thickness of the barrel likewise diminishes by about 25%. The lubrication response is usually delayed although exceptions were noted. In the three cases that Masters and Johnson were able to document that had had uninterrupted weekly coital activity throughout their maturing years, no delay occurred despite postmenopausal status and atrophic vaginal mucosa. Although the excitement phase expansion of the vaginal barrel is reduced with advancing years, direct penile stimulation produces more expansion than masturbation does. The orgasmic contraction phase is identical in quality but its frequency is reduced, from an average of 5 to 10 orgasmic contractions in the young woman to 3 to 5 contractions in the older woman.[77] The cervix diminishes with the steroid decline as well.

Because of the delay in vaginal lubrication it can be very helpful to explain to the patient the need for extended foreplay before sexual intercourse in order to facilitate lubrication. According to Masters and Johnson it may take up to 5 minutes of "non-demanding sex play" for any degree of lubrication response in the 50+ woman. One notes that this is similar to the male's delayed onset of erection with advancing age and although the arousal mechanisms take longer to achieve, the quality of the experience is not necessarily diminished.[78] In fact, it can be easily enhanced. Sensuous experience is not confined to the mechanical response capacities.

The true source of the vaginal lubrication has been a subject of study but remains unresolved.[18,76,100] Masters and Johnson, using a transparent penis, described the rapid lubricative response to sexual stimulation.[76] Preti and co-workers noted no consistent alterations in the organic compounds of vaginal secretion caused by sexual arousal but a clear change in quantity of fluid.[100] Cutler and García discussed a potential for cervical contribution to coital lubrication if estrogen levels are adequate.[18] Semmons described the vaginal function in postmenopausal women who were estrogen deprived as being deficient and showed a return to more youthful levels of vaginal blood flow, vaginal fluid, vaginal pH, and transvaginal potential difference to the perimenopausal level in women given estrogen replacement therapy.[111] See Table 3–1. The literature is consistent in showing declines in vaginal function and lubrication response to sexual arousal that

TABLE 3-1. Baseline values for study subjects at beginning of study and at 1, 3, and 6 months after administration of conjugated estrogens

	Estrogen Administration, months					
	0 (N=13)	1 (N=12)*	3 (N=11)	6 (N=13)	SD	p
Vaginal blood flow, mW†	208 b	236 a	244 a	225 ab	22.9	0.004
Vaginal fluid, g†	0.08 b	0.11 ab	0.14 a	0.10 b	0.4	0.001
Vaginal pH†	5.4 a	4.8 b	4.6 b	4.7 b	0.5	0.006
Transvaginal potential difference, mV†	22.7 b	28.8 b	36.0 a	27.0 b	7.2	0.001

*Except in the test for vaginal fluid, in which there were 11 subjects
†Any two mean values above the same letter are not significantly different ($p > 0.05$).
Semmens JP, Wagner G 1982, JAMA 248:445–448; copyright 1966–79, 1981–82, American Medical Association

directly reflect the levels of estrogen. However, even when estrogen levels are equivalent, in age-matched postmenopausal women 50 to 65 years old, sexually active women show less vaginal atrophy than their inactive counterparts.[72]

The potential for cervical stimulation (received from deep coital thrusting) to promote a uterine orgasm has been discussed in the literature.[18, 59a, 125] The changes in the cervix with the menopausal declines in estrogen[10,77,78] have provided further suggestions for a general decline in such a putative orgasmic capacity with advancing years.

DYSPAREUNIA

The thinning of the vaginal mucosa as well as the tendency for diminished lubricative response increases the potential for dyspareunia that occurs with the diminution of estrogen levels. This also increases the probability of developing vaginitis, particularly followed by unlubricated coitus. The Stanford Menopause Study, which was jointly founded by one of us (and Dr. Julian Davidson), originally enrolled several hundred women as they were entering their menopausal transition and continued to follow them through the years. Twenty-five percent of the perimenopausal women in The Stanford Menopause Study reported a lubricative deficit at least half the time they have coitus (Fig. 3–1). One notes the apparent lack of relationship between lubricative dryness and overall symptomatology. The K score, developed by Kupperman and colleagues, is a composite score that quantifies the severity (by a factor loading number) for the 11 common menopause distress symptoms. Higher scores denote greater levels of distress. The age distribution of the sample is shown in Figure 3–2. Dyspareunia is a less frequent complaint in this group of women (Fig. 3–3). Dyspareunia is a common complaint in menopausal women who are having sporadic sexual activity, although it is common in young women as well (sexual activity not reported).[68] For menopausal or climacteric dyspareunia, estrogen replacement therapy is reported to be effective in providing relief.[25,26,56,93,110] Semmens noted that estrogen-responsive dyspareunia may actually precede any physical evidence of vaginal atrophy.[110] Furthermore, although cytologic

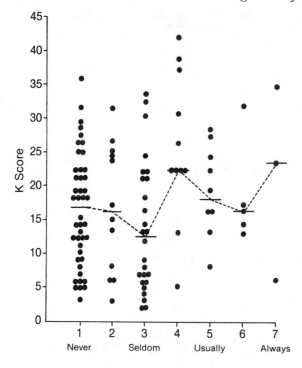

FIG. 3-1. The Stanford Menopause Study—Perimenopausal women's sexual lubrication response. Participants responded to the question, "Do you currently suffer from lack of vaginal lubrication (wetness) during sex?"

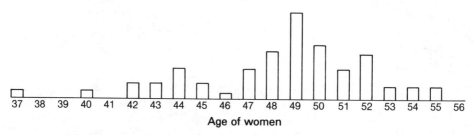

FIG. 3-2. Age distribution of the Stanford Menopause Study women

improvement is rapid when estrogens are prescribed, recovery from painful intercourse can easily take many more months to achieve. The improvement is progressive and was continuing at the 18-month checkup. Progestins were not considered effective, because they failed to produce adequate cornification of vaginal epithelia.[25,56] Moreover, they are also antiestrogenic.

SEXUAL LIFE AFTER ABSTINENCE

It has been noted that sporadic sexual activity may disrupt the maintenance of a vaginal ruggor.[72] The patient is well cautioned to carefully resume sexual activity after a period of abstinence. Painful abrasions caused by coitus can be avoided. If resumption is gradual so that the vaginal barrel has an opportunity to respond to the new friction and dilatation pressure, within several weeks the propensity for abrasions should diminish. If coitus is

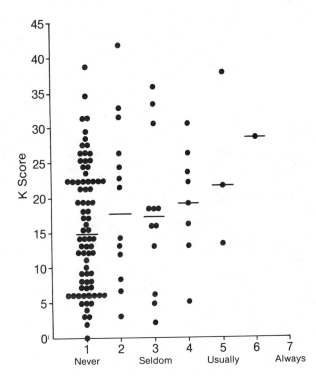

FIG. 3-3. Dyspareunia incidence among perimenopausal women asked, "Do you currently suffer from dyspareunia (pain during intercourse)?"

resumed too vigorously after a period of abstinence, the trauma to the tissues is likely to increase the dyspareunia and the couple may give up on sex altogether. The clinician, armed with this knowledge, should be able to help the couple to enjoy a sexual life well into old age. Sensitively offered explanations of this physiological pattern should be routine.

The effect of steroid hormones on the buccal mucosa of menopausal women provides some insight into the mechanisms involved. Pisantry and colleagues compared postmenopausal dental patients who were complaining of oral dryness, burning sensation, and unpleasant viscosity of saliva with age-matched, noncomplaining controls. Regular gingival massage, whether with estrogen cream, progesterone and estrogen cream, or placebo, *all* yielded restoration of the mucosa by inducing proliferative changes in the buccal epithelia. The regular massage also induced an increase in saliva.[99] This oral mechanism is probably mirrored in a vaginal tissue response to penile massage as well as to masturbation.

LIBIDINAL CHANGES WITH AGE IN WOMEN

Hormone changes, advancing age, and loss of partner produce very variable libidinal effects.[38,42,43,52,57,90] Although the power of a new relationship to increase libido is well acknowledged and sex interest sometimes does increase, a libidinal increase is reported in less than 25% of perimenopausal women.[90] Figure 3-4 shows the tendency to experience sexual fantasy (libido) in relation to the amount of menopausal distress a climacteric woman was experiencing (Kupperman score). One notes a wide range of libido scores and no obvious relationship between libido and menopausal distress score.

In Figure 3–5 this same population answered whether their libidinal status had changed since the onset of climacteric changes in menstruation pattern. One notes that the overwhelming majority (average age 49) have not observed a change in their libidinal life. One further notes that there was a small percentage that did show a decline as well as a small percentage that did show an increase. Again the change in fantasy shows no obvious relationship to the amount of menopausal distress the woman is experiencing. Others have also evaluated sexual behavior patterns in the early menopausal years. Gruis and Wagner reviewed the literature with regard to sexual functioning and sexual appetite for men and for women. They noted an overwhelming trend toward decline with the passage of time (for both sexes).[45] Others have also observed a clear decline with the passage of years.[46,50,98] The effect is noted in *both* men and women.

While libidinal changes are based on reported data and are considered "soft," nonetheless a significant pattern is demonstrable. Thus, it would appear that the sexual responses gradually decline with age and that these declines occur simultaneously with the diminution in steroid levels. In addition, there appears to be an influence of a woman's earlier sexual satisfaction on the postmenopausal frequency of coital activity.[13] Women who were sexually active in their 20s tend to seek sexual activity in the menopause.

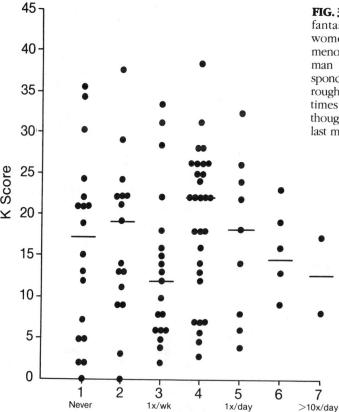

FIG. 3-4. Frequency of sexual fantasy in perimenopausal women and their incident menopausal distress (Kupperman score). Participants responded to statement "Give a rough estimate of how many times you have had sexual thoughts or fantasies during the last month."

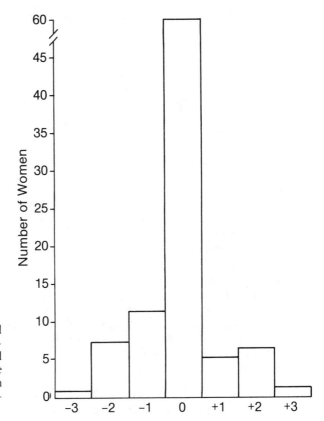

FIG. 3-5. Change in sexual fantasy (premenopausal transition) during the menopausal transition years. Overall change in libido: current compared with the years before menstrual cycles became irregular.

SEXUAL LIFE AFTER GYNECOLOGIC OPERATIONS

By 1983, the Centers for Disease Control had provided data to show that 50% of women can be expected to have been hysterectomized by the age of 45. With such an increasing incidence of gynecologic surgery in the United States, it becomes imperative for the clinician to be sensitive to the potential these surgeries have for modifying sexual response. The short-term effects, that is, abdominal and vaginal soreness, pass after several months.[4] The long-term effects are often more critical.[26]

For women who are accustomed to deriving sexual pleasure from cervical stimulation or for women who regularly experience uterine contractions at orgasm, it is reasonable to question what the loss of these tissues and their associated neural afferents would do to the sexual life of the couple. These questions have recently been raised in the literature.[18,59a,125] In brief, the potential neural afferent network is present in the cervix, as well as the efferent neural innervation to the uterine smooth muscle, to support the potential for a reflex orgasmic loop between cervical stimulation and subsequent uterine contraction at orgasm.[16,61,75,79,116] Cervical procedures that interfere with such a putative orgasmic pathway would be expected to diminish the capacity for full sexual response in those women who experience uterine orgasm. It is commonly reported that 25% to 45% of posthysterectomy patients notice a deficit in libido that does not recover.[26,121,122] It has been suggested that the women at greatest risk for this subsequent loss of libido may be those individuals who are accustomed to a cervical/uterine orgasm.

THE BRAIN AS A MEDIATOR OF HORMONES AND BEHAVIOR

GENERAL CONSIDERATIONS

Intriguing puzzles about the relationships between hormones and behavior consume the energy of countless scientists, and no clear or complete answers have yet evolved. Money, in 1961, was discussing sex hormones and other variables in human eroticism. He concluded that there are three coordinates to sexual function: local genital surfaces, the brain, and the hormones. None was indispensable. For example, vulvectomized women are still sexual beings; hypogonadal men receiving androgen therapy show increased sexual behavior with diminution following decrease in therapy; androgen therapy in women has been reported to increase sexual desire;[83] and androstenedione levels were shown to be positively correlated with levels of sexual desire in younger[95] and postmenopausal women.[72] Answers to the puzzle of how these various situations combine to form a mechanistic system will probably never be achieved. The complex involvement of the human cortex in perceptual processes is far from simple. McEwen has addressed the question of endocrine effects on the brain and their relationships to behavior.[81] He described the relationship between hormones and receptors, saying that a putative receptor could only be confirmed when a series of criteria could be met. These include their presence in hormone-responsive tissues or brain regions, their absence from nonresponsive ones, and the ability to bind steroids that are either active agonists or effective antagonists of the hormone and not to bind steroids that are inactive in either sense. Even when these conditions have been met and hormones and receptors are thereby known to be interacting, the way in which the stimulation of nucleic acid synthesis and the subsequent production of protein could ultimately be mediated to produce behavior and emotion is one of the great puzzles of psychoneuro-endocrinology. Obtaining these data in humans poses logistic and ethical problems. One must, perforce, turn to animal models for information, realizing that not all of the data are transferable to understanding humans. Particularly intriguing, in the sexual spheres, are early studies in rats that showed that removing the testes on the day of birth produces an adult animal that shows more feminine behavior in response to an estrogen injection than intact males; also, testosterone administration to infant females on the day of birth with subsequent ovariectomy as adults produces adult females that are more masculine in behavior when given testosterone injections than intact untreated adult females. The clear important of sex hormones in sexually displayed behaviors continues to baffle rather than elucidate. It is apparent from the animal data that profound influences do exist. How these apply to the human is questionable, but the hypothesis is intriguing.

PHEROMONES

Several recent studies have examined the possibility that interpersonal relationships between women may affect menstrual synchrony while interactions between men and women may influence cycle length. These studies suggest that a common mediating factor is body aroma. McClintock provided evidence that women who spend extensive time together experience synchronization of the onset of the time of menses.[80] This phenomenon has been replicated and is well accepted. The hypothesis that menstrual synchrony might be mediated by axillary substances was recently supported by the study of Russell and colleagues[104] and more recently by our own experiments.[16a] In the Russell study, axillary secretions from a single female donor rubbed above the upper lip of subjects shifted the mean difference of onset of bleeding from 9.3 days in the pretreatment month to 3.4 days after 4 months of treatment. Women given the "pheromone" showed a menstrual synchrony with the donor of the "perfume" even though they had no direct contact with the donor. In the Cutler and colleagues' study,[16a] 3 male donors supplied axillary secretions that, when compared to placebos, were associated with increased frequency of normal length luteal-phase menstrual cycles.

Chemical analysis of the substances found in the human axillary follicles showed compounds of exogenous origin interacting with two androgen steroids (dehydro-epiandrosterone sulfate and androsterone sulfate).[65,66] Subsequent attempts to apply androstenol to naive subjects to search for a pheromonal effect produced no obvious results[9] nor did another attempt to locate a pheromonal influence on human sexual behavior by using synthetic aliphatic acids.[88] We are thus left with a potential pheromonal influence on human sexual behavior whose nature and mechanism remain unresolved. The implications that a pheromonal influence would have on the decline in sexual behavior in aging populations will no doubt eventually be revealed.

Although so many pieces of the puzzle are missing that neat precise discussions of human sexuality cannot begin to be formulated, some research into particular areas of hormone and sexual behavior is available. Young men and women have been studied, and older ones as well, as will be detailed in what follows.

HORMONES AND SEXUAL BEHAVIOR IN MEN AND WOMEN

CYCLIC VARIATION IN CYCLING WOMEN

Studies of young couples demonstrate a small but significant increase in female-initiated sex behavior at ovulation with perhaps another peak at the mid-luteal phase.[2] Pill users (oral contraceptives) did not show these effects. The distribution of coitus in the menstrual cycle was also reported.[87,119] A mid-cycle peak in coital activity in women who did not take oral contraceptives appeared to exist but such a peak was absent among women who took oral contraceptives that suppressed ovulation. Subsequently, however, the same investigators reported that the probability of coitus and orgasm was no greater the day before the LH surge than at any other time of the cycle. It has been suggested that the occasional failure to find a cyclic activity is a result of the dynamics between the man and the woman. If there is an increase in female initiated activity at midcycle there could be a concomitant reluctance for a male response.[2] If this is the case, the overall activity of the couple may appear to be noncyclic even in the face of the woman's cyclic desire for sex as a function of hormone level.

Attempts to identify a cyclic variation in vaginal response—using self-reports, vaginal blood volume, vaginal pulse amplitude and labial temperature in response to a laboratory experiment with erotic and neutral tapes—yielded no cyclic variation. Whether such absence of positive results would be replicated in a more natural setting remains to be tested. A cyclic variation in the shape and diameter of the cervix has been described[74] as has a cyclic variation in the quantity and characteristics of vaginal fluids.[44,100] The accompanying profound changes in the amount of cervical secretions during the periovulatory phases of the cycle are well known. Lactic acid in the vagina and blood estrogens showed a significant correlation among women who do not use oral contraceptives; the greater the plasma estrogen, the greater the lactic acid concentration in the vagina.[8] Studies of cyclic variations in aliphatic acids in the vagina have also been positive.[82] Cyclic variation in the capacity for uterine contraction has also been characterized. The estrogen-dominated uterine smooth muscle contracts as a syncitium; the progesterone-dominated muscle can only contract in specific focal areas—a phenomenon that has been suggested as a mechanism for preventing fetal expulsion during pregnancy.[18]

Hormonal variation in estrogens and progesterone during the menstrual cycle are so well accepted that they need not be characterized in detail here. However, a brief statement is appropriate. Estrogen varies as a function of follicular development in the follicular phase and of corpus luteum development in the luteal phase of the menstrual cycle. Predictable peaks in estrogen levels can be expected at approximately days 12 through 14 (in a typical 29.5 day cycle) as well as again in mid-luteal phase approximately 7 days before menses. Likewise the plasma progesterone concentration peaks at the middle of the luteal phase (approximately 7 days before menses). See Figure 3–6 to review these relationships.

Androgen also shows a cyclic variation in many women with peak levels of dehydroepiandrosterone in plasma showing in the early follicular and ovulatory phases as contrasted with lower levels in the luteal phase.[37] Likewise, testosterone peaked at ovulation[39] and again at mid-luteal phase in those women for whom a cycle was apparent.[96] Urinary testosterone secretion showed a cyclic variation in 5 of 7 normally menstruating women with peaks throughout the luteal phase.[55] However, the issue of whether or not there is a consistent testosterone cycle in young cycling women remains unresolved. No regular variation could be shown—either according to time of day or time of cycle—in one other report in which cycles were not normalized to an LH peak (and may have failed to show the phenomenon because of this experimental design). One can conclude that there is some evidence for a testosterone variation in some women, but the effect is not universally demonstrated.

SEXUAL BEHAVIOR AND ENDOCRINE MILIEU IN WOMEN

A series of studies have provided information that combines to suggest a relationship between a woman's sexual behavior and her endocrine milieu. Infertile women tended to have later first coital ages than women who were fertile.[19] Among the infertility patients, those who had never conceived presented a later first coital age than those who had previously conceived. Routine gynecologic patients reported the youngest first coital ages of the groups studied. (Fig. 3–7).

Sexual behavior frequency and menstrual cycle length were also shown to carry replicable relationships. Women who had regular weekly sexual intercourse with men had menstrual cycles, the average duration of which was 29 days ±3 while women with less frequent behavioral interactions tended to have more extreme cycle lengths (Fig. 3–8).[20,23] The effect was noted consistently in college women but also occurred in infertile and perimenopausal women. Aberrant menstrual cycle lengths (greater than 33 days or less than 26 days) tend to associate with subfertile endocrine milieus.[20,23] Among women who showed sporadic sexual behavior, those who had greater quantities of sporadic behavior were more likely to show extreme cycle lengths than those sporadically active women who had lower frequency of coital activity.[21] From that study it appeared that the stability of sexual behavior patterns was associated with stable endocrine milieu. Further studies showed that women with luteal phase defects,

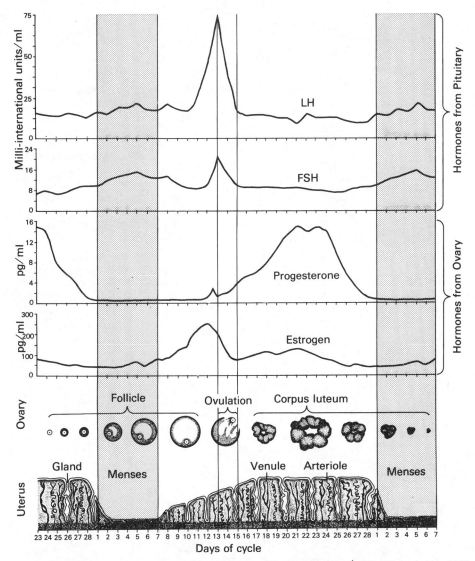

FIG. 3-6. Cyclic variation in reproductive system (Cutler WB, García CR, Edwards DA, 1983, *Menopause: A Guide for Women and the Men Who Love Them,* New York, WW Norton & Co

determined by hyperthermal phase lengths of less than 12 days, tended to have sporadic sexual activity during the luteal phase of their menstrual cycles.[22]

Relationships between sexual behavior and endocrine milieu were also studied in the Stanford Menopause Study. Perimenopausal women (average age 49) who had regular weekly intercourse with men tended to have either *no* hot flashes or a much lower incidence than perimenopausal women who were less sexually active (Table 3-2).[17] The women with regular sexual activity had higher levels of estrogen than women with sporadic sexual activity (Fig. 3-9) Despite the fact that the mean values of plasma

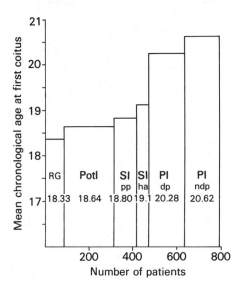

FIG. 3-7. First coital age and tendency toward infertility. RG = routine gynecological; PotI = pathology other than infertility; SI = secondary infertility; PI = primary infertility; pp = prior parity; ha = habitual aborter; dp = detectable pathology; ndp = no detectable pathology (Cutler WB, García CR, Krieger A, 1979, J Biosci Sci 11:425–432)

FIG. 3-8. Frequency of intercourse and menstrual cycle length (Cutler WB, García CR, Krieger AM, 1980, Horm Behav 14:163–172

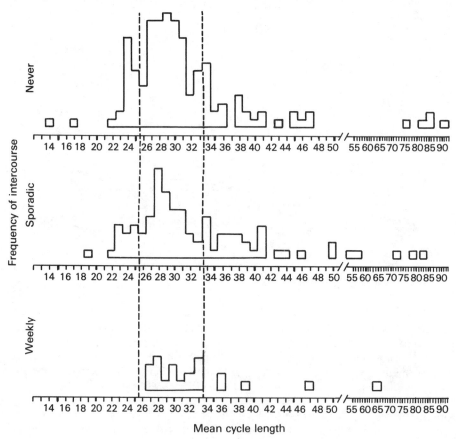

TABLE 3-2.   Current coital frequency and hot flashes

A. Phase 2, Interview 1

	Sexual Activity		
	Sporadic	Weekly	TOTAL
Hot Flashes: Present	24	6	30
Absent	12	18	30
TOTAL	36	24	60

One notes that of the 30 women with hot flashes, 80% were
sporadically active
of the 30 women without flashes, 40% were
sporadically active

Or expressed another way:

of the 36 women with sporadic sexual activity, 66% had hot
flashes
of the 24 women with weekly sexual activity, 25% had hot
flashes

B. Phase 2, Interview 2*

	Sexual Activity		
	Sporadic	Weekly	Total
Hot Flashes: Present	24	6	30
Absent	9	17	26
TOTAL	33	23	56

One notes that of the 30 women with hot flashes, 80% were
sporadically active
of the 26 women without flashes, 35% were
sporadically active

Or expressed another way:

of the 33 women with sporadic sexual activity, 73% had hot
flashes
of the 23 women with weekly sexual activity, 26% had hot
flashes

estradiol fell to within 50 to 80 pg/ml, the distribution of the values varied from 15 to over 100 pg/ml. One sees that the women with sporadic sexual activity show lower estrogen levels and that 3 months later the estrogen levels had declined more precipitously than levels of estrogen in sexually active women (Table 3-3). Figure 3-9 provides the individual data of estradiol, age, and sexual behavior. One notes the age trends in both sexual activity and estrogen level as well as the tendency for weekly sex to be associated

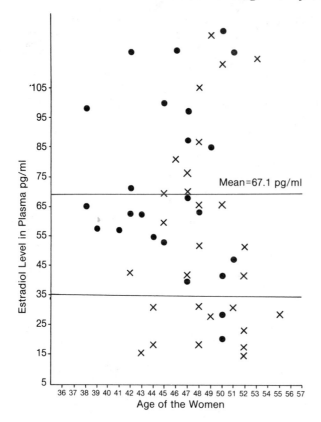

FIG. 3-9. Perimenopausal women: estrogen, sexual frequency, and age. x = sporadic sex; ● = weekly sex.

with higher estrogen levels. Attention should be directed to the fact that Treloar observed a delayed onset of menopause in those women taking premenopausal estrogen therapy (see Fig. 1-20).

Although questions of whether the hormonal milieu promotes the behavior or *vice versa* remain unresolved, it seems likely that the interaction is circular and that alteration in either hormone or sexual behavior could predictably influence the other component.

FEMALE SEXUAL BEHAVIOR AND CARDIOVASCULAR FUNCTION

There appears to be a relationship between sexual life and various aspects of heart function. The issues are far from resolved, but two studies offer intriguing evidence for a role. Abramov compared 100 myocardial infarction patients with 100 hospitalized controls. He noted an earlier menopause in the myocardial infarction patients.[1] He then defined the term "frigidity" as either a failure to achieve orgasm "(thereby producing frustration)" or as never having "enjoyed" sex. He found there was significantly higher incidence of "sexual frigidity" with myocardial infarction patients than with the controls. There was no significant difference between age at menopause and frigidity or between married and unmarried women. What mechanism could account for such a finding? The answer is unclear. Gillan and Brindley, studying women using a vibrator on the clitoris, recorded heart rate increases that were smoothly accelerating through the period of

TABLE 3-3. Estradiol concentration (pg/ml) in plasma of perimenopausal women as a function of level of sexual activity

	Sexual Activity			
	Sporadic	Weekly	t	p
Phase 2 Interview 2	57.65 +/− 7.53	77.94 +/− 8.08	1.84	<0.01
Phase 2 Interview 3	50.00 +/− 8.40	76.57 +/− 18.06	1.33	0.10

Women with regular weekly coital activity show higher estrogen levels than women with sporadic (less than weekly) coital activity.

Three months later, weekly active women show estrogen levels similar to those observed 3 months earlier. Sporadically active women show lower estrogen levels.

vibration, with a slight further increase during orgasm and a fall to approximately resting level within 10 seconds of the end of orgasm.[38] They also reported a large deceleration in heart rate during the 10 seconds after orgasm. These heart rate changes are consistent with those reported by Masters and Johnson during the sexual response cycle.[77]

The role of sexual activity in stimulating healthy heart function is probably a critical one, although other forms of aerobic exercise would probably be equally effective in maintaining the heart.

CYCLIC VARIATION IN SEX HORMONES OF MEN

The potential for a regular repeated variation in the male level of testosterone has been evaluated in several different ways. A circadian and circannual rhythm in sexual activity and plasma hormones was also demonstrated in human males.[102] Baker reported annual variation in testosterone concentration with consistent elevations in the autumn.[5] Another study showed that there are individual variations that repeat themselves over time in plasma testosterone cycles.[27] Different men showed different cycle patterns, ranging from several days in length to much longer spans. Thus, there are both male and female cyclic variations in hormones. The potential for hormones to induce alterations in sexual behavior (or *vice versa*) creates an intriguing yet unsolved puzzle concerning the nature of human sexuality and hormones. Changes occur with age as well.

AGING CHANGES IN REPRODUCTIVE HORMONES OF MEN

Testosterone levels in men show a general tendency to decline with age.[3,5,24,123] Although there is a wide variation in individual testosterone levels, the general trend is unmistakable. Figure 3–10 shows cross-sectional data of testosterone levels gathered from males ranging from 10 through 90 years of age.[123] Total and free testosterone levels decline with advancing ages although the free testosterone concentration declines more than the total testosterone concentration (Fig. 3–11).[24] Prolactin and estrogen levels did not change with age while gonadotropin levels increased (Fig. 3–12).[24]

It appears that a testosterone decline with advancing age is neither inevitable nor random.[47] In the Baltimore Longitudinal Study, which followed exceptionally healthy men for 2 years, there was no tendency for a progressive decline in testosterone with age.

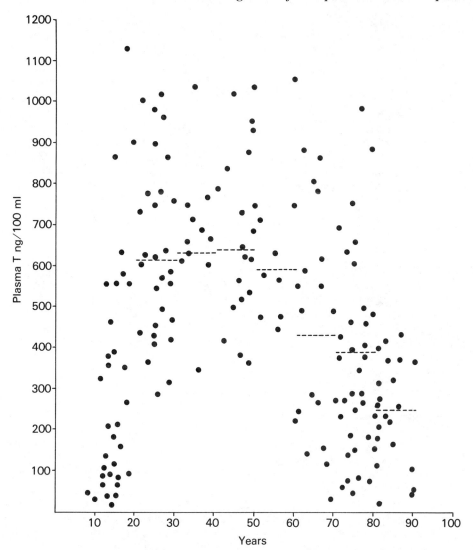

FIG. 3-10. Plasma testosterone levels in men throughout life (Vermeulen A, Rubens R, Verdonck L, 1970, J Clin Endocrinol Metab 34:730)

The men were selected on the basis of good health: being nonobese, not using excess alcohol, having no chronic illness, nothing more than a mild prostatic hypertrophy, no prostate surgery history, and no medication to interfere with hormonal balance. Moreover, the subjects of this study were also self-selected; only 40% of those who qualified agreed to participate in the study. Because of these factors, one cannot be certain whether the declining levels of testosterone so consistently reported elsewhere are a function of a general tendency of aging and failure to exercise regularly or whether the absence of the decline in this one study was exceptional in itself.

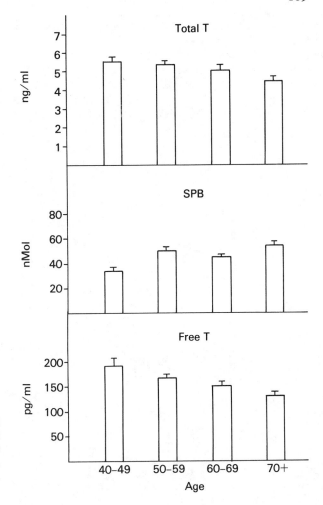

FIG. 3-11. Age-related changes in male steroid and serum-binding protein levels (Davidson JM, Chen JJ, Crapo L, Gray GD, et al, 1983, J Clin Endocronol Metab 57:41–93)

As described earlier, there is a clear tendency for decline in sexual activity in both men and women with advancing age. Both men and women tend to attribute this declining sex frequency to the male. More women are without available sex partners than men because women live longer than men. A sexual deficit for many women is quite real.

GONADOTROPINS, RELEASING HORMONES, AND COITUS IN MEN AND WOMEN

Coitus does not appear to produce any detectable changes in gonadotropin levels although there is some suggestion of increases after sexual arousal. Stearns and colleagues, studying married couples, before and then 10 minutes after coitus, could find no change in gonadotropin levels. They did note a postcoital increase in prolactin in one-third of the couples.[115] Lee and co-workers studied plasma related to coital acts before, 10 minutes after, 30 minutes after, and then hourly for 7 consecutive samplings.[69]

About three-quarters of the men did not show differences in gonadotropins or in testosterone in relation to coitus.

In contrast to these findings were results of male patients who were known to have hypopituitary conditions (but whose plasma levels of gonadotropins were not reported) and who all reported behavioral tendencies that caused the researchers to label them hypoerotic.[14] Furthermore, in one study, sexual arousal in normal males resulted in elevated levels of gonadotropins, but no change was observed in the releasing hormone.[67]

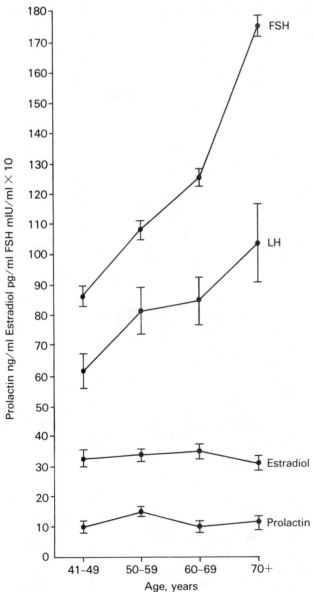

FIG. 3-12. Age-related changes in male levels of FSH, LH, estradiol, and prolactin (Davidson JM, Chen JJ, Crapo L, Gray GD et al, 1983, J Clin Endocrinol Metab 57:41–93)

Thus, there may be some relationship between the gonadotropins and sexual function in men, but the nature of such a relationship remains elusive. Nonetheless, Moss and co-workers, from their studies in rodents extrapolated to humans, concluded that LHRH-induced copulatory behavior is dependent upon estrogen in women and testosterone in men.[89]

Dream sleep and elevated steroid levels are related in both men and women. REM sleep is known to be reflective of the dream state. In male subjects, Schiazi and co-workers showed an abrupt elevation of testosterone as well as of LH, that, when looking at individual pulses, appeared unrelated to the stages of sleep. However, when testosterone levels were averaged for the entire collection period of REM sleep with penile tumescence, testosterone was then noted to be consistently higher during those periods of sleep than during the periods free of REM.[106] Thompson has reported tight coupling in women between estrogen and REM sleep as well, as was described in Chapter 1. For both men and women the steroids appear to provide more predictive information about sexual function than the peptides.

ANDROGENS AND SEXUAL BEHAVIOR IN MEN AND WOMEN

It has long been thought that there is a relationship between androgen levels and some aspect of sexuality. Although the issues are far from resolved, relationships between libido and testosterone have been frequently suggested.

Helen Singer Kaplan has commented that, theoretically, unopposed androgens should lead to increased libido.[57] Greenblatt has concluded that testosterone determines or produces sex drive in women and in men.[42] He sees sex drive as a "chemical test tube equation" that may be affected by psychic overtones and noted that over-libidinous men responded to estrogen with a reduction in their sex drive.

In Women

Other studies of testosterone and sex drive have been consistent in women, albeit sparse. Salmon and Geist, as early as 1943, reported that testosterone improves libido.[105] More recently, Studd and co-workers reported successful treatment of women with libido problems who had relatively stable marriages. Hormone implants of 50 mg estrogen with 100 mg testosterone were tested in 76 women.[118] Three months of daily checklist monitoring showed libido increases. Significant improvement in libido was reported for 80% of those who had suffered a loss.[118] Because no placebos were used, causality can only be intimated in this report. Since then, Bancroft and co-workers studied androgens and sexual behavior in women who were using oral contraceptives.[6] In their study of 40 women on the pill, 20 of whom had sexual problems, they noted that total androgens were low in both groups. They further reported that only in the group without these sexual problems was testosterone and estrogen a correlative factor with measures of sexual interest.[6] Exogenous androstenedione, given in a double-blind fashion, failed to improve sexual function. They also noted that most pill-users show a rise in androgen and estradiol on the pill-free week and concurrently showed increased sexuality then.[6] In a recent report of 52 postmenopausal women, both androstenedione and testosterone levels were positively associated with level of desire for sexual activity.[72]

In women with polycystic ovary disease, of which one characteristic is increased testosterone levels, patients recorded higher sexual initiation scores when compared with age-matched control groups.[40] In that population, the degree of hirsutism (presumably a reflection of testosterone level) did not show any clear relationship to retrospective interview scores of sexual drive, initiation, or frequency. Polycystic ovary patients were not different from control women on any of the other measures of presumed androgenization: play preference, energy expenditure, interest in dress and appearance, career vs. family preference, or sexual arousal to a narrative and visual stimuli. Only the sexual initiative was higher in polycystic ovary syndrome patients than age-matched controls.

Thus, in these studies of women, there does appear to be some evidence for relationships between androgen levels and sexual drive.

In Men

In men, studies of relationships between testosterone and sexuality have also offered some positive results. However, ambiguity exists here as well. According to some studies, sexual activity increases plasma testosterone levels. Relationships between testosterone levels and both penile tumescence and REM sleep in men have also been studied—with positive results.

Bancroft and Skakkebaeck reported the use of exogenous androgens given to people with impaired sexual response.[7] There was no clear improvement. More recently, Schwartz and co-workers studied the plasma testosterone of men with sexual dysfunction and compared these levels to those of men married to sexually dysfunctional women but whom, themselves, were presumably normal.[108] The plasma testosterone concentrations were not related to therapy outcome, although they were negatively correlated with the age of the subject, as would be expected from other reports.[108] However, Kwan and colleagues, in studies of hypogonadal men (<1.7 ng/ml testosterone) found clear erectile improvements in response to testosterone (200- and 400-mg doses of testosterone ethanate). Steroid or placebo injections were administered at monthly intervals. They concluded that "the major androgen action on (hypogonadal) male sexuality involves libido factors (i.e., sexual motivation/interest)." Moreover, both sleeping and spontaneous waking erections were increased on testosterone therapy.[64]

Other studies do report relationships between endogenous milieu and sexuality. Legros and co-workers were able to distinguish prediabetic from normals in a "psychogenically impotent" population to show that—only among the prediabetics—testosterone levels and sexual interest were positively associated.[70] Persky and colleagues found that a maximum value of testosterone for each man (in stable marriages) tended to occur 7 days after his wife's ovulation.[96] The phenomenon was noted in 78% of the cycles that were studied. It is noted that the wives showed two peaks of testosterone each cycle: one at ovulation and one 7 days afterward (mid luteal). The concomitant male increase in testosterone during his wife's mid-luteal phase could be his steroidal response to increased sexual activity at that time. This is especially likely considering the work of Ismael who showed, in only two subjects however, that testosterone was lower during periods of abstinence than when copulating.[54] Support for a steroid response to coitus is provided by a report by Fox and co-workers, in which prolonged study of one subject showed that testosterone levels during and after coitus were significantly higher than under control conditions.[31]

Should it be the case that sexual activity does lead to an increase in testosterone it becomes interesting to note that, according to studies of Fox and co-workers, masturbation usually does not appear to influence or be influenced by testosterone, although heterosexual sex is related.[31] Support for that finding is found in the more recent work of Davidson and colleagues in which close linking between a variety of measures of sexual behavior and testosterone levels across life spans were noted but in which masturbation was irrelevant to the androgen level association.[24] However, elsewhere, endocrine effects of masturbation have been reported for male volunteers in the army.[101] All the plasma steroids (pregnenolene, DHA, androstenedione, testosterone, DHT, estrone, estradiol, and cortisol) were significantly increased in that army sample after masturbation. Although no alteration was noted in LH levels, seminal plasma showed a significant positive response. Testosterone concentrations were increased in both seminal plasma and peripheral blood.[101] Thus, the literature leaves unresolved questions related to self-stimulation and testosterone. Vitamin E, in comparison with placebo, showed no association with measures of human sexual function.[51]

Studies of the male decline in sexual behavior have recently allowed some wider perspectives. Davidson and co-workers, in their studies of men aged 41 to 93 years, showed a clear decline in steroid levels that was highly correlated with sexual declines in activity, libido, and potency measures.[24] They concluded that these changes in testosterone with advancing age roughly parallel a decline in sexual function, which affects all components of male sexuality *except for* the perception of enjoyment. Figure 3–13 shows an age-dependent decline in frequency of orgasm, morning erections, sexual thoughts, and sexual enjoyment. One notes the much sharper declines in the physical (orgasm and erections) than the mental processes (thoughts and enjoyment).[24] Lief has described the chief sexual problems of couples after 50 to lie in the man's inability to maintain an erection.[73] The incidence, etiology, diagnostic approaches to, and

FIG. 3-13. Decline in male sexuality with age (Davidson JM, Chen JJ, Crapo L, Gray GD et al, 1983, J Clin Endocrinol Metab 57:41–93)

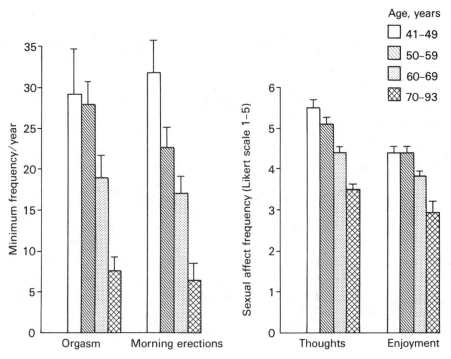

treatment of this male impotence have, recently, been sporadically reported in the literature.

IMPOTENCE

The initial problem in dealing with impotence is the embarrassment and ignorance with which both patients and some clinicians may approach the problem. There is a long history of the perspective that discussions of sexual matters are mired in impropriety, even on the part of physicians.[58,71] The need for objective facts is critical. The incidence of impotence appears to be somewhere between 35% and 40% of men over age 40.[113,117] Of 1200 men in a medical clinical outpatient Veterans Administration Hospital who were screened for a wide variety of health factors, fully 34% acknowledged that impotence was a problem for them.[113] The age distribution of men with sexual dysfunction appears to rest most heavily in the 50- to 59-year-old age group, with some further heavy incidence in men 10 years younger and older than this span.[84] The age variation in morphological characteristics of post-thaw sperm motility also corresponds somewhat to this general age distribution pattern.[107] Post-thaw motility declines significantly after age 36, although the variation is not significant for sperm count, semen volume, and total number of spermatozoa in older men.[107]

Female impotence exists as well, taking the form of a failure to achieve orgasm. Recently, the Grabers have shown that the capacity for orgasm is related to the strength of the pubococcygeal muscles.[41] For this reason, as well as to correct problems of urinary stress incontinence,[63] Maly has suggested that clinicians be aware of and routinely suggest practice to strengthen these muscles.[73a]

ETIOLOGY

Although, even quite recently, the cause of male impotence has been attributed at least 90% of the time to psychological influences,[12,117] more recent and rigorous research has indicated a different etiology.[15,86,91,92,103,113,114] Among medical clinic outpatients who, incidentally answering a questionnaire, acknowledged impotence and requested treatment for it, a thorough workup and diagnosis showed the following array of causes:

25% medication effect
14% psychogenic
7% neurologic
6% urologic
10% primary hypergonadism
9% secondary hypogonadism
9% diabetes mellitus
5% hypothyroidism
1% hyperthyroidism

In that sample the mean age was 59 years.[113] A number of different organic diseases can lead to impotence. Most common are the following:

- Diabetes, which leads to microvasculature declines, leading to neuropathy, which then leads to interference of neurology (impotence occurs in approximately 50% of such patients who maintain normal plasma testosterone)
- Renal failure, yielding gonadal dysfunction

- Cirrhosis of the liver, yielding loss of virility and hypogonadism, often with elevated estrogens
- Sickle cell anemia, leading to impairment of skeletal and sexual maturation, often with zinc deficiencies
- Paraplegia, yielding a decreased testicular function, although generally accompanied by normal testosterone levels
- Thyroid disorders, both hypo and hyper
- Coronary heart disease, inhibiting sexual activity in many patients, generally out of fear that such activity could be lethal
- Altered endocrine milieu
  hypogonadism, with or without hypogonadotrophic evidence
  hyperprolactinemia (mechanism is unknown, effect is often impotence)[15,86,114]

Burger has pointed out the variety of drug therapies that can produce impotence.[12] A partial list includes the following:

Antihypertension agents (alpha methyl dopa, bethanidine, fertilium, guanethidine)
Tricyclic antidepressants
Thinothiazines

Morley has noted the high incidence of use of diuretics among impotent men, reaching 60% of impotent men studied.[113] Vascular incompetency has been studied and found to be an additional cause of impotence. In addition, arterial inflow disturbances have been described as one of the etiologies common in aging men's impotence.[91,92]

Recent investigations of the arterial venous system of erection have shown that some of the old perceptions may be inaccurate.[91,92,103] There is a lack of evidence for a venous outflow restriction to be necessary for erection in spite of anatomical searches for the phenomenon.[91] Flow studies of erection help the vascular surgeon treat impotence, and these studies have shown that autonomic nervous system involvement, long considered to be involved in the erection mechanism, is not proved.[91]

DIAGNOSIS

Segraves and co-workers have described two distinct populations of male patients who approached the medical system for help in dealing with impotence: those who go to a urologist and those who go to some form of sex therapist. The results showed that those who were urology-based had a much lower incidence of psychogenic impotence, and the authors commented that the urology patients showed a "remarkable naivete about the impact of interpersonal forces on sexual function."[109] These two populations can probably be most efficiently treated by considering their entry point into the medical care system since the likelihood is that those who enter at the urology level have a problem that can be dealt with organically. Normal limits of testosterone, gonadotropins, prolactin, T4, and T3 have been listed by Spark and co-workers and deficiencies in any of these can associate with impotence, a condition which is often correctable.[114]

Thus, until an appropriate diagnostic procedure has been employed, the clinician should not assume that the menopausal woman's partner has been adequately evaluated. Clinical tests include a complete sexual history including a general medical history, with particular reference to a review of all medications, illicit drug use, and alcohol. Clinical data to be collected commonly include glucose tolerance tests, serum testosterone, and consultation with a psychiatrist who is also a sex therapist. Penile systolic blood pressure with evaluation for vascular insufficiency is considered to form a natural part of an appropriate workup as well as measures of bladder function as an indirect neurological test of sexual function.[84] Significantly important is the fact that almost half of impotence patients in one sample[84] and even more in another[113] were able to be effectively treated once the source of the precipitating factor of impotence had been revealed through these organic studies. Future refinements should improve the prognosis even more.

Diagnosis is further complicated by our lack of understanding, which is rapidly changing. For example, anatomical errors in the description of penile arterial arrays have recently been discovered;[92] moreover, the presence of morning erections in an impotent man is now shown to be insufficient evidence for a diagnosis of psychogenic impotence.[11,30,114] The diagnostic value of any workup therefore is limited by many factors that are beyond the control of the clinician treating his menopausal patient. Nonetheless, it is useful to know that there has been a period of rapid change and improvement in the diagnostic capacity of impotent men and we look forward to a continuation of this trend.

TREATMENT

Effective treatments have included psychotherapy or sexual counseling,[109,117] surgery to correct vascular disease,[91,92] penile prosthesis,[12] androgen therapies and/or gonadotropin therapy,[12] and nonhormonal pharmacological manipulations (Yohimbine, an α-adrenergic antagonist).[85] All have been claimed effective with varying degrees of success. The clinician should be alert to future changes in this area.

REPRODUCTIVE HORMONES AND ERECTION AND AROUSAL IN MEN

There has been some suggestion of a gonadotropin influence on the maintenance of erection. Evans and Distiller evaluated the effects of luteinizing hormone-releasing hormone (LRH) on sexual response in normal men.[29] They reported a consistently greater onset of erection, maximum degree of erection, and overall level of tumescence following LRH administration than when compared with saline placebo. Although the differences did not reach statistical significance, the consistency of the trend was unmistakable. The effect was suggested as being due to the gonadal effects triggered by the hypothalamic–pituitary interaction because, after erotic stimulation, a small incremental increase in LRH was noted. LaFerla and co-workers also concluded that sexual arousal in normal men may result in elevated levels of circulating LH and FSH.[67]

The potential for a gonadotropin or releasing hormone therapy to reverse erectile dysfunction remains to be rigorously studied and reported.

Some reported studies do show that sex steroids and sexual behavior have intricate interrelationships with each other. Particularly, one can expect the androgens to be responsive to sexual activity and, perhaps, to be responsible for certain tendencies in sexual activity. Whether testosterone replacement therapy or therapy that stimulates testosterone will be effective in restoring declining sexual function remains to be resolved. One potential difficulty with such treatment lies in the resulting suppression of gonadotropins with subsequent testicular atrophy. For aging men, the benefits may override the detriments. Nonetheless, the issues are unresolved.

CONCLUSIONS

One is left with a clear picture of a declining male physical sexuality that is not necessarily reflected in the mental processes. Nonetheless this physical alteration often influences the couple and appears to be largely responsible for the declining sexual opportunity of aging women. Although there is some confidence that individual treatment approaches are effective, the complexity of the etiology and the confusing contradictions in the recent literature combine to delay their solution. Vigorous research in this biomedical specialty should improve the picture. For the menopausal woman, hormonal and educational help for her, as needed, should be combined with help for her partner when indicated. To maintain and promote good health, these sexual issues should be reviewed within the general examination routine and procedures.

REFERENCES

1. Abramov LA (1976) Sexual life and frigidity among women developing acute myocardial infarction. *Psychosom Med* 38:6:418–425.

2. Adams DB, Gold AR, Burt AD (1978) Rise in female-initiated sexual activity at ovulation and its suppression by oral contraceptives. *N Engl J Med* 299:1145–1150.

3. Albeaux-Fernet M, Bohler C, Karpas A (1978) Testicular function in the aging male. In: *Geriatric Endocrinology*. Greenblatt, RB (eds). New York, Raven Press.

4. Amias AG (1975) Sexual life after gynaecological operations-I. *Br Med J* 2:5971:608–609.

5. Baker HWG, Burger HG, deKretser DM, Hudson B, O'Connor S, Wange C, Mirovics A, Court J, Dunlop M, Rennie GC (1976) Changes in the pituitary-testicular system with age. *Clin Endocrinol* 5:349–372.

6. Bancroft J, Davidson DW, Warner P, Tyrer G (1979) Androgens and sexual behavior in women using oral contraceptives. *Clin Endocrinol* 12:327–340.

7. Bancroft J, Skakkebaek NS (1978) Androgens and human sexual behavior. Ciba Foundation Symposium number 62, Sex Hormones and Behavior, pp. 209–220, Excerpta Medica, Amsterdam.

8. Bauman J, Kolodny RC, Webster SK (1982) Vaginal organic acids and hormonal changes in the menstrual cycle. *Fertil Steril* 38:572–579.

9. Black SL, Biron C (1982) Androstenol as a human pheromone: no effect on perceived physical attractiveness. *Behav Neural Biol* 34:326–330.

10. Blandau RJ, Moghissi K (1973) *The Biology of the Cervix*. Chicago, University of Chicago Press.

11. Bohlen JG (1981) Sleep erection monitoring in the evaluation of male erectile failure. *Urol Clin North Am* 8:119–134.

12. Burger H, Rose N (1979) Sexual impotence. *Med J Aust* 2:24–26.

13. Christenson CV, Johnson AB (1973) Sexual patterns in a group of older never married women. *J Geriatr Psychiatry* 7:80–98.

14. Clopper RP (1976) Postpubertal psychosexual function in males with hypopituitarism. *Progress in Sexology*, pp 69–71. Gemne R, Wheeler CC (eds). New York, Plenum Press.

15. Colp R, Colp CR (1981) One of the "least understood areas of sexuality." *Arch Intern Med* 141:424–425.

16. Csapo A (1959) Function and regulation of the myometrium. *Ann NY Acad Sci* 75:790–808.

16a. Cutler WB, Preti G, Huggins G, Garcia CR (1984) Sexual behavior frequency and fertile-type menstrual cycles. In preparation.

17. Cutler WB, Davidson JM, McCoy N (1983) Sexual behavior, steroids and hot flashes are associated during the perimenopause. Neuroendocrinology letters 5(3)185.

18. Cutler WB, Garcia CR, Edwards DA (1983) *Menopause: A Guide for Women and the Men Who Love Them*. WW Norton & Co. New York.

19. Cutler WB, Garcia CR, Krieger A (1979) Infertility and age at first coitus: a possible association. *J Biosoc Sci* 11:425–432.

20. Cutler WB, Garcia CR, Krieger A (1979) Sexual behavior frequency and menstrual cycle length in mature premenopausal women. *Psychoneuroendocrinology* 4:297–309.

21. Cutler WB, Garcia CR, Krieger AM (1980) Sporadic sexual behavior and menstrual cycle length in women. *Horm Behav* 14:163–172.

22. Cutler WB, Garcia CR, Krieger AM (1979) Luteal phase defects: a possible relationship between short hyperthermic phase and sporadic sexual behavior in women. *Horm Behav* 13:214–218.

23. Cutler WB, Preti G, Huggins J, Erickson B, Garcia CR (1984) Sexual behavior, frequency and fertile type menstrual cycles. In preparation.

24. Davidson JM, Chen JJ, Crapo L, Gray GD, Greenleaf WJ, Catania JA (1983) Hormonal changes and sexual function in aging men. *J Clin Endocrinol Metab* 57:41–93.

25. Dennerstein L, Burrows G, Wood C, Hyman G (1980) Hormones and sexuality: effect of estrogen and progestogen. *Obstet Gynecol* 56:316–322.

26. Dennerstein L, Wood D, Burrows G (1977) Sexual response following hysterectomy and oophorectomy. *Obstet Gynecol* 49:92–96.

27. Doering C et al (1975) A cycle of plasma testosterone in the human male. *J Clin Endocrinol Metab* 40:497.

28. Easley EB (1978) Sex problems after the menopause. *Clin Obstet Gynecol* 21:1:269–277.

29. Evans IM, Distiller LA (1979) Effects of luteinizing hormone-releasing hormone on sexual arousal in normal men. *Arch Sex Behav* 8:5:385–395.

30. Fisher C, Schiavi RC, Edwards A (1979) Evaluation of nocturnal penile tumescence in the differential diagnosis of sexual impotence. *Arch Gen Psychiatry* 36:431–437.

31. Fox CA, Ismail AAA, Love DN, Kirkham KE, Loraine JA (1972) Studies on the relationship between plasma testosterone levels and human sexual activity. *J Endocrinol* 52:51–58.

32. Geer JH, Morokoff P, Greenwood P (1974) Sexual arousal in women: the development of a measurement device for vaginal blood volume. *Arch Sex Behav* 3:6:559–564.

33. Geer JH (1975) Direct measurements of genital responding. *Am Psychol* 30:3:415–418.

34. Geer JH (1976) Genital measures: comments on their role in understanding human sexuality. *J Sex Marital Ther* 2:3:165–172.

35. Geer JH (1978) Letter to the Editor. *Arch Sex Behav* 7:511–512.

36. Geer JH, Quartararo (1976) Vaginal blood volume responses during masturbation. *Arch Sex Behav* 5:403–414.

37. Genazzani AR, Devoto MC, Cianchetti C, Pintor C, Facchinetti F, Mangoni A, Fioretti P (1978) Possible correlation between plasma androgen variations during the menstrual cycle and sexual behavior in the human female. In: *Clinical Psychoneuroendocrinology in Reproduction* Carenza L (ed). London, Academic Press.

38. Gillan P, Brindley GS (1979) Vaginal and pelvic floor response to sexual stimulation. *Psychophysiology* 16:471–481.

39. Goebelsmann U, Arce H, Thorneycroft IH, Mishell DR (1974) Serum testosterone concentrations in women throughout the menstrual cycle and following HCG administration. *Am J Obstet Gynecol* 19:445–452.

40. Gorzynski G, Katz J (1977) The polycystic ovary syndrome: psychosexual correlates. *Arch Sex Behav* 6:215–222.

41. Graber B, Kline-Graber G (1979) Female orgasm: Role of the pubococcygeus muscle. *J Clin Psychiatry* 40:348–351.

41a. Grafenberg E (1950) The role of the urethra in female orgasm. Intern J Sexology 3:145–148.

42. Greenblatt RB, Leng J-J (1972) Factors influencing sexual behavior. *J Am Geriatr Soc* 20:49–54.

43. Greenblatt RB, Perez D (1974) Problems of libido in the elderly. In: *The Menopausal Syndrome.* New York, Medcom Press.

44. Gregoire AT, Lang WR, Ward K (1960) The human vagina: the qualitative identification of free amino acids in human vaginal fluid. *Ann NY Acad Sci* 83:185–188.

45. Gruis ML, Wagner NN (1979) Sexuality during the climacteric. *Postgrad Med J* 65:5:197–207.

46. Hallstrom T (1977) Sexuality in the climacteric. *Clin Obstet Gynaecol* 4:227–239.

47. Harman SM, Tsitouras PD (1980) Reproductive hormones in aging men. 1. Measurement of sex steroids, basal luteinizing hormone, and leydig cell response to human chorionic gonadotropin. *J Clin Endocrinol Metab* 51:35–40.

48. Hatch JP (1979) Vaginal photoplethysmography: methodologic considerations. *Arch Sex Behav* 8:4:357–374.

49. Heiman JR (1976) Issues in the use of psychophysiology to assess female sexual dysfunction. *J Sex Marital Ther* 2:3:197–204.

50. Henker FC (1977) A male climacteric syndrome. Sexual psychic, and physical complaints in 50 middle aged men. *Psychosomatics* 18:5:23–27.

51. Herold E, Mottin J, Sabry Z (1979) Effect of vitamin E on human sexual functioning. *Arch Sexual Behav* 8:397–403.

52. Hoon PW, Bruce K, Kinchloe B (1982) Does the menstrual cycle play a role in sexual arousal? *Psychophysiology* 19:21–26.

53. Hoon PW, Wincze JP, Hoon EF (1976) Physiological assessment of sexual arousal in women. *Psychophysiology* 13:196–204.

54. Ismail AAA, Harkness RA (1967) Urinary testosterone excretion in men in normal and pathological conditions. *Acta Endocrinol* (Copenh) 56:469–480.

55. Ismail AAA, Harkness RA, Loraine JA (1968) Some observations on the urinary excretion of testosterone during the normal menstrual cycle. *Acta Endocrinol* (Copenh) 58:685–695.

56. Jones GS (1966) Sexual difficulties after 50. *Obstet Gynecol Surv* 21:628.

57. Kaplan HS (1974) *The New Sex Therapy* New York, Brunner Mazel.

58. Kaplan HS (1980) Sexual medicine, a progress report. *Arch Intern Med* 140:1575–1576.

59. Kent S (1975) Sex after 45. *Geriatrics* 30:142–144.

59a. Kilkku P, Gronroos M, Hirvonen T, Rauramo L (1983) Supravaginal uterine amputation versus hysterectomy: effects on libido and orgasm. *Acta Obstet Gynecol Scand* 62:147–151.

60. Kinsey A, Pomeroy W, Martin C (1953) *Sexual Behavior in the Human Female* Philadelphia, Saunders.

61. Krantz KE (1959) Innervation of the human uterus. *Ann NY Acad Sci* 75:770–784.

62. Krantz KE (1960) The gross and microscopic anatomy of the human vagina. *Ann NY Acad Sci* 83:89–100.

63. Kegel AM (1951) Physiologic therapy for urinary stress incontinence. *JAMA* 146:915–917.

64. Kwan M, Greenleaf WJ, Mann J, Crapo L, Davidson JM (1983) The nature of androgen action on male sexuality: a combined laboratory—self report study on hypogonadal men. *J Clin Endocrinol Metab* 57:557–562.

65. Labows J, Preti G, Hoelzle E, Leyden J, Kligman A (1979) Analysis of axillary volatiles: compounds of exogenous origin. *J Chromatogr* 163:294–299.

66. Labows J, Preti G, Hoelzle E, Leyden J, Kligman A (1979) Steroid analysis of human apocrine secretion. *Steroids* 34:3:249–258.

67. LaFerla JJ, Anderson DL, Schalch DS (1976) Psychoendocrine response to visual erotic stimulation in human males. *Psychosom Med* 38:1:62–63.

68. Lamont JA (1980) Female dyspareunia. *Am J Obstet Gynecol* 136:282–285.

69. Lee PA, Jaffe RB, Midgley AR, Jr. (1974) Lack of alteration of serum gonadotropins in men and women following sexual intercourse. *Am J Obstet Gynecol* 120:985–987.

70. Legros JJ, Mormont C, Servais J (1978) A psychoneuroendocrinological study of erectile psychogenic impotence. In: *Clinical Psychoneuroendocrinlogy in Reproduction,* pp 301–319. Carenza L, Pancheri P, Ziche L (eds). New York, Academic Press.

71. Lewis D (1983) The gynecologic consideration of the sexual act. *JAMA* 250:222–227.

72. Lieblum S, Bachmann G, Kemmann E, Colburn D, Swartzman L (1983) Vaginal atrophy in the postmenopausal woman: the importance of sexual activity and hormones. *JAMA* 2:249:2195–2198.

73. Lief HI (1968) Roundtable: sex after 50. *Med Aspects Human Sexuality* 41–45.

73a. Maly BJ (1980) Rehabilitation principle in the care of gynecologic and obstetric patients. *Arch Phys Med Rehab* 6T:78–81.

74. Mann EC, McLarn WD, Hayt DB (1961) The physiology and clinical significance of the uterine isthmus. *Am J Obstet Gynecol* 81:209–222.

75. Marshall JM (1970) Adrenergic innervation of the female reproductive tract. *Rev Physiol* 62:6–67.

76. Masters WH (1959) The sexual response cycle of the human female: vaginal lubrication. *Ann NY Acad Sci* 83:301–317.

77. Masters WH, Johnson V (1966) *Human Sexual Response.* Boston, Little, Brown & Co.

78. Masters WH, Johnson V (1970) *Human Sexual Inadequacy.* Boston, Little, Brown & Co.

79. Mattingly R, TeLinde R (1977) Presacral Neurectomy. In: *Telinde's Operative Gynecology,* 5th edition. Philadelphia, JB Lippincott.

80. McClintock M (1971) Menstrual synchrony and suppression. *Nature* 229:244–245.

81. McEwen BS (1977) Endocrine effects on the brain and their relationship to behavior. *Basic Neurochemistry,* 2nd edition. Siegel G, Albers, Katzman and Agranoff (eds). Boston, Little, Brown & Co.

82. Michael RP, Bonsall RW, Warner P (1974) Human vaginal secretions: volatile fatty acid content. *Science* 186:1217–1219.

83. Money J (1961) Sex hormones and other variables in human eroticism. In *Sex and Internal Secretions,* Vol II, 3rd Edition, pp 1383-1400. Young WC (ed). Williams and Wilkins.

84. Montague DK, James RE, DeWolf, VG, et al (1979) Diagnostic evaluation, classification and treatment of men with sexual dysfunction. *Urology* 14:545-548.

85. Morales A, Surridge HC, Marshall PG, Fenemore J (1982) Nonhormonal pharmacological treatment of organic impotence. *J Urol* 128:45-47.

86. Morley JE, Melmed S (1979) Gonadal dysfunction in systemic disorders. *Metabolism* 28:1051-1073.

87. Morris N, Udry J, Underwood LE (1977) Study of the relationship between coitus and LH surge. *Fertil Steril* 28:440-442.

88. Morris NM, Udry JR (1978) Pheromonal influences on human sexual behavior: an experimental search. *J Biosoc Sci* 10:147-157.

89. Moss RL, Riskind P, Dudley CA (1978) Effects of LH-RH on sexual activities in animals and man. In *Central Nervous System Effects of Hypothalamic Hormones.* Coll R (ed), New York, Raven.

90. Neugarten BL, Wood V, Kraines RJ, Loomis B (1963) Women's attitudes toward the menopause. *Vita Humana* 6:140-151.

91. Newman HF, Northup JD (1981) The mechanism of human penile erection—an overview. *Urology* 17:399-408.

92. Newman HF, Reiss HF (1982) Method for exposure of cavernous artery. *Urology* 19:61-62.

93. Notelovitz M (1978) Gynecologic problems of menopausal women: Part 3. Changes in extragenital tissues and sexuality. *Geriatrics* Oct.:51-58.

94. Perry JD, Whipple B (1981) Pelvic muscle strength of female ejaculators: evidence in support of a new theory of orgasm. *J Sex Res* 17:22-39.

95. Persky H, Dreisbach L, Miller W, O'Brien CP (1982) The relation of plasma androgen levels to sexual behaviors and attitudes of women. *Psychosom Med* 44:305-319.

96. Persky H, Lief H, O'Brien C, Strauss D (1977) Reproductive hormone levels and sexual behaviors of young couples during the menstrual cycle. In *Progress in Sexology.* Gemme R, Wheeler CC, (eds). New York, Plenum Press.

97. Persky H, Lief H, Strauss D, Miller W, O'Brien C (1978) Plasma testosterone level and sexual behavior of couples. *Arch Sex Behav* 7:157-173.

98. Pfeiffer E, Verwoerdt A, Davis G (1972) Sexual behavior in middle life. *Am J Psychiatry* 128:1262-1267.

99. Pisantry S, Rafaely B, Polishuk W (1975) The effect of steroid hormones on buccal mucosa of menopausal women. *Oral Surg* 40:3:346-353.

100. Preti G, Huggins GR, Silverberg GD (1979) Alterations in the organic compounds of vaginal secretions caused by sexual arousal. *Fertil Steril* 32:47-54.

101. Purvis K, Landgren BM, Cekan Z, Diczfalusy E (1976) Endocrine effects of masturbation in men. *J Endocrinol* 70:439-444.

102. Reinberg A, Lagoguey M (1978) Circadian and circannual rhythms in sexual activity and plasma hormones (FSH, LH, testosterone) of five human males. *Arch Sex Behav* 7:13-30.

103. Reiss HF, Newman HF, Zorgniotti A (1982) Artificial erection by perfusion of penile arteries. *Urology* 20:284-288.

104. Russell MJ, Switz GM, Thompson K (1980) Olfactory influences on the human menstrual cycle. *Pharmacol Biochem Behav* 13:737-738.

105. Salmon UJ, Geist SH (1943) Effect of androgens upon libido in women. *J Clin Endocrinol* 3:235-238.

106. Schiavi R, Davis D, Fogel M, White D, Edwards A, Igel G, Szechterr Fisher C (1977) Luteinizing hormone and testosterone during nocturnal sleep: relation to penile tumescent cycles. *Arch Sex Behav* 6:97-104.

107. Schwartz D, Mayaux MJ, Spira A, Moscato ML, Jouannet P, Czyglik F, David G (1983) Semen characteristics as a function of age in 833 fertile men. *Fertil Steril* 39:4:530-535.

108. Schwartz M, Kolodny R, Masters W (1980) Plasma testosterone levels of sexually functional and dysfunctional men. *Arch Sex Beh* 9:355-366.

109. Segraves RT, Schoenberg HW, Zarins CK et al (1981) Characteristics of erectile dysfunction as a function of medical care system entry point. *Psychosom Med* 43:227-234.

110. Semmens JP (1982) In reply to Wulf Utian's letter to the editor. *JAMA* 294:195.

111. Semmens JP, Wagner G (1982) Estrogen deprivation and vaginal function in postmenopausal women. *JAMA* 248:445-448.

112. Sintchak G, Geer JH (1975) A vaginal plethysmograph system. *Psychophysiology* 12:113-115.

113. Slag MF, Morley JE, Elson MK, Trence DL, Nelson CJ, Nelson AE, Kinlaw WB, Beyer HS, Nuttall FQ, Shafer RB (1983) Impotence in medical clinic outpatients. *JAMA* 249:1736–1740.

114. Spark RF, White RA, Connolly PB (1980) Impotence is not always psychogenic: newer insights into hypothalamic-pituitary-gonadal dysfunction. *JAMA* 243:750–755.

115. Stearns EL, Winter JSD, Faiman C (1973) Effects of coitus on gonadotropin, prolactin and sex steroid levels in man. *J Clin Endocrinol Metab* 37:687–691.

116. Steer C (1959) Electrohysterography. *Ann NY Acad Sci* 75:809–812.

117. Strauss EB (1950) Impotence from a psychiatric standpoint. *Br Med J* 1:697–699.

118. Studd JWW, Collins WP, Chakravarti S, Newton JR, Oram D, Parsons A (1977) Oestradiol and testosterone implants in the treatment of psychosexual problems in the postmenopausal woman. *Br J Obstet Gynaecol* 84:314–316.

119. Udry JR, Morris NM (1968) Distribution of coitus in the menstrual cycle. *Nature* 220:593–596.

120. Reference deleted.

121. Utian WH (1975) Definitive symptoms of postmenopause—incorporating use of vaginal parabasal cell index. *Front Horm Res* 3:74–93.

122. Utian WH (1975) Effect of hysterectomy, oophorectomy and estrogen therapy on libido. *Int J Obstet Gynecol* 13:97–100.

123. Vermeulen A, Rubens R, Verdonck L (1970) Testosterone secretion and metabolism in male senescence. *J Clin Endocrinol Metab* 34:730–735.

124. Weinman J (1967) Photoplethysmography. In *A Manual of Psychophysiological Methods* pp 185–217. Venables PH, Martin I (eds). Amsterdam, North Holland Publishing Company.

125. Zussman L, Zussman S, Sunley R, Bjornson E (1981) Sexual response after hysterectomy-oophorectomy: Recent studies and reconsideration of psychogenesis. *Am J Obstet Gynecol* 140:725–729.

4

Hormone Replacement Therapy:
An Introduction

HISTORICAL BACKGROUND

Among the early "scientific" demonstrations of hormones in the human are those of Bayliss and Starling, who reported on secretin as a specific chemical substance, produced in an organ or tissue, liberated and carried into the blood, to affect another organ situated at a distance. The actual concept of hormones can be found very early in different writings. Records are poor, but the consistency of the reporting lends some credence to them. The use of testicular and placental tissue as early as 1100 AD (from humans and other animals) for medicinal purposes to rejuvenate, produce sons, and treat infertility, has been described.[57] Descriptions of fractionation of urine and subsequently drinking it whole for a variety of medicinal purposes are found in ancient writings on Taoism, with records dating to the year 200 AD.[57] Although it is likely that such "medicinal" uses for urine and glandular tissue occurred before recorded history, it was not until the modern capacity to measure, extract, and synthesize hormones that the vast acceleration in hormone replacement therapy could begin to have occurred.

In the 17th century, only 28% of women were said to have lived to experience menopause and a mere 5% to have survived to age 75.[74] Such statistics contrast greatly with more recent ones in developed countries, where 95% of women can expect to experience menopause and 50% to reach age 75.[74] The classical symptoms of menopause are described in Chapter 1. They include the following:

- Vasomotor instability (hot flushes and night sweats)
- Loss of well-being
- Dyspareunia
- Insomnia
- Lethargy
- Loss of motivation
- Diminished concentration
- Depression
- Loss of libido
- Atrophic vaginal changes
- Osteoporosis

Hormone replacement therapy may ameliorate all of these symptoms.

The intricate interrelationships between gonadal steroids and adrenal steroids, hypothalamic-releasing hormones and endogenous opiates, and the gonadotropins with all of the above were discussed in Chapter 1. Moreover, emerging relationships between the steroids and endogenous opiate secretion into pituitary stalk blood of primates suggest another potential advantage to the affective milieu of the woman. Some of the implications of these relationships may not be fully appreciated at the present time.

The basic underlying etiology of menopausal symptoms is the decline of plasma estrogen. Logically, estrogen replacement therapy has been the most commonly studied and reported treatment. The estrogens, 17-beta estradiol, estrone, and estriol and the pharmacological modifications of these, have all been studied, albeit some more than others. The use of progesterone alone has also been reported as has the use of combinations of estrogen and progestins. Other treatments have also been able to effect relief from certain symptoms, but do not correct the basic underlying problem—estrogen deprivation.

In Chapter 7, the various doses and responses that have been reported in the literature are reviewed. In this chapter, hormone therapies are considered with respect to routes of administration, effectiveness, potential complications, potential benefits outside the reproductive system, and contraindications to their use.

KINDS OF HORMONE REPLACEMENT THERAPIES

Estrogens are administered by a variety of routes. Injections are effective although somewhat cumbersome and, moreover, the patient must repeatedly return for continuation of therapy. Oral tablets, administered in one or another regimen, are probably the simplest, but absorption through the gastrointestinal tract implies hepatic transport. Vaginal absorption circumvents the gastrointestinal tract but may be resisted by the patient because of its messiness, higher cost, or other inconvenience. Some mention of vaginal insertion of oral tablets has appeared but remains to be systematically tested. Preliminary studies support the effectiveness of the latter method, which also avoids the messiness associated with the cream. Sublingual tablets would appear to offer the benefits of the vaginal route without its messiness and minimize the gastrointestinal absorption. Unfortunately the literature offers very few studies of the sublingual approach. Recent studies support the transdermal route as a potentially effective approach.[49]

Recent evidence tends to favor a nonoral route for steroid administration. Unless *low* doses of estrogen are used, the least risks accrue to vaginal creams and potentially to the sublinguals, as will be discussed later in this and the next three chapters.

Recent clinical experience supports a protective effect of progestin administered sequentially with the estrogens. Progestin supplementation is rapidly gaining acceptability among the medical community as well as among patients.[31] There is some resistance to this approach since the progestin administration often causes uterine bleeding and, in some, also a mild suggestion of hot flashes during the tailend of the progestin course. However, recent studies have confirmed the protective value of progesterone opposition to estrogen in preventing endometrial and breast neoplasms.

Details on the values and risks of estrogens and progestins are reviewed in this chapter as well as in the chapters on hormones and cancer (Chap. 5) and hormones and coronary heart disease (Chap. 6). This chapter focuses on the routes, effectiveness, and potential complications, balanced against benefits to allow the reader to form a realistic appraisal of appropriate use and contraindications.

EFFECTIVENESS

At appropriate doses, estrogen replacement therapy is highly effective in eliminating or, at the very least, ameliorating the symptoms of hot flashes, vaginal atrophy, and certain kinds of depression. The prevention of further acceleration of bone resorption plus new bone deposition is a positive attribute of the hormone replacement therapy.

SYMPTOM RELIEF

Hot Flashes and Night Sweats

Hormone replacement therapy usually eliminates hot flashes and night sweats. Clinical evaluations support the supposition that women who are experiencing hot flashes are more likely to have lower estradiol levels than women who are not, and they probably have elevated FSH and perhaps LH levels. Premarin (1.25 mg/day, administered 3 weeks out of 4 each month) was effective; 85% were totally relieved of their flashes. Pretreatment estrogen levels in the women with hot flashes were lower than those in the women without hot flashes (76.6 pmol/1 vs. 200.8 pmol/1). By the end of the treatment period, the level rose (157 pmol/1 vs. 210 pmol/1). Gonadotropin levels concomitantly declined—from 37.9 U/I (units international) vs. 5.4 U/I (pretreatment) to 14.8 vs. 4.4 (posttreatment).[14]

Although the most effective dose appears to vary from woman to woman and to reflect her own degree of estrogen deprivation, it is clear that most patients can be relieved. Higher doses of estrogen may be necessary for women who have more hot flashes. In one study 5 flashes per day was defined as "more" in differentiating the effective dose to prescribe; only 4% did not find adequate relief on adjusted doses of micronized estradiol.[12] Micronization is a physical process that reduces the particle size, leading to an increased absorption of the hormone. Among patients who reported hot flashes, 76% of these experienced a total disappearance of flashes within several months. Tingling, a symptom apparently akin to other vasomotor distress, was relieved in 94% of the patients who experienced it.[12] Table 4–1 shows the relative response to a variety of regimens.[50] One notes the general failure of placebo as well as the dose-dependent success of each of the estrogen regimens.

Estriol is the main metabolite of both estradiol and estrone. It has a weaker therapeutic effect on hot flashes and sweating than has estradiol.[80] However, if effective, it may be the most desirable because it has very weak effects on the endometrium (the main tissue at risk). Elsewhere two estrogenic compounds, 0.05 mg ethinyl estradiol and 1.25 mg conjugated equine estrogens, produced 70% to 90% relief of symptoms in double-blind studies that were crossed over with placebo.[48] Ethinyl estradiol is probably a less desirable hormone to prescribe because of potential cardiovascular (see Chapter 6) and glucose metabolic side effects. Details of several representative studies follow.

Dennerstein and co-workers evaluated oophorectomized, hysterectomized women who had hot flashes.[22] Placebos were ineffective, estrogen (ethinyl estradiol, 0.05 mg a day) was most effective, and combined estrogen plus D-norgestrel was midway—more effective than placebo but not as good as the estrogen alone—in providing comfort. Progesterone alone was a less effective ameliorative of hot flashes. However, Albrecht and colleagues, in their study of menopausal women 2 to 4 years after the last menstrual period, reported that medroxyprogesterone acetate did reduce the average 1-hour total of all flashes to 15% of the control level. LH was reduced to about 50% of the control level, and these results were significantly lower than both the placebo and the control values;

TABLE 4-1. Estrogen therapies relieve menopausal symptoms

Complaints	No. of Patients with Complaints Before Therapy (=100%)	Remaining Complaints After 8 Weeks Therapy, %			
		Conjugated Estrogens, 1.25 mg/day	Placebo (Lactose)	Estriol	
				1.0 mg/day	2.0 mg/day
Hot flushes	122	3	87	12	2
Sweating	120	4	90	8	4
Vertigo	103	3	94	6	5
Palpitation	94	10	92	14	7
Irritability	87	6	88	8	4
Anxiety	63	8	97	10	6
Insomnia	56	14	90	13	10
Depression	46	6	95	9	5
Headaches	33	13	97	17	9

Estriol 1 mg/placebo all complaints p<0.001
Estriol 2 mg/placebo all complaints p<0.001
Conjugated estrogens 1.25 mg/placebo all complaints p<0.001
Lauritzen C, 1973, Front Horm Res 2:2–21, S Karger A.G., Basel

the placebo reduced flashes to only 70% of the control value short-term.[3] Thus the effect of placebo was minor, and short-term; in fact, the author suggested it was equivalent to the acknowledged influence of posthypnotic suggestion. Schiff also found medroxyprogesterone acetate 20 mg p.o. to be effective. Figure 4–1 shows the effectiveness of progestin on relief of vasomotor flushes as compared to placebo. One notes that in crossover to placebo a loss of effectiveness is apparent and immediate.[66] Lobo and colleagues more recently reported that 150 mg of depo-medroxyprogesterone acetate by injection 25 days per month was highly effective.[52a]

Progestins are not the treatment of choice because they have antiestrogenic properties. Atrophic vaginitis is not reversed by progestins.[42]

Vitamin E was no better than placebo in double-blind studies.[50] Elsewhere, the short-term placebo effects that did occur were not maintained over the long run.[3]

Hot flashes have also been treated with nonsteroidal approaches, but these methods have been less successful. Clonidine, an antihypertensive drug that in small doses helps prevent migraine headaches without inducing a blood pressure change, has been investigated in three double-blind trials for its effect on menopausal flushes.[16,51,62] Clonidine was slightly better than placebo, but not nearly as effective as estrogen (as shown in other studies). Although clonidine, in a 9-week, double-blind crossover with placebo, was reported to be "significantly" more effective than placebo in reducing the hot flush frequency, a close look at the results showed that it was never more effective than reducing the flushes to half the incidence they had been. Results such as these compare poorly with hormone therapies. Salmi and Punnonen also studied clonidine treatment in double-blind crossover design with placebo. In that study, both were equally effective in producing a mild reduction in hot flushes. The most severe flushes

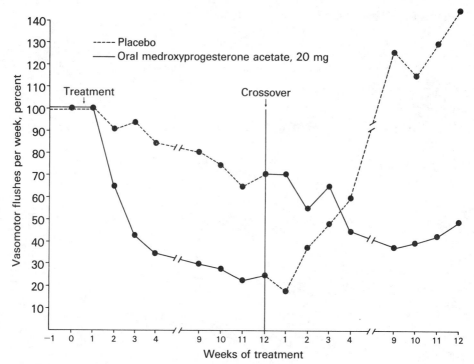

FIG. 4-1. Effectiveness of medroxyprogesterone vs. placebo on relief of vasomotor flushes (Schiff I, Tulchinsky D, Cramer D, 1980, JAMA 244:1443) Copyright © 1966–79, 1981–82, American Medical Association.

were responsive to clonidine.[62] Clonidine has also failed to show good responsive effects in another study.[51]

The effectiveness of propranolol, a drug that blocks peripheral and central beta receptors, was evaluated in a double-blind randomized comparison with placebo.[17] Both propranolol and placebo were equally effective in reducing hot flashes. The slight response to both treatments appears to be the natural placebo effect so commonly reported. Therefore, neither clonidine nor propranolol can be recommended as a useful treatment for hot flashes when hormone therapies are available and so much more effective.

Estrogen replacement therapy is effective in relieving hot flushes. Progesterone also appears to have beneficial effects on hot flashes and is probably a useful treatment when estrogen is contraindicated. This should be balanced against the antiestrogenic effects of the progestational agents. Night sweats were described and characterized in Chapter 1. Sleep disturbances and night flashes were evaluated in menopausal women in a sleep laboratory. Figure 4–2 is a graphic illustration of the relief from night sweats that can be achieved with estrogen therapy.[24] One notes that "wake time" during the night was not much altered by hormone therapy for this one patient. One further notes the absence of night sweats associated with these wake times when estrogen therapy was used.[24]

Genitourinary Complaints

Estrogen deficiencies are associated with atrophic vaginitis and denerative changes in the urethra and urinary bladder.[54,80] Good responsiveness is generally noted on estrogen therapies.[6,12,13,42,48,54,80] Callantine reported an 88% reversal of genital atrophy.[12] Campbell and Whitehead have reported a highly significant placebo effect on vaginal dryness as well as on urinary frequency and coital satisfaction, but conjugated equine estrogens were significantly better than placebo in providing relief.[13] Cervical secretions increase with estrogen therapy.[6,69] A daily dosage of 0.1 mg estradiol in a cream is sufficient to maintain vaginal normalcy.[37] Discontinuation of this therapy led to a complete relapse of dyspareunia, itching, and membrane thinning in the women who participated in this double-blind experiment. Atrophic vaginitis appears to require continual therapy throughout the menopause.

Vaginal relaxation in elderly women appears not be responsive to estrogen therapy. In one double-blind crossover study, the influence of estrogens on pelvic floor tone could not be demonstrated in women who received 1.25 mg conjugated equine estrogen for 8 weeks.[73] However, future, long-term evaluations are needed because some clinical experience not carefully detailed seems to support the contrary.

Affective Symptoms

The relief of affective symptoms—depression, insomnia, irritability, and loss of concentration—is elusive. Some investigators have shown excellent response to hormone therapy. Others have not. There are many reasons for depression and the other

FIG. 4-2. Effectiveness of ethinyl estradiol in relieving night sweats; * = night flashes; W = awake; R = rapid eye movement (Erlik Y, Tataryn IV, Meldrium DR, Lomax P, Bajorek JG, Judd HL, 1981, JAMA 245:1741–1744) Copyright © 1966–79, 1981–82 American Medical Association.

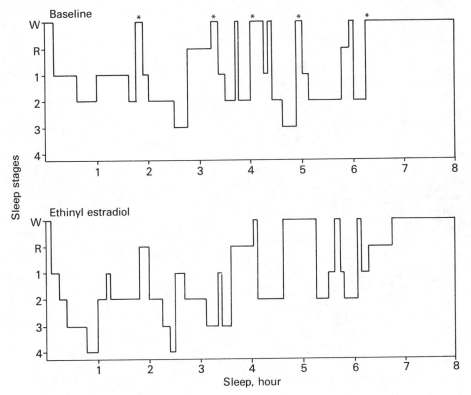

affective symptoms, and when these are related to an altered endocrine milieu, one can expect a positive response to hormone therapies. The critical question for the clinician is to determine the causes and the relative components involved in the affective problems. Only time with the patient and patience and understanding are likely to yield that information.

One should recall the discussion in Chapter 1 that showed the increasingly wider and wider swings from high to low in estrogen concentration as the menopause approaches. During this transition, the plasma estrogen levels during the follicular phase reach their highest lifetime peak whereas premenstrual phase estrogen levels are at the lowest of the reproductive years. Thus, with age, the highs get higher and the lows get lower. The coincidence of depression in the years when the swings are the greatest is worthy of note.

Improvement in a variety of assessments of well-being was demonstrated in a double-blind crossover with placebo study.[25] Plasma estrogen levels increased gradually throughout the period of study. Behavioral and emotional scales indicated that women who took hormones became less neurotic with the passage of time, more extroverted, less depressed, and that their concentration improved. Estrogen (estradiol 17-beta valerianate, 1 mg, 27 days per cycle: D-norgestrel 30 μg days 13–22) had a positive effect in improving libido, sexual activity, satisfaction, fantasy, and capacity for orgasm.[25] Placebos were not helpful but hormonal therapy was. As time passed the placebo group deteriorated slightly on all scales of affect and sexual response that were measured. Because the study was double-blind and the members of the group given placebos were told they were taking hormones, the positive changes in those on hormone therapies were particularly noteworthy. Other investigators have shown similar positive responses. Dennerstein and co-workers found that estrogen and progestogen had a pharmacological effect on mood, anxiety, irritability, and insomnia.[23] All improved on ethinyl estradiol therapy (0.050 mg/day for 3 months). Progestins (levonorgestrel, 0.025 mg per day) initially produced less favorable results, but the initial problems with progestins diminished by the third therapy month.[23] In another study, a research team of a psychiatrist, a gynecologist, and a psychologist followed climacteric women with symptomatic problems (45–55 years old) during a period of 4 years.[56] They evaluated the response to estradiol and testosterone therapies for hot flashes, night sweats, and sleep disturbances. They noticed a marked reduction in all three complaints.[56] More recently, symptomatic women at a climacteric clinic were compared with asymptomatic postmenopausal women. The effects of unopposed estrogen (several different regimens were used) were significantly better than placebo on all subjective parameters of anxiety and depression, including objective tests and self-reports. The clonidine-treated group reported feeling significantly better in health and energy, but found no significant difference on the other five parameters (of depression and well-being).[34]

One of the aspects of well-being appears to relate to the amount of time an individual spends dreaming. In sleep laboratories, patients showed marked improvement in all parameters of sleep during estrogen therapies.[77] Dream-stage sleep tended to increase on estrogen therapies and sleep disruptions during the night tended to decrease. Although many details remain unknown, a number of human and other studies of mammals have shown that dream-sleep loss and various suboptimal psychological functions are associated. Rapid eye movement (REM) sleep deprivation does not produce psychotic behavior but it does increase anxiety, irritability, and reduce the person's capacity for concentration.[20] Hartmann has suggested that REM sleep serves to restore the capacity to focus attention and considers catecholamine involvement in REM sleep a fruitful area for study.[38] It may be that one of the influences of estrogen on well-being is to increase the amount of time an individual can be dreaming and thereby, in some as yet undefined way, improve well-being during the daytime. Schiff and colleagues have quantified some of these aspects. They noted that estrogens increased REM time from 16.5% to 21.7% of sleep time in their sleep laboratory experiments of hypogonadal women given estrogen replacement therapy (0.625 conjugated equine or placebo), and the estrogen users fell asleep faster.[65]

These issues are controversial. Some studies of the effects of estrogens on psychometric measures find improvements whereas others do not.[18] It is likely that this failure in the face of such clear positive results from several well-designed studies rests more in the research design employed. For example, in the study in which REM sleep was shown to increase, a term of "aggression" was ascribed to women who fit the characteristics of boastful, forceful, sarcastic, and rude.[65] Such adjectives can be applied in different ways. "Forceful" may express an individual who is competent and achieving or one who is offensively aggressive. The ambiguity intrinsic to such adjectives probably contributes to the confusion in the literature.[65] However, on those issues where clear objective measurement is available, as in a quantifiable measure like percentage of REM sleep, there is no ambiguity. Estrogens increase dream sleep as measured by REM monitoring. Whether estrogens increase or decrease the amount of boastfulness will probably never be solved in an objective way.

Potential Biochemical Mechanisms for Affective Symptoms, Their Relationship To Steroids. Although much information is missing, there does appear to be a growing body of knowledge to support a biochemical basis for the putative effects on well-being that have been reported for estrogen.

A *catecholamine hypothesis* of affective disorders has been considered. Some depressions are associated with absolute or relative decreases in levels of catecholamines, especially norepinephrine, that are available at central adrenergic receptor sites.[67] The opposite emotion, elation, is considered to be associated with an excess of such amines. The beneficial effects of antidepressants are thought by some to be mediated through the catecholamines. Monoamine oxidase inhibitors increase brain concentrations of norepinephrine. Imiprimine-like agents potentiate the physical effects of norepinephrine. Although this hypothesis could not be confirmed absolutely, the available body of knowledge does provide support for its essential value. Reduced levels of monoamine oxidase do lead to increases in norepinephrine.[46,47] Daily administration of estrogen (5 mg/day Premarin) reduced the elevated plasma monoamine oxidase activity in a group of moderately depressed outpatients.[46] Monoamine oxidase activity was examined in different estrogen-deficiency states, during the menstrual cycle and after treatment with estrogen replacement therapy (5 mg/day Premarin for 25 days with 10 mg Provera for the last 5 days). States that are characteristic of low estrogen simultaneously showed high monoamine oxidase (MAO).[47] Because this high MAO is postulated to decrease central catecholamines, a biochemical explanation for depression in estrogen-depleted women is plausible. Estrogen therapy significantly reduced MAO activity in amenorrheic and in postmenopausal women. Estrogen and progesterone combined significantly increased MAO activity over estrogen alone, but not nearly as much as for those without any hormone therapy.[47] Although the sample size was very small, such significant results provide compelling evidence for a relationship.

Tryptophan and monoamine oxidase inhibitors have been reported to reduce depression elsewhere as well.[9] Depressed subjects have reduced levels of tryptophan as shown in Table 4–2. One notes that the free tryptophan level of the depressed subjects was significantly lower than that of either control subjects or recovered depressives.[85] Furthermore, perimenopausal aged women also show the lowest levels of free plasma tryptophan.[85] Table 4-3 arrays these data for the women from whom plasma was collected.[85] One notes that the women between 47 and 56 years old, the menopausal transition years, show levels of free plasma tryptophan that are significantly lower than those of younger or older women.[85] Furthermore, when estrogen therapy was given to lithium-treated depressives there was a significant increase in the level of free tryptophan.[85] Paradoxically, abnormal tryptophan metabolism was found in all those who used conjugated estrogens for more than 1 year, but the metabolic defect could be easily corrected by vitamin B_6.[39] That study expressed abnormal tryptophan metabolism as increased xanthurenic acid excretion. Conjugated estrogens (Premarin) had the same effect, reported by others, as oral contraceptives in creating a vitamin B_6 deficiency.[39] Vitamin B_6 deficiency produces depression, emotional instability, loss of libido, fatigue, concentration disturbances, and sleep disturbances. These authors suggested that women who are given estrogen therapies may find vitamin B_6 supplements helpful since the vitamin did prevent these problems. They recommend a 250-mg tablet the last week of each month on the hormone-free week. Their experiment, however, tested 100-mg tablets every day for a month, and this regimen was effective.[1] There is, therefore, a

TABLE 4-2.   Depression and free plasma tryptophan are related

Depression	N	Age	Plasma Tryptophan	
			Total	Free
Control Subjects	51	47.7 ± 1.47	58.8 ± 1.47	6.71 ± 0.25
Depressed	50	55.1 ± 1.90	59.8 ± 1.47	4.07 ± 0.20*
Recovered Depressives	17	53.1 ± 3.20	58.8 ± 1.96	5.54 ± 0.34
Recovered Depressives on Lithium	14	52.1 ± 2.50	51.01 ± 1.96	5.39 ± 0.29

* Depressed patients have significantly less free plasma tryptophan than controls.
   Wood K, Coppen A, 1978, In: *The Role of Estrogen/Progesterone in the Management of the Menopause,* Cooke ID, ed, Baltimore, University Park Press, pp. 29–38

TABLE 4-3.   Age and tryptophan concentration are inversely related

Age	N	Plasma Tryptophan (μmol/liter)	
		Total	Free
<46	20	58.2 ± 2.3	7.06 ± 0.49
47–55	20	58.7 ± 1.8	6.18 ± 0.25*
>56	11	59.7 ± 2.6	7.25 ± 0.59

*Perimenopausal group had significantly lower plasma-free tryptophan than pre- and postmenopausal groups.
   Wood K, Coppen A, 1978, In: *The Role of Estrogen/Progesterone in the Management of Menopause* Cooke ID, ed, Baltimore, University Park Press, pp. 29–38

growing body of evidence to suggest that altered tryptophan metabolism may be one element in estrogen-associated depression. One notes that estrogen deficiencies as well as estrogen excesses can apparently influence depression. Further study would be desirable on these issues. Until that happens, the clinician would probably be wise to be alert to the development of a depression *after* long-term estrogen use and in that case to prescribe vitamin B$_6$—pyrodoxine, 100 mg per day.

The influence of estrogen, as well as estrogen combined with progesterone, on the endogenous opiates has also been reported. These studies also are beginning to indicate an intricate relationship between steroid levels and beta endorphins in primates.[29,82,83] Hypothalamic B endorphin levels (in venous effluent of portal blood) are undetectable at times of the cycle when plasma concentrations of estrogens are low and highest when steroid secretions are high in the nonhuman primate.[82] Ovariectomy is followed by a severe deficit in pituitary stalk beta endorphin.[83] Estrogen replacement therapy yields a minor restoration in half the monkeys.[82] However, replacement therapy with estrogens *and* progestins to physiologic levels restores the hypophyseal portal blood levels.[82] Moreover, ovariectomized rhesus monkeys showed a significant decrease in circulating gonadotropins for 4 to 5 hours after a 9-mg injection of morphine.[29] Because estrogen with progesterone so clearly has been shown to be associated with high levels of pituitary stalk beta endorphin and because ovariectomy results in undetectable levels, it is reasonable to assume that menopausal women are probably deficient in pituitary stalk beta endorphin. Since those studies showed that estrogen, by itself, had little influence in increasing beta endorphin levels, but that estrogen cycled with progesterone increased these levels by a factor of 10, it is also reasonable to assume that a steroid replacement program that uses estrogen and progesterone can be expected to, in time, maximize endogenous opiate levels in menopausal women. The fact that endogenous opiate levels may be implicated in a sense of well-being (as appears to be the case in "jogger's high") is increasingly plausible albeit unproved.

Conclusions on Affective Symptoms and Hormones.   Mechanisms notwithstanding, several investigators have been able to demonstrate clear improvements (in recovery from depression) among menopausally depressed women.[13,23,34,68,78] Campbell and Whitehead showed, in their double-blind study comparing Premarin (1.25 mg) and placebo, a significantly better sense of general well-being among the hormone users.[13] Dennerstein and colleagues, in their double-blind study, reported that estrogen plus progesterone had a pharmacological effect upon mood, anxiety, irritability, and insomnia.[23] Their regimen used ethinyl estradiol (0.05 mg/day) combined with levonorgestrel (0.25 mg/day). Gerdes and co-workers comparing regimens of opposed estrogens to clonidine in a double-blind study, reported a significant improvement in all subjective parameters of anxiety and depression for the hormone users.[34] Schneider and colleagues, evaluating the effect of exogenous estrogens on depression in menopausal women, dichotomized, by the Beck Depression Inventory, those women who showed severe psychiatric depresson from those who were mildly depressed.[68] They noted that estrogens improved the prognosis for those who were mildly depressed but were ineffective in the severe psychiatric cases. From results such as these one might consider that there are different components of depression and that, when a severe psychiatric source exists, estrogens probably will not help. Utian, evaluating posthysterectomized, postoophorectomized women aged 45 to 55 in a double-blind crossover study with placebo, noted that while there was a 20% placebo response in terms of improved well-being, the response to hormones was significantly higher.[78]

With these many different studies finding a positive effect on well-being after hormone therapies, it does seem that there are at least a subset of women who will find a general improvement in their affective milieu if they are given hormone therapies.

Backache

Low backaches have been suggestive of the first sign of osteoporosis; indeed backaches are common in the perimenopausal period. Backaches that occur at the base of the spine without any radiating pain have been suggested to reflect a deteriorating spongy bone. The reader is referred to Chapter 2, Osteoporosis, for details.

POTENTIAL COMPLICATIONS

DOSE-DEPENDENT NONNEOPLASTIC SIDE-EFFECTS

A number of side-effects have been reported, and, with the refinement of dosing, most side-effects tended to be reduced to the level of the placebo. Most common is mastalgia, followed by edema, and bleeding (withdrawal or breakthrough), and in some cases headaches.[6,12,13] In the woman deprived of estrogen for more than 2 years, the initiation of hormonal replacement may awaken mastalgic symptoms similar to those of the adolescent. These are usually transient and do not reflect an excessive dose.

Mastalgia as well as unscheduled bleeding appeared to have dose-dependent effects with relationships to estrogen; both were diminished at the lower estrogen doses. Table 4–4 shows the results of one large study in which two different regimens of estrogen were used. Both regimens of estrogen were also evaluated with a 10-day course of 1 mg progestin (norethisterone acetate) opposition.[6] The age distribution was skewed toward the younger age group:

    20% were under age 49
    65% were between ages 49 and 56
    15% were over 56 years of age

One notes from Table 4–4 that approximately 18% of the patients given the high dose of estrogen experienced mastalgia whereas only 3% of the patients treated with the lower dose had the problem. The addition of progestin did not decrease the mastalgia. Callantine and co-workers described mastalgia as being a common side-effect before dosages were lowered.[12] In their study, 24% reported breast tenderness and 31% reported edema. They did note that these symptoms tended to be dose dependent and by reducing the doses the incidence was diminished. Van Keep and colleagues stated that breast tenderness on hormone replacement therapy is best treated by the addition of a progestin, and they emphasized that breast tenderness can be corrected with an antiestrogen.[80] However, the results of Borglin, represented in Table 4–4, do not support this approach. It appears rather that estrogen overdosing may cause the breast tenderness, and a reduction of incidence is seen when estrogen doses are lowered.

Withdrawal and breakthrough bleeding have been a subject of considerable confusion in the literature. Bleeding while on medication is characterized as "planned" (withdrawal bleeding), occurring during the hormone-free period of the cycle or after progestin addition when continuous estrogen therapy is taken; "breakthrough" bleeding is any visible blood when not expected. Whether or not a withdrawal type bleed is cause for concern is currently unresolved. In 1983 the AMA Council on Scientific Affairs stated,

TABLE 4-4. Side-effects in women on hormone replacement therapy

			Incidence of Bleeding		Incidence of Mastalgia	
			% of Patients	% of Cycles	% of Patients	% of Cycles
Regimen 1	28 days	3–7 days	51%	16%	18%	5%
	4 mg E2	hormone				
	2 mg E3	free				
Regimen 2	28 days	3–7 days	28%	7%	3%	1%
	2 mg E2	hormone				
	1 mg E3	free				
Regimen 3	12 days	10 days	6 days	10%	2%	18%	6%
	4 mg E2	4 mg E2	1 mg E2			
	2 mg E3	2 mg E3	0.5 mg E3			
		1 mg NEA				
Regimen 4	12 days	10 days	6 days	17%	4%	11%	6%
	2 mg E2	2 mg E2	1 mg E2			
	1 mg E3	1 mg E3	0.5 mg E3			
		1 mg NEA				

Borglin NE, Staland B, Acta Obstet Gynecol Scand 43:3–11

"Any vaginal bleeding in the postmenopausal patient must be investigated promptly." [19] Although they state this, actual data to support the validity appear to be lacking. While *unexpected midcycle bleeding* is reasonable cause for concern and should be investigated promptly, a withdrawal *bleed* in a postmenopausal woman is far more common and probably not indicative of pathology. In Borglin's study, data of unexpected bleeding were provided that showed that 51% of the patients who were given high doses of unopposed estrogen and only 17% of those who were opposed with progestin ever had breakthrough bleeding.[6] Those given lower doses of estrogen had a lower incidence: 28% on estrogen alone showed some breakthrough bleeding whereas 17% of those on low-dose estrogen opposed with progestin showed breakthrough bleeding. Although the percentage of patients who showed any evidence of unexpected bleeding appears high, a different statistic shows the phenomenon to be much lower. The actual number of cycles with which women will expect to have some unexpected bleeding appears to be always less than 17%—even for the most pronounced effect.[6]

There is some confusion in the literature that appears to revolve around the ambiguity in differentiating unexpected from withdrawal type bleeding. Bates, in reviewing the literature, revealed that progestin, while effective in relieving hot flushes, also led to abnormal bleeding in 43% of users.[5] Eighteen percent of the intact patients in Callantine's series experienced some withdrawal bleeding.[12] Lauritzen evaluated the incidence of uterine bleeding during the administration of various oral estrogens in the postmenopause.[50] Conjugated estrogens produced an incidence of uterine bleeding of less than 1% of cycles and in less than 12% of patients did it ever occur. The phenomenon was dose dependent, occurring much more often with the 1.25 mg dose than in the 0.6 mg dose. Likewise other estrogens showed dose-dependent incidences of uterine bleeding, with estradiol valerate (2.0 mg) producing uterine bleeding in 0.3% of cycles while half the dose of the estrogen yielded one-third the incidence of uterine bleeding. Estriol appears to be a much weaker inducer of bleeding. The 2.0-mg dose yielded bleeding in 0.03% of cycles, the 0.1-mg dose yielded bleeding in 0.015% of cycles as did the 0.5 mg dose.[50] Gambrell has, through the development of the Progestin Challenge Test, established a case for beneficial effects of withdrawal bleeding in the prevention of cystic glandular hyperplasia. His data support that the withdrawal bleeding produced by the replacement therapy in response to the progestin is benign. These issues are detailed in Chapter 8.

The relationship between headaches and hormone replacement therapy has been considered but there is no clear resolution. Dennerstein and colleagues, reporting on heterosexually active, hysterectomized, oophorectomized women found an increase in headache frequency when the concentration of medication fell.[21] That is, there were more headaches in the estrogen-free period or when shifting from estrogen to placebo. Utian, considering a similar question, could find no association between estrogen withdrawal as produced by oophorectomy, or cessation of estrogen therapy in ovariectomized women, or by exogenous estrogen therapy and the symptom of headache.[79] However, in a group of women after hysterectomy he did note an increase in headaches among the women studied—from an initial incidence of 22% of the subjects to 50% of the subjects by 2 years after hysterectomy.[79] Headaches, then, remain an uncertain phenomenon with respect to hormones.

Leg cramps have been mentioned as a potential side-effect of overdoses of estrogen.[13] In double-blind comparisons of Premarin (1.25 mg) to placebo, a 21% incidence of leg cramps occurred on Premarin versus 5% on placebo. Others, also, considered leg cramps to be a dose-dependent side-effect that could be relieved by reducing the dose of estrogen.[2,50]

HEPATIC EFFECTS

The liver responds to oral estrogen by an increase in sex hormone binding globulin (SHBG).[4] Particularly relevant to the role of estrogens in liver function are intimations that estrogens given orally may affect the liver's excretory functions and in some undefined way increase the incidence of gallstones.[7,35,45,53,70] A closer look suggests that the obesity factor is a more critical component in the development of cholesterol gallstones in older women who take estrogen. Although the Boston Collaborative Drug Surveillance Program created some stir with its 1974 report that the risk for gall bladder disease in postmenopausal women who were users of conjugated estrogens was 2.5, factors such as age, parity, obesity, or prior hysterectomy were not clearly presented.[7] Cholesterol cholelithiasis in more common in women than in men in every geographical area studied thus far (Malmo, Prague, United States, and Pima).[45] For this reason, estrogen would appear to be a likely candidate, and in fact one study showed that when gallstone patients were compared with controls, there was always a higher incidence of either oral contraceptive use or estrogen replacement therapy use among the symptomatic patients than among controls.

Cholesterol gallstones occur when the cholesterol fraction of bile exceeds its usual safe range. Bile is normally made up of bile acids (70%–85%), lecithin (10%–25%), and cholesterol (5%–10%).[45] When the cholesterol exceeds 10% of the fraction, it tends to be supersaturated and precipitate, creating seeds or crystals that precipitate gallstone formation. Shaffer has shown that there are two kinds of gallstone patients with two different mechanisms causing the disease. In grossly obese patients the gallstones are caused by increased cholesterol synthesis and excretion. In the nonobese, gallstones are caused by a reduced secretion rate of bile salt and phospholipid.[64] Sturdevant presented a clear case for the risk of cholesterol-lowering diets (in men who were enrolled in an atherosclerosis prevention program) in increasing the formation of gallstones.[75] The mechanism involved remains unclear.

However, altered gallbladder function in response to estrogen therapy has been incompletely studied and seems much more a reflection of the amount of fat an individual has than the amount of estrogen she takes. For example, Honore, in a paper entitled "Increased incidence of symptomatic cholesterol cholelithiasis in perimenopausal women receiving estrogen replacement therapy" showed that cholelithiasis patients had a 3.73 greater use of estrogen replacement therapy when compared to a control population.[40] However, obesity was found in 71% of the gallstone patients compared to 46% of the controls. Estrogen replacement use was found in fewer than 10% of the patients versus 2% of the controls. Moreover, of the 25 estrogen replacement therapy users, 17 were overweight in the patient group. Because of the much greater influence of obesity on gallstone formation it is critical that the clinician be aware of the role of obesity. Although the incidence of gallstones appears to be higher in estrogen users, the removal of obese patients from estrogen therapy groups would probably alter the statistics drastically and thereby produce a much lower risk ratio.

Gallstones appear to occur more frequently in silent form. Of one population screened, 5.1% were shown (after oral cholecystography) to have gallstones present.[63] Silent cases occurred twice as often as diagnosed cases. The diet was not significantly different in those with and those without gallstones: There was no significant difference in calories ingested or in composition of the diet with respect to protein, fat, or carbohydrates. That study did not reveal the overall weight variation among gallstone patients. There is, also, an increased risk of myocardial infarction in women with a prior history of gallbladder disease, although how this might interact with the use of hormones is currently undefined.[59]

We are thus left with an incomplete picture—one that at first suggests that oral estrogen therapies may increase the risk from a very low level to a somewhat higher but still low level. A closer look reveals that obesity is a more critical factor, and for the patient who is not obese, estrogen therapy will probably not have much effect. Nonetheless, there are profound increases in CBG, binding capacity (bc), SHBG bc, and angiotensinogen with the synthetic hormones showing 200- to 1000-fold greater potency than the natural estrogens in their commonly prescribed oral doses.[53] See Chapter 7 for further details of dosing equivalencies. Synthetic hormones (ethinyl estradiol) appear to be particularly likely to affect the liver when hormones are taken orally.

NEOPLASMS

Endometrial Cancer

Endometrial cancer remains a real concern of unopposed high-dose estrogen therapy.[84] Chapter 5 reviews the studies and shows the overall beneficial effect that is apparently gained from appropriate durations of low-dose progestin opposition to estrogen.

Breast Cancer

Breast cancer has also been discussed in the literature. In 1983 the AMA Council on Scientific Affairs concluded that estrogen replacement therapy is specifically contraindicated in those patients "with an estrogen dependent neoplasm of the breast or a history of such a lesion." [19] The recent discoveries of two apparently different forms of breast cancer, one estrogen-dependent and the other not, would appear to make such a precaution sensible. Most studies report up to an 80% response if the tumor had a high estrogen receptor content (3–100 fentomoles/mg) and, in contrast, less than 6% chance of response to hormonal manipulation in breast cancer patients who have estrogen receptor concentrations (in tumor) lower than a certain cutoff point (3 fmol/mg cytosol protein).[15,52,58] Eighty percent response rates have also been reported for tumors when progesterone receptors were measured instead of estrogen receptors. Nisker and Siiteri concluded that the assessment of the cytoplasmic progesterone receptor may be easier and more predictive of those who will benefit from hormonal therapy.[58] In general, however, hormone replacement therapies and breast cancer tend not to be associated in any negative way. Furthermore, adequate progestin duration may protect against neoplasia.[33,36] A review of the literature follows.

Burch and co-workers in 1975 reported a nonsignificant difference in breast cancer between hormone users and nonhormone users, after evaluating over 11,000 patient years in hysterectomized women.[8] Two years later, the same team published further details.[11] They noted there was a marked decline in deaths from all causes due mainly to reduced myocardial infarction and cancer mortality. However, there was a slightly increased incidence of breast carcinoma (nonfatal) that declines to less than 1 after 10 years of estrogen use. A closer look enabled them to discern those at risk for breast cancer as being those who are nulliparous and mothers who have their first child after the age of 20 and who begin estrogen support after the age of 53.[11] That combination seemed to form a special subgroup who were at excess risk of breast cancer. Hoover and colleagues reviewed data of 1900 women given conjugated equine estrogens for more than 6 months in one 30-year practice.[41] Comparing their own data to those of the Second and Third National Cancer Surveys, they found 49 cancer cases compared with an expected incidence of 39.1, producing a relative risk of 1.3. The highest risk occurred in users of doses of conjugated equine estrogen that exceeded 0.625 mg/day.[41] Benign breast disease that developed after hormone replacement therapy onset was a risk factor for subsequent breast cancer.[41,61] Further details of this study led them to conclude that menopausal estrogen "does not protect against nor is indicated in causing breast cancer." Other studies have shown less dangerous results. Table 4–5 shows the

TABLE 4-5.   Incidence of breast cancer: hormone users vs. nonusers

	Patient Years of Observation	Cancers	Incidence
Estrogen users	7263	13	1.8:1000
Estrogen + Progesterone users	3855	6	1.6:1000
Other hormones	994	1	1.0:1000
Untreated women	2436	28	11.5:1000
Total	14,548	48	3.3:1000

Van Keep PA, Serr DM, Greenblatt RB, Kopera H, Workshop report in: *Female and Male Climacteric: Current Opinion 1978* Baltimore, University Park Press incidence of breast cancer at Wilford Hall USAF. Estrogen users, after more than 7000 patient years of observation, had a 1.8 per 1000 risk of breast cancer. Untreated women had an incidence more than 5 times higher than this.[80] Hormone therapies appear to reduce the risk of death due to breast cancer. In 1983 Bush and colleagues showed that estrogen use reduced the risk of all-cause mortality significantly.[10]

Ross and co-workers evaluated two retirement communities for a population sample of 30,000 and drew two control subjects for each breast cancer case. They concluded:

- Family history of breast cancer was not a risk factor
- Young age at menopause conveyed lower risk
- A slightly increased risk of breast cancer was noted in certain subgroups of estrogen users, *i.e.,* those who had a total dose of high estrogen over long duration (at least 1.25 mg daily for 3 years unopposed with a progestin). In that case the overall risk of breast cancer was 2.5.
- Low dose unopposed estrogen (0.625 or less) was not a risk factor
- Benign breast disease when combined with hormone therapy accounts for most of the risk of estrogens associating with breast cancer
- In the absence of benign breast disease the occurrence of breast cancer is lower for those who take hormonal replacement therapy than for those who do not. Control subjects were two times more likely to have taken estrogen than those with cancer.
- Ovariectomized women showed no increased risk of breast cancer when they used estrogen.[61]

More recently, Gambrell published his study of the role of hormones in the etiology and prevention of endometrial and breast cancer (1982) that updated and expanded data from Table 4-5. The trend continued. Breast cancer in hormone users was lower than National Cancer Survey rates and lowest among those currently using hormones at menopause.[32] Estrogen/progestin users appeared even more protected than users of unopposed estrogens.[33] Moreover, death from breast cancer was half the rate in hormone users than in nonusers (14.9% vs. 29.8%). Women with potential risks for breast cancer tended to be excluded from the hormone replacement therapy subgroups.

Ovarian Cancer

There is no evidence to demonstrate an increased risk of ovarian cancer among hormone replacement therapy users. Chapter 8 reviews the literature as it relates to hysterectomy and ovariectomy.

CARBOHYDRATE METABOLISM

Several studies have evaluated relationships between hormone therapies and carbohydrate metabolism.[43,44,71,72,76] No consistent changes in glucose tolerance or insulin level that can be attributed to estrogens were found in a study of hysterectomized women before and then after any of 4 hormone replacement therapy regimens (Premarin, 1.25 mg; mestranol, 0.08 mg; ethinyl estradiol, 0.05 mg; or ethinyl estradiol, 0.5 mg).[72] There was an increase in growth hormone in response to ethinyl estradiol and to mestranol but not in response to Premarin.[72] Estradiol valerate (2 mg/day, 20 of every 28 days) produced no significant changes in response to glucose tolerance tests in postmenopausal subjects tested 4 months later.[60]

Thom and colleagues found things to be somewhat different in their studies of glucose tolerance in postmenopausal women.[76] They noted that two synthetic hormones, ethinyl estradiol and mestranol, did, while conjugated equine estrogens (1.25 mg 3 weeks out of

4, or estrogen valerianate, 2 mg) did not, impair glucose tolerance in some of the 50 symptomatic postmenopausal women studied. Even in those cases in which there was an impaired glucose tolerance, all results were within the normal limits anyway. Nonetheless, it is relevant to note that the natural estrogens seem to be somewhat safer than the synthetics.[76] Barret-Conner and colleagues studied 1500 menopausal women and found no association between fasting blood glucose and use of hormones in age-matched comparisons. Investigators have also considered progestin as a potential mediator of altered glucose tolerance. Reviewing the literature and citing his own work, Spellacy concluded that alterations in glucose and plasma insulin after oral contraceptives are real and that estrogens are not responsible; progestins are.[71] In that literature review, he noted that norgestrel consistently showed a tendency for a marked effect on increased insulin and increased glucose to test doses of glucose and that, although norethindrone sometimes induced some small changes, these were not as consistent nor as profound as those of norgestrel.[71] Ethynodiol diacetate also increased glucose and insulin. Because medroxyprogesterone acetate (a principal menopausal progestin) is not used in oral contraceptives, the relative effect of this hormone was not reported. Spellacy concluded that the rate of development of diabetes probably is a function more of the other risk factors (weight and genetics), but that it is still sensible to be prudent and be aware.[71] Others have also considered the potential for progesterone to have influences on carbohydrate metabolism.[44,86] However, one consistently notes that obesity is a more profound risk than any hormone variation.[43]

The new lower doses of progestin that are currently being recommended are far below the levels used in the studies that showed carbohydrate risks; they are unlikely to produce significant changes in carbohydrate metabolism. Nonetheless, the issue is currently unreported.

POTENTIAL BENEFITS OUTSIDE THE REPRODUCTIVE SYSTEM

Although the principal reason for considering hormone replacement therapy is the response to the particular symptoms that occur as a function of declining reproductive potential, in fact a variety of studies has shown a number of benefits to the overall health and well-being of women who take hormones. There appears to be positive responses in the immune system, the cardiovascular system, bones, skin, and longevity.

THE IMMUNE SYSTEM

There is some suggestion, based on animal studies, that estrogens but not progestins have profound influences on the immune system. For example, 17-β estradiol given at successively later stages of immunization (to an immunoglobulin G challenge) prevented the usual postimmunization antibody titer decay in guinea pigs and reduced the rate of rise and magnitude of peak titer.[28] Estrogens also reduced the rate at which antibody titer decayed, thus facilitating the prolonged maintenance of antibody in circulation.[26] These estrogen effects appear to interact with vitamin C.[27,30] Although at present the details remain elusive, the implications are wide reaching.

THE CARDIOVASCULAR SYSTEM

There are profound beneficial influences on the cardiovascular system derived from natural estrogens in replacement therapy. Chapter 6 reviews the literature on the various aspects of cardiovascular system responses to exogenous hormone therapy. One example indicates the kind of result found. A review of ten North American lipid research clinics provided data from large samplings culled from 70% to 90% participation. Menopausal estrogen users showed significant reductions in levels of low-density lipoprotein in serum cholesterol and significant increases in those of high-density lipoprotein cholesterol in comparisons with nonusers after adjustments for age.[81] Both of these changes in blood lipids reflect improved cardiovascular health. Many intricate studies of the various components in the lipoprotein, triglyceride, blood pressure, and atherosclerotic potential have been reported. Not all hormones are beneficial. See Chapter 6.

BONES

The beneficial influence of hormone therapies on bone physiology, morphology, and osteoporosis is also a major one. Chapter 2 is devoted to the subject.

SKIN

The positive and beneficial response of skin to estrogen therapies has been described in Chapter 1. Estrogen replacement therapy induces a series of changes in skin tending toward a longer retention of youthful appearance.

INCREASED LONGEVITY

After Hysterectomy and Oophorectomy

Long-term estrogen administration to women following hysterectomy was reviewed in a study of 1016 cases for over 11,000 patient years of observation. Results indicated a marked drop in deaths from all causes (80% of expected). This was due mainly to reductions in heart attack and cancer mortality.[8,11] Nonhormone type deaths, for example automobile accidents, were equivalent to general population norms. Since the major risk of estrogen therapy has been shown to be that of potentially inducing endometrial cancer, the use of estrogen therapy in hysterectomized women should be and actually appears to be significantly beneficial.

All-cause Mortality

All-cause mortality was reviewed in the Lipid Research Clinic's prevalence study of cardiovascular disease.[10] Of 2269 white women ranging from 40 to 69 years, viewed over 5 years (1971–1976), a total of 72 died of all causes. The relative risk of death was lower for estrogen replacement therapy users than for nonusers:

   0.54 in gynecologically intact women
   0.34 in hysterectomized women
   0.12 in bilaterally oophorectomized women[10]

In a 10-year prospective study by Nachtigall and co-workers, a similar relationship was reported.[55]

It would therefore seem that there are profound benefits to be derived from estrogen replacement therapy. Following the appropriate precautions, hormonal therapies offer a real advantage for health-care programs for women.

CONTRAINDICATIONS TO HORMONE REPLACEMENT THERAPY

Various authors have, at different times, expressed opinions as to the relevant contraindications to hormone replacement therapy. Van Keep and co-workers considered the contraindications to be the following: a history of venous thrombosis, a family history of or treated breast cancer, liver dysfunction or chronic gallbladder disease, familial hypercholesterolemia, and porphyrinuria.[80] As cited previously, the AMA Council on Scientific Affairs in 1983 concluded that estrogen replacement therapy was "specifically contraindicated in those patients with an estrogen-dependent neoplasm of the breast or a history of such a lesion."[19] Although liver dysfunction would seem to contraindicate oral estrogens, low doses of vaginally applied estrogen creams would not seem to be contraindicated because this route of administration would be less likely to overload the liver. The delicate balance of competing influences needs careful review. Then a full and frank discussion with the patient follows, so that, together, the physician and patient can make an informed decision. The ensuing chapters review details of studies with respect to hormones and endometrial cancer (Chap. 5) and hormones and the cardiovascular system (Chap. 6). Chapter 7, the final hormone replacement chapter, contains a review of the dosages and regimens so far reported in order to suggest acceptable guidelines for patient care.

CONCLUSIONS

Hormone replacement therapy, appropriately dosed and judiciously used, is highly effective in relieving the symptoms of menopausal distress, preventing or halting the degeneration of bone that afflicts 60% of untreated white women, and improving the sense of well-being. Potential complications are minimal when appropriate dosage is observed. The benefits that accrue to the women, incidental to the hormone/menopause relationships, include cardiovascular health improvements, enhancement of the skin, potential improvements in the immune system, and an overall reduction in all-cause mortality. Appropriately screened candidates for hormonal replacement therapy live longer and enjoy a generally improved state of overall health. One must be alert in health screening and aware of the contraindications to its use and to inappropriate dosing.

REFERENCES

1. Adams PW, Rose DP, Folkard J, et al (1973) Effect of vitamin B6 upon depression associated with oral contraception. *Lancet* 1:897–904.
2. Aitken JM, Hart DM, Lindsay R (1973) Oestrogen replacement therapy for prevention of osteoporosis after oophorectomy. *Br Med J* 3:515–518.
3. Albrecht BH, Schiff I, Tulchinsky D, Ryan K (1981) Objective evidence that placebo and oral medroxyprogesterone acetate therapy diminish menopausal vasomotor flushes. *Am J Obstet Gynecol* 139:631–635.
4. Anderson DC (1976) The role of sex hormone binding globulin in health and disease. In *The Endocrine Function of the Human Ovary*, p 141–158. James VHT, Serio M, Giusti G, London: Academic Press.
5. Bates GW (1981) On the nature of the hot flash. *Clin Obstet Gynecol* 24:231–241.
6. Borglin NE & Staland B (1975) Oral treatment of menopausal symptoms with natural oestrogens. *Acta Obstet Gynecol Scand* (suppl) 43:3–11.
7. Boston Collaborative (1974) Surgically confirmed gallbladder disease, venous thromboembolism, and breast tumors in relation to postmenopausal estrogen therapy: A report from the *Boston Collaborative Drug Surveillance Program*. Boston University Medical Center. *N Eng J Med* 290:15–19.

8. Burch JC, Byrd BF, Vaughn WK (1975) The effects of long-term estrogen administration to women following hysterectomy. *Front Horm Res* 3:208–214.

9. Burns DD, Mendels J (1979) Serotonin and affective disorders. In: *Current Developments in Psychopharmacology,* Vol 5, pp. 293–359. Easman WB, Valzelli L (eds). New York, SP Medical and Scientific Books.

10. Bush TL, Cowan LD, Barret-Connor E, Criqui MH, Karon JM, Wallace RB, Tyroler HA, Rifkind BM (1983) Estrogen use and all-cause mortality. *JAMA* 249:903–906.

11. Byrd BF Jr, Burch JC, Vaughn WK (1977) The impact of long term estrogen support after hysterectomy. A report of 1016 cases. *Ann Surg* 185:5:574–580.

12. Callantine MR, Martin PL, Bolding OT, Warner PO, Greaney MO Jr (Jul 1975) Micronized 17 Beta-Estradiol for oral estrogen therapy in menopausal women. *Obstet Gynecol* 46:1:37–41.

13. Campbell S, Whitehead M (1977) Oestrogen therapy and the menopausal syndrome. *Clin Obstet Gynecol* 4:1:31–47.

14. Chakravarti S, Collins WP, Thom MH, Studd JWW (1979) Relation between plasma hormone profiles, symptoms, and response to oestrogen treatment in women approaching the menopause. *Br Med J* 1:6169:983–985.

15. Clark GM, McGuire WL, Hubay CA, Pearson DH, Marshall JS (1983) Progesterone receptors as a prognostic factor in stage II breast cancer. *New Eng J Med* 309:22:1343–1347.

16. Claydon JR, Bell JY, Pollard P (1974) Menopausal flushing: double blind trial of a non-hormonal medication. *Br Med J* 1:409–412.

17. Coope J, Williams S, Patterson JS (1978) A study of the effectiveness of propanolol in menopausal hot flushes. *Br J Obstet Gynaecol* 85:6:472–475

18. Coulam CB (1981) Age, estrogens and the psyche. *Clin Obstet Gynecol* 24:291–229.

19. Council on Scientific Affairs (1983) Estrogen replacement in the menopause. *JAMA* 249:359–361.

20. Dement WC (1974) *Some Must Watch While Others Must Sleep.* San Francisco, WH Freeman & Co.

21. Dennerstein L, Laby B, Burrows G, Hyman G (1978) Headache and sex hormone therapy. *Headache* 18:146–153.

22. Dennerstein L, Burrows G, Hyman G (1978) Menopausal hot flushes: a double blind comparison of placebo, ethinyl oestradiol and norgesterel. *Br J Obstet Gynaecol* 85:852–856.

23. Dennerstein L, Burrows G, Hyman G (1979) Hormone therapy and affect. *Maturitas* 1:247–259.

24. Erlik Y, Tataryn IV, Meldrium DR, Lomax P, Bajorek JG, Judd HL (1981) Association of waking episodes with menopausal hot flushes. *JAMA* 245:1741–1744.

25. Fedor-Freybergh P (1977) The influence of estrogens on the well-being and mental performance in climacteric and postmenopausal women. *Acta Obstet Gynecol Scand* (suppl). 64:1–66.

26. Feigen GA, Fraser RC, Peterson NS (1978) Sex hormones and the immune response. II. Perturbation of antibody production by estradiol 17B. *Int Arch Allergy Appl Immunol* 57:488–497.

27. Feigen G, Fraser R, Dix C, Flynn C, Taylor K, Peterson N, Grant R (1980) Manipulation of the immune response by Na ascorbate and estradiol 17B. *Abstract of 4th International Congress of Immunology,* Paris, July 21–26, 1980.

28. Feigen G, Smith B, Fraser R, Dix C, Flynn C, Peterson N (1980) Ascorbate, estradiol and the immune response in guinea pigs. *Int J Immunopharmacology* 2:227.

29. Ferin M, Wehrenberg WB, Lam NY, Alston EJ, Vande Wiele RL (1982) Effects and site of action of morphine on gonadotropin secretion in the female rhesus monkey. *Endocrinology* 111:1652–1656.

30. Fraser RC, Pavlovic S, Kurahara OG, Murata A, Peterson NS, Taylor KB & Feigen GA (1980) The effect of variations in vitamin C intake on the cellular immune response of guinea pigs. *Am J Clin Nutr* 33:839–847.

31. Gambrell RD (1982) The menopause: benefits and risks of estrogen-progestogen replacement therapy. *Fertil Steril* 4:457–474.

32. Gambrell RD (1982) Roles of hormones in the etiology and prevention of endometrial and breast cancer. *Acta Obstet Gynecol Scand Suppl* 106:37–46.

33. Gambrell RD, Maier RC, Sanders BI (1983) Decreased incidence of breast cancer in postmenopausal estrogen-progestogen users. *Obstet Gynecol* 62:435–443.

34. Gerdes LC, Sonnendecker EWW, Polakow ES (1982) Psychological changes effected by estrogen-progesteron and clonidine treatment in climacteric women. *Am J Obstet Gynecol* 142:98–104.

35. Glenn F (1978) An update on our epidemic of gall stones. *Med Times* 106:38–43.

36. Gonzalez ER citing Coulan CB, Anngers JP (1983) Chronic anovulation may increase postmenopausal breast cancer risk. *JAMA* 249:445–446.

37. Gordon WE, Hermann HW, Hunter DC (1979) Treatment of atrophic vaginitis in post-menopausal women with micronized estradiol cream—a follow-up study. *J Ky Med Assoc* 77:7:337–339.

38. Hartman EL (1973) *The Functions of Sleep.* New Haven, Yale University Press.

39. Haspels AA, Coelingh Bennink HJT, Schreurs WHP (1978) Disturbance of tryptophan metabolism and its correction during oestrogen treatment in postmenopausal women. *Maturitas* 1:15–20.

40. Honore LH (1980) Increased incidence of symptomatic cholesterol cholelithiasis in perimenopausal women receiving estrogen replacement therapy. *J Reprod Med* 25:187–190.

41. Hoover R, Gray LA, Cole P, MacMahom B (1976) Menopausal estrogens and breast cancer. *New Eng J Med* 295:8:401–405.

42. Jones GS (1966) Sexual difficulties after 50. *Obstet Gynecol Surv* 21:628.

43. Judd HL, Davidson BJ, Frumar AM, Shamonki IM, Lagasse LD, Ballon SC (1980) Serum androgens and estrogens in postmenopausal women with and without endometrial cancer. *Am J Obstet Gynecol* 136:859–871.

44. Kalkhoff RK (1982) Metabolic effects of progesterone. *Am J Obstet Gynecol* 142:735–738.

45. Kern F (1978) Cholesterol gallstones. *Clinical Conference* 75:514–522.

46. Klaiber EL, Broverman DM, Vogel W, Kobayashi Y, Moriarty D (1972) Effects of estrogen therapy on plasma MAO activity and EEG driving response in depressed women. *Am J Psychiatry* 128:1492–1498.

47. Klaiber EL, Kobayashi Y, Broverman DM, Hall F (1971) Plasma monoamine oxidase activity in regularly menstruating women and in amenorrheic women receiving cyclic treatment with estrogens and a progestin. *J Clin Endocrinol Metab* 33:630–638.

48. Kupperman HS, Wetchler BB, Blatt MHG (1959) Contemporary therapy of the menopausal syndrome. *JAMA* 171:1627–1637.

49. Laufer LR, DeFazio JL, Lu JK, Meldrum DR, Eggena P, Sambhi MP, Hershman JM, Judd HL (1983) Estrogen replacement therapy by transdermal estradiol administration. *Am J Obstet Gynecol* 146:533–540.

50. Lauritzen C (1973) The management of the premenopausal and the postmenopausal patient. *Front Horm Res* 2:2–21.

51. Lindsay R, Hart DM (1978) Failure of response of menopausal vasomotor symptoms to clonidine. *Maturitas* 1:21–25.

52. Manni A (1983) Hormone receptors and breast cancer. *New Eng J Med* 309:22:1383–1384.

52a. Lobo RA, McCormick M, Singer F, Roy S (1984) Depo-medroxyprogesterone acetate compared with conjugated estrogens for the treatment of postmenopausal women. *Obstet Gynecol* 63:1–5.

53. Maschak CA, Lobo RA, Dozono TR, Eggena P, Nakamura RH, Brenner PF, Mishell DR (1982) Comparison of pharmacodynamic properties of various estrogen formulations. *Am J Obstet Gynecol* 144:511–518.

54. Masters WH, Johnson VE (1970) *Human Sexual Inadequacy.* Boston, Little, Brown & Co.

55. Nachtigall LE, Nachtigall RH, Nachtigall RD, Beckman EM (1979) Estrogen replacement therapy II: a prospective study in the relationship to carcinoma and cardiovascular and metabolic problems. *Obstet Gynecol* 54:74–79.

56. Navratil J, Novakova D, Pichner J (1975) The treatment of climacteric disorders with a combination of estradiol and testosterone—an outline of the pathogenesis of psychic symptoms in the climacterium. *Activ Nerv Supp (Praha)* 17:4:307–308.

57. Needham J, Gwei-Djen L (1968) Sex hormones in the Middle Ages. *Endeavor* 27:130–132.

58. Nisker JA, Siiteri PK (1981) Estrogens and breast cancer. *Clin Obstet Gynecol* 24:301–322.

59. Petitti DB, Wingerd J, Pellegrin F, Ramcharan S (1979) Risk of vascular disease in women: smoking, oral contraceptives, non-contraceptive estrogens and other factors. *JAMA* 242:1150–1154.

60. Pyonala T (1976) The effect of synthetic and natural estrogens on glucose tolerance, plasma insulin, and lipid metabolism in postmenopausal women. In: *The Management of the Menopause and Postmenopausal Years,* pp 195–210. Campbell S (ed). Lancaster, England, MTP Press.

61. Ross RK, Paganini-Hill A, Gerkins VR, Mack TM, Pfeffer R, Arthur M, Henderson BE (1980) A case control study of menopausal estrogen therapy and breast cancer. *JAMA* 243:1635–1639.

62. Salmi T, Punnonen R (1979) Clonidine in the treatment of menopausal symptoms. *Int J Gynaecol Obstet* 16:422–426.

63. Sarles H, Gerolami A, Cros RC (1978) Diet and cholesterol gallstones: a further study. *Digestion* 17:128–134.

64. Shaffer EA, Small DH (1977) Biliary lipid secretion in cholesterol gallstone disease. *J Clin Invest* 59:828–840.

65. Schiff I, Regestein Q, Tulchinsky D, Ryan KJ (1979) Effects of estrogens on psychological state of hypogonadal women. *JAMA* 242:2405–2407.

66. Schiff I, Tulchinsky D, Cramer D (1980) Oral medoxyprogesterone in the treatment of postmenopausal symptoms. *JAMA* 244:1443.

67. Schildkraut JJ (1965) The catecholamine hypothesis of affective disorders: a review of supporting evidence. *Am J Psychiatry* 122:509–522.

68. Schneider MA, Brotherton PL, Hailes J (1977) The effect of exogenous oestrogens on depression in menopausal women. *Med J Aust* 2:5:162–163.

69. Semmens JP, Wagner G (1982) Estrogen deprivation and vaginal function in postmenopausal women. *JAMA* 248:445–448.

70. Shoemaker ES, Forney DP, MacDonald PC (1977) Estrogen treatment of postmenopausal women: benefits and risks. *JAMA* 238:1524–1530.

71. Spellacy WN (1982) Carbohydrate metabolism during treatment with estrogen, progestogen and low dose oral contraceptives. *Am J Obstet Gynecol* 142:732–734.

72. Spellacy WN, Buhi WC, Birk SA (1972) The effect of estrogens on carbohydrate metabolism: glucose, insulin and growth hormone studies on one hundred and seventy-one women ingesting Premarin, mestranol, and ethinyl estradiol for six months. *Am J Obstet Gynecol* 114:378–392.

73. Stark M, Adonia A, Milwidsky A, Gilon G, Palti Z (1978) Can estrogens be useful for treatment of vaginal relaxation in elderly women? *Am J Obstet Gynecol* 131:585–586.

74. Studd JWW, Chakravarti S, Oram D (1976) Practical problems of the treatment of the climacteric syndrome. *Postgrad Med J* 52 (Suppl 6) 60–64.

75. Sturdevant RAL, Pearce ML, Dayton S (1973) Increased incidence of cholelithiasis in men ingesting a serum-cholesterol-lowering diet. *New Eng J Med* 288:24–27.

76. Thom M, Chakravarti S, Oram DH, Studd JWW (1976) Effect of hormone replacement therapy on glucose tolerance in postmenopausal women. *Br J Obstet Gynaecol* 84:776–783.

77. Thomson J, Oswald I (1977) Effect of oestrogen on the sleep, mood and anxiety of menopausal women. *Br Med J* 2:6098:317–319.

78. Utian WH (1972) The mental tonic effect of oestrogens administered to oophorectomized females. *S Afr Med J* 46:1079.

79. Utian WH (1974) Oestrogen, headache and oral contraceptives. *S Afr Med J* 48:2105–2108.

80. VanKeep PA, Serr DM, Greenblatt RB, Kopera H (1978) Effects, side-effects and dosage schemes of various sex hormones in the peri- and post menopause. Workshop Report in *Female and Male Climacteric: Current Opinion 1978* Baltimore, University Park Press.

81. Wallace RB, Hoover J, Barrett-Conner E, et al (1979) Altered plasma lipid and lipo-protein level associated with oral contraceptive and oestrogen use. *Lancet* 1979, ii:112–114.

82. Wardlaw SL, Wehrenberg WB, Ferin M, Antunes JL, Frantz AG (1982) Effect of sex steroids on B-endorphin in hypophyseal portal blood. *J Clin Endocrinol Metab* 55:877–881.

83. Wehrenberg WB, Wardlaw SL, Frantz AG, Ferin M (1982) B-endorphin in hypophyseal portal blood: variations throughout the menstrual cycle. *Endocrinology* 111:879–881.

84. Whitehead MI, McQueen J, Minardi J, Campbell S (1978) Clinical considerations in the management of the menopause: the endometrium. *Postgrad Med J* 54:69–73.

85. Wood K, Coppen A (1978) The effect of estrogens on plasma tryptophan and adrenergic function in patients treated with lithium. In: *The Role of Estrogen/Progestogen in the Management of the Menopause*, pp 29–38. Cooke ID (ed). Baltimore, University Park Press.

86. Wynn V (1982) Effect of duration of low dose oral contraceptive administration on carbohydrate metabolism. *Am J Obstet Gynecol* 142:739–746.

5

The Endometrial Cancer Risk

As was described in the preceding chapters, hormone replacement therapy is so clearly beneficial to so many systems that it was a common prescription for many years. Hormones were prescribed before assays were available to test the plasma levels that had been achieved by different dosages. With our current knowledge, it has become clear that the original prescription dosages were much too high. These high dosages of unopposed estrogens significantly increased the risk of endometrial carcinoma in certain women.

This chapter on the risk of endometrial carcinoma includes a review of both the epidemiologic and the morphological studies. The results of these studies combine to establish a relationship between high doses of unopposed estrogen and the increased incidence of endometrial carcinoma. The literature also shows that, with appropriate dosages of steroids, the incidence of endometrial carcinoma is lower among women who use hormones in the menopausal years than among those who do not. The association with endometrial carcinoma is a critical consideration in selecting a sequential combination with progestin as a replacement hormone regimen, the goal being to avoid the increased likelihood of this malignancy.

UTERINE CARCINOMA AND ITS RELATIONSHIP TO HYPERPLASIAS

The histology of uterine adenocarcinoma has been described by Reagan and Ng.[54] Hyperplasia of the endometrium denotes an abnormal proliferation that varies from the normal one. Hyperplasia has three distinct classifications: cystic hyperplasia, adenomatous hyperplasia, and atypical hyperplasia. There is a progressive transition from adenomatous hyperplasia to atypical hyperplasia and to endometrial carcinoma.

Reagan notes that more differentiated tumors are less serious and that the differentiation reflects a similarity to the parent tissue. A grading system from I to IV reflects the percentage of undifferentiated mass. The greatest danger is that tumor cells will spread via the blood or lymphatic systems or by distant displacement of cancerous tissue through the oviducts into the peritoneal cavity.[54] Accuracy of detection of endometrial carcinoma has been improving since the late 1940s, reaching 88% in the Cleveland hospitals among the gynecological staff, who were using a common sampling method.[54]

Although it is commonly considered that there is a developmental progression from cystic hyperplasia to the more complex adenomatous hyperplasia to the more progressed atypical hyperplasia, and onward to carcinoma, there is some controversy in the literature. Cystic hyperplasia apparently has a very low progression rate to the adenomatous stage.[43] McBride traced and followed up long-term 544 patients with cystic glandular hyperplasia; he found that fewer than 1% subsequently developed endometrial carcinoma.[43] This finding may reflect a prolonged latent period that exceeds the length of the study. This low progression rate for cystic hyperplasia contrasts with that of adenomatous hyperplasia.[21] Among patients not treated for adenomatous hyperplasia, 18.5% with a short follow-up, and 35% followed up for at least 10 years, subsequently developed endometrial carcinoma.[21] Gusberg has long held the opinion that cystic hyperplasia is not necessarily a precarcinomatous condition but that the adenomatous hyperplasia represents an ominous condition.[22]

SURVIVAL RATE AND PROGNOSIS

The age distribution of endometrial carcinoma patients is depicted in Figure 5-1. One notes the heaviest occurrence during the menopausal years, beginning at about age 50 and continuing through age 75.[75] The average age of detection, according to Ng, who evaluated consecutive endometrial carcinomas in patients over a 20-year period at the University Hospital of Cleveland, was 59.7 with a range of 21 to 89 years.[50] The 5-year survival rate, 69.7%, varied as a function of the extent of the tumor. Survival was better when tumors were well differentiated and low grade, with the lowest grade yielding the highest survival rate (86.7%). The highest grade, grade IV, yielded the lowest 5-year survival rate (32.9%).[50] These data are in general agreement with those of Mickal in which the overall 5-year survival rate averaged 62.6%.[46] Menczer and co-workers also noted that the 5-year survival was higher in the lower stage but further described that younger women had a much higher survival rate than older ones. In their sample of premenopausal and postmenopausal women, 92.9% of the younger but 60.3% of the older survived 5 years after the diagnosis of endometrial adenocarcinoma.[45] More than 80% of those with Stage I carcinoma survived, whereas fewer than 11% of those with more advanced stages in the postmenopausal group survived 5 years.[45]

FIG. 5-1. Age distribution of endometrial cancer patients (Wynder EL, Escher GC, Mantel N, 1966, Cancer 19:489–520)

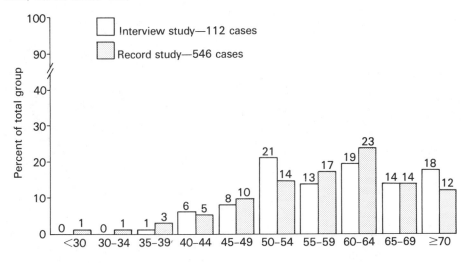

We are thus presented with a picture of endometrial carcinoma that is bleak in the older patient as well as in the advanced stages but relatively more benign in its early stages of identification as well as in the younger patient.

INCIDENCE OF ENDOMETRIAL DISEASES

Although abnormal bleeding is the most common presenting symptom,[45] endometrial disease can present itself in silent form as well.

AVAILABLE DATA ABOUT THOSE WHO BLEED

Mantalenakis, in a retrospective study of over 1000 dilatation and curettage patients covering 14 years at the Alexandria Maternity Hospital, studied women over age 50. Bleeding ranged from severe to mild, blood-stained discharge. In this population of predominantly Greek women, estrogen replacement therapy was rare. Bleeding at older ages was more prognostic of malignancy than was bleeding occurring at earlier ages.[42] Endometrial carcinoma was the most common malignant tumor. The overall malignancy rate for any form of abnormal bleeding was 22.7% in that series. Figure 5-2 shows the relationship between age of the patient and rate of malignancy.

Every one of the patients who developed menstrual irregularities or postmenopausal bleeding or spotting and who was not suspected of being pregnant was biopsied. Hofmeister also performed routine endometrial biopsies in over 20,000 patients spanning the years 1949 to 1973.[25,26] He defined the biopsy as a complete evaluation of the endocervix and complete circumferential evaluation of the uterus. The absolute detection rate of endometrial carcinoma was 0.9%, and he noted that in the general population it would be lower because his sample was somewhat skewed by the presence

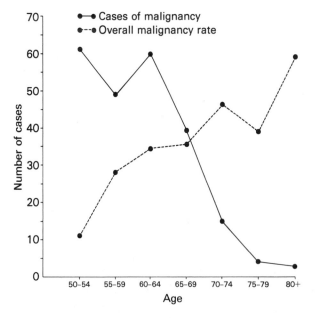

FIG. 5-2. Overall malignancy rate in relation to age among women with abnormal bleeding (Mantalenakis SJ, Papapostolon MG, 1977, International Surgery, the Journal of the International College of Surgeons 62: 103–105)

of bleeding abnormalities.[25] In a separate report, he evaluated 4400 routine endometrial samplings and found 25 cases of endometrial carcinoma.[26] Six of the 25, or roughly 25% of the endometrial carcinomas, were asymptomatic.[26]

SILENT HYPERPLASIA AND ENDOMETRIAL CARCINOMA

Pretreatment screening of endometrial tissue has yielded hyperplasia incidences of 2.5%[3] and 4.9%[8] among peri- and postmenopausal candidates for hormone replacement therapy. Campbell and co-workers detected 4.9% endometrial hyperplasia in pretreatment screening of perimenopausal patients, with 40% being totally asymptomatic.[8] These women had never used hormone replacement therapy. Undetected cystic hyperplasia was also evaluated by Vanderick and colleagues in 1348 endometrial biopsies during some 5000 cycles. They noted that, in the majority of cases, endometrial hyperplasia remained asymptomatic.[64] Callantine's group noted that endometrial biopsies of 32 "normal" candidates for hormone replacement therapy revealed 4 cases of cystic glandular and 7 of adenomatous hyperplasia.[7] In a particularly definitive study, Horwitz and co-workers evaluated all the necropsies at the Yale–New Haven Hospital and the Massachusetts General Hospital for the period 1918 to 1978 and 1952 to 1978, respectively. They noted that undetected endometrial carcinoma was much higher than had been expected.[28] Evaluating the postmenopausal women's records showed the following:

1. At the Yale-New Haven Hospital, 67% of the endometrial carcinomas were unsuspected before necropsy whereas 52% were unsuspected at the Massachusetts General Hospital.
2. The degree of "detection bias" is substantial, since the rate of detection at necropsy is about 4 to 6 times greater than the detection rate during life.
3. The endometrial carcinoma frequently exists in symptomless form.
4. Vaginal bleeding had not occurred in any of the 24 cases (combined from both hospitals) that were first diagnosed at necropsy (probably why they were not diagnosed before then).
5. Estrogen use was mentioned in only 1 of these 24 records.

Table 5–1 provides these data with appropriate percentages.[28] In view of these significant data, one must review epidemiologic studies with care, keeping in mind this unsuspected potential for bias.

EPIDEMIOLOGIC STUDIES POINTING TO ESTROGEN REPLACEMENT THERAPY AND ENDOMETRIAL CARCINOMA

THE STUDIES

In the early 1970s, investigators became aware that there was an increasing incidence of endometrial carcinoma in the United States and considered that this might reflect the increased incidence of estrogen replacement therapy. In 1975 several studies were published.[57,66,76] Weiss stated that the probability of untreated postmenopausal women developing endometrial carcinoma was, then, 1 per 1000 per year.[66] Smith and colleagues evaluated an association of exogenous estrogen and endometrial carcinoma.[57] They compared 317 endometrial carcinoma patients to 317 hospitalized

TABLE 5-1. Necropsy detection of endometrial cancer in women aged 45
years or more with intact uteri

	Yale- New Haven Hospital (1918-1978)	Massachusetts General Hospital (1952-1978)
Eligible necropsy population	4636	4462
Patients with endometrial cancer	15	27
Patients whose cancer was first diagnosed at necropsy	10	14
Unsuspected cancers (%)	67	52
Rate of endometrial cancer first detected at necropsy (per 10,000)	22	31
Rate of detected endometrial cancer estimated by CSTR (per 10,000)	4.7 (1935-1974)	5.5 (1950-1974)

Horwitz RI, Feinstein AR, Horwitz SM, Robboy SJ, 1981, Lancet July 11:66-67

controls (206 with cervical carcinoma, 88 with ovarian carcinoma, and 23 with vulvar carcinoma). One hundred fifty-two of the endometrial carcinoma patients were estrogen users; 54 of the other carcinoma patients were estrogen users. The type and duration of estrogen replacement therapy were not evaluated in this report. It appeared that there was a higher incidence of estrogen use in endometrial carcinoma patients than in the other sample used, but it is important to note that the "other carcinoma" patients were probably less likely to be estrogen replacement therapy users than women in the general population. The results may therefore have been somewhat skewed in the direction of the trend.[57] Ziel evaluated the increased incidence of endometrial carcinoma among users of conjugated estrogens.[76] He estimated a "risk-ratio" of 7.6 for conjugated estrogen use associating with carcinoma that the "risk-ratio" had increased as the duration of exposure increased (from a "risk-ratio" of 5.6 for less than 5 years of estrogen replacement therapy exposure to 13.9 for 7 or more years of exposure).[76] In 1976, Weiss and co-workers noted the increasing incidence of carcinoma of the uterine corpus from 1969 to 1973 in a variety of United States cities.[68] They commented about the simultaneous increases in estrogen replacement therapy use. Gordon and colleagues, identifying 66 cases in which carcinoma was concurrently diagnosed by several pathologists and noting that 40 of those women were users of conjugated estrogens, evaluated the "risk-ratio" to conclude that conjugated estrogens carried an 8.1 relative "risk-ratio" for endometrial carcinoma in their double-blind studies.[17] Neither dosage nor duration of the estrogen therapy used was evaluated or reported.

By 1980 there was little doubt that unopposed estrogen replacement therapy was associated with an increased incidence of endometrial carcinoma.[30,44,69] However, others were noting the effective role of progestin in reducing or even reversing this trend.[58] For example, Stahl was among those who had, before 1975, made such statements:[58]

> While there is little doubt that unopposed estrogen can be an endometrial carcinogenic stimulus, in some women, it is also clear that progestogens in adequate doses can reverse these hyperplastic changes. Thus by inducing maturing tissue and subsequent 'bleeds' carcinoma can be prevented.

Meanwhile, other studies were beginning to appear that showed a definite dose–response relationship between estrogen use and endometrial carcinoma.[3,52,63,67] Aylward and colleagues, in a prospective study in which patients were assigned to either high or low doses of estrogen replacement therapy in accordance with the severity of their menopausal symptoms, provided meaningful evidence of a dose–response relationship.[3] Four of the 13 who were given cyclic "high-dose" estrogens presented cystic glandular hyperplasia within 10 months after the start of therapy. High-dose regimens included ethinyl estradiol, 0.03 mg daily, conjugated equine estrogens, 1.25 mg daily, oestrone piperazine sulfate, 3.0 mg daily, or estradiol valerate, 2.0 mg daily. "Low-dose" regimens were set at half these levels. Similar trends with much larger samples were reported by Paterson and colleagues.[52] Low-dose regimens of estrogens were compared to high-dose regimens of proportions similar to those of the previously mentioned study. The type of estrogen did not affect the rate of cystic hyperplasia, but the dose of the estrogen did.[52] Van Campehout and co-workers reviewed their own and other data to show that *all* of the reported young patients with endometrial carcinoma had a history of use of very high doses of estrogens, which, in most instances, were unopposed by progestins.[63] They also noted that among patients with endometrial hyperplasia, 84% had received unopposed estrogen for a number of years.

Vanderick and colleagues provided a clear demonstration of a dose–response relationship between increasing estrogen dose (several regimens of ethinyl estradiol) and the development of cystic hyperplasia as evaluated by morphologic criteria.[64] Endometrial hyperplasia occurred in 48% of those patients who had a total dose of ethinyl estradiol per cycle that exceeded 2.8 mg.

The duration of estrogen use was also evaluated with respect to frequency and occurrence of endometrial carcinoma.[24,30,44,69] Studies made it clear that the longer that unopposed estrogen replacement therapy was used, the greater the likelihood was for an increased risk of endometrial carcinoma. Hulka noted that estrogen use of 3.5 years or more increased the likelihood of developing endometrial carcinoma of early stage and low grade. These are the cancers that have the best prognosis.[30] She also noted that in comparison to chemical carcinogens from which latency periods of 15 to 30 years have been reported, latency periods of only 3 to 6 years were common with estrogen replacement therapy use. The frequency of occurrence of carcinoma dropped to that of non-estrogen users after a 2-year, estrogen-free interval. Such short latency and easy recovery are most unusual among carcinogens.[30] This finding suggested that the estrogens' influence on potential carcinoma was more a potentiation of an underlying propensity than a unique stimulus. Other studies also provided convincing evidence of an increased risk of endometrial carcinoma in those women who took unopposed estrogen replacement therapy.[1,24,32,56] Moreover, there was a suggestion that the association decreased for estrogen users in the later years.[32]

LOGISTICAL PROBLEMS

Although there is no reasonable doubt that estrogen therapy increased the incidence of endometrial carcinoma, there are logistical problems with the studies just described. Kay pointed these out.[35] In an elegant mathematical discussion, she showed that the minimum number of woman-years that would be necessary to evaluate the effect of estrogen hormone replacement therapy on increasing the incidence of endometrial carcinoma by a factor of 2 at a 1% probability level, would be about 50,000. This would require the cooperation of about 1000 practitioners, a phenomenon that would be difficult to achieve. Although each of the studies pointing to an increased association did go a long way in building a case, the numbers were so small that they did not begin to approach this 50,000 woman-years requirement.

Horwitz and Feinstein used alternate analytic methods for case control studies of estrogen and endometrial carcinoma to conclude that the epidemiologic estimates were grossly overstated.[27] They believed that women with uterine carcinoma "who take estrogens are more likely than non-takers to bleed and to be referred to hospital for diagnosis." This detection bias disproportionately weights the hormone use in carcinoma patients and thereby artificially elevates the "risk-ratio." According to their recast "risk-ratio"s, a 1.8 increased jeopardy of endometrial carcinoma in estrogen replacement therapy users would be a more reasonable estimate.[27] Their arguments were not universally accepted.[31] In 1981, Horwitz and co-workers, then published their actual studies that attempted to prove a detection bias.[28] As described in Table 5-1, they reviewed all reports at the Yale–New Haven Hospital and the Massachusetts General Hospital in which the body was examined after the death of the individual (necropsy). At the Yale–New Haven Hospital, the records span the years 1918 to 1978; at the Massachusetts General Hospital, 1952 to 1978. Their data supported their contentions. The rate of endometrial carcinoma that was first detected at necropsy was 2.2 per 1000 in the Yale–New Haven population and 3.1 per 1000 in the Massachusetts General Hospital. Since the undetected rate of endometrial carcinoma was high, actually as high as some of the elevated risk estimates for hormones inducing carcinoma, their point is worthy of note. Judd and co-workers also describe a 25% to 50% incidence of asymptomatic endometrial carcinoma cases.[33]

Conclusions

These studies combine to suggest that unopposed estrogen replacement therapy of long duration and high dose is associated with an increased incidence of endometrial carcinoma. Such an association appears to be considerably lower than the first reports indicated, and the role of progestin opposition seems to vastly improve the safety of estrogen replacement therapy.

PROGESTIN OPPOSITION TO ESTROGEN: REDUCING THE VULNERABILITY

As the awareness of the danger of unopposed high-dose estrogen was growing, a number of investigators began publishing opinions and studies showing the beneficial role of progestin.[2,3,5,15,67,69] Discussions of the appropriate dose and duration of progestin also followed.

The early suggestions were that at least 7 days of progestin would be necessary to be protective.[2,8] In the study of Campbell and colleagues, although the increasing dosages of unopposed estrogen were associated with an increased incidence of cystic hyperplasia, it was also noted that those women who took at least 7 days of progestin with their estrogen therapy had a much lower frequency of development of any form of hyperplasia.[8] Data showed that those women who took sequential estrogen with progestin had a 92% rate of normal endometrium, which contrasted with a 75% rate of normal endometrium for those taking the low-dose unopposed estrogen and a 65% normal endometrium rate for those taking the high-dose, unopposed estrogen.[8] Weiss, one of the earlier proponents of the risk of estrogen therapy in endometrial carcinoma, had by 1980 reached the point that he had suggested that there was a delicate balance between estrogen and progestin in determining the safety of hormone replacement therapy.[67]

A number of studies of comparative treatments for menopausal symptoms compared different regimens of estrogen with and without progestin opposition. There was a general consistency in the results. Although estrogen therapies, unopposed, tended to be associated with an increased incidence of hyperplasia and carcinoma, the progestin opposition reduced this proportion to figures even lower than population norms. Hammond showed that synthetic progestin opposition to estrogen therapy provided significant protection. Of the 72 women who were treated with progestin opposition to 0.625 mg of Premarin, none had endometrial malignancy.[24] Nachtigall and colleagues, in their 10-year, double-blind, prospective study of 84 pairs of menopausal women, found that a 10-mg per day medroxyprogesterone acetate course for 7 days each month was very effective.[48] They paired this progestin dose to a high (2.5 mg) daily dose of conjugated estrogen and reported that there was no case of endometrial carcinoma. There was one case in the control group.[48] Paterson and colleagues confirmed the value of taking 7 to 10 days of progestin and noted that, in their samples, the endometrial disease incidence for progestin users was actually lower than that in the general population figures.[52] Van Campehout and colleagues also provided confirmatory evidence in their use of progestin for at least 7 to 10 days.[63] Others did as well.[8,14,23,59] Van Keep and co-workers clearly demonstrate this protective effect (Table 5-2).[65] One notes the higher incidence of endometrial carcinoma among estrogen users and the fact that those who used estrogen with progestin had a lower frequency than untreated women.[65] These epidemiologic studies and clinical observations are strongly supported by the receptor studies in endometrial tissue that are discussed later in this chapter.

PROGESTIN THERAPY CAN REVERSE ENDOMETRIAL HYPERPLASIA

Evidence has been mounting convincingly that cystic hyperplasia can often be reversed with appropriately dosed progestin therapy.[8,14,37,70] Kistner first reported this. Kelley and Baker presented data of 8366 cases from 27 clinics. They noted that the overall 5-year survival rate was 54.3% after carcinoma of the uterus had been diagnosed and that the most common remote metastasis was to the pulmonary site.[37] In this investigation the authors chose progestational agents for trial of far advanced endometrial carcinoma. Six of the 21 patients showed objective regressions lasting for 9 months to 4.5 years.[37] In 1974, Wentz showed that progestin therapy was fully able to

TABLE 5-2. Incidence of endometrial cancer at Wilford Hall USAF Medical Center, 1975-1977

	Patient Years of Observation	Cancer Cases	Incidence
Estrogen	2088	8	3.8 per 1000
Estrogen + progestin	3792	1	.3 per 1000
Other hormones	775	1	1.3 per 1000
Untreated women	1515	3	2.0 per 1000
TOTAL	8170	13	1.6 per 1000

Van Keep PA, Ser DM, Greenblatt RB, Kopera H, 1978, Workshop Report, In: *Female and Male Climacteric: Current Opinion.* Baltimore, University Park Press reverse the adenomatous and the atypical hyperplasia in both premenopausal and postmenopausal women (Table 5-3).[70] One notes that high dosages of progestins (20 mg oral megesterol acetate per day for 6 weeks, or 100 mg dimethisterone per day for 6 weeks) clearly reversed these hyperplasias. Campbell and co-workers provided similar results. They presented data of 16 women with pretreatment hyperplasia and 25 women who developed hyperplasias after cyclic estrogen therapies.[8] In all cases but one, progestin reversed the hyperplastic condition within 6 months to yield normal endometrial histology. Because they had noted a dose-dependent hyperplasia incidence and a reversal on progestin, their phenomenon was in accord with that of Wentz. Gambrell also reported the beneficial effects of progestin.[14] Table 5-4 shows the beneficial effects of 19 norprogestins on endometrial hyperplasia.[14] Of the 60 women with varying endometrial pathologic conditions before therapy, one notes the elimination of 59 hyperplastic conditions after 3 months of a combined ethinyl estradiol and norgestrel therapy. Gambrell concluded that 19 nortestosterone derivatives (such as norethindrone and norgestrel) were superior to other progestins for preventing and treating endometrial hyperplasias. He also noted that progestogen therapy was superior to curettage alone in treating the endometrial hyperplasia because the pathology persisted in 50% of cases treated only with curettage. In none of the patients treated with progestins had it recurred after 18 months.[14]

TABLE 5-3. Reversal of persistent endometrial hyperplasia by oral progestin therapy (oral megesterol acetate 20 mg progestin/d for 6 weeks)

	N	Length of Follow-up (yr)			Recurrence
		1	3	5	
Adenomatous hyperplasia	80 (27–53)*	10	38	32	0
Atypical hyperplasia	30 (5–25)*	5	8	17	0

*Numbers in parentheses indicate pre- and postmenopausal patients, respectively.
Wentz WB, 1974, Gynecol Oncol 2:363–367

TABLE 5-4. Effects of 19-nor progestogens on endometrial hyperplasia

Pathology Before Therapy	N	Endometrium After Therapy	N
Benign hyperplasia	42	Proliferative	30
Cystic hyperplasia	9	Secretory	13
Adenomatous hyperplasia	5	Atrophic	11
Atypical adenomatous hyperplasia	4	Dyssynchronous maturation	5
		Benign hyperplasia	1
Total patients	60	Total patients	60

Gambrell RD, 1977, Clin Obstet Gynaecol 4:129–143

THE PROGESTIN CHALLENGE TEST

These results led Gambrell to suggest the use of a "Progestin Challenge Test." He states that if 3 months of progestin opposition yields no withdrawal bleeding in estrogen and progestin regimens, then it is safe to discontinue the progestin for 6 months or so. After each 6 months have passed in which unopposed estrogen is used, The Progestin Challenge Test should be repeated.

Sturdee and co-workers, in comprehensive studies, have concluded that both cyclic unopposed estrogen and constant estrogen were equally unsafe in relation to endometrial hyperplasia risk.[60] Paterson and colleagues showed clearly that duration of treatment had a profound influence on the likelihood of abnormal histology in the case of conjugated equine estrogen 1.25 mg daily.[52] They showed that after 6 months of such unopposed treatment, 8.8% of the women who had had satisfactory pretherapy endometrial biopsy specimens showed abnormalities. This percentage increased at 1 year to 12%, by a year and a half to 13%, and by 2 years to 42%. The predominant abnormality was cystic hyperplasia. The use of the Progestin Challenge Test is considered to prevent such a sequence.

HORMONE LEVELS OF CARCINOMA PATIENTS DIFFER

Investigators have questioned whether women with endometrial carcinoma have different plasma levels of various steroids. Their results are mixed. Androstenedione was reported not to be different in a sample of 35 women with adenocarcinoma of the endometrium at an average number of 12.5 years post menopause (503 ± 34 pg/ml).[34] In contrast, Calanog[6] and Carlstrom[9] each reported a significantly elevated level of plasma androstenedione in patients with endometrial carcinoma. Calanog found that 14 carcinoma patients had a mean plasma level of 996 pg/ml vs. 880 pg/ml in the 5 controls.[6] Carstrom showed, among 18 women with endometrial carcinoma (average age 74.1), a plasma level of dehydroepiandrosterone of 2010 ± 195 nmol; this contrasted with 40 healthy women whose average level was 1299 ± 117 nmol.[9] Plasma estrone levels were reported not different in Judd's population (38.7 ± 3.6 pg/ml).[34] In contrast, one other investigator did report differences. The Carlstrom study showed elevated estrone levels of 2.38 ± 0.24 nmol vs. the 40 healthy women whose level averaged 1.36 ± 0.11.[9] The Calanog study showed no differences in estrone, which is consistent with Judd's data.

It would thus appear that there is some evidence for an elevated steroid level in endometrial carcinoma patients. However, the picture is not consistent.

UTERINE STUDIES *IN VITRO*

A number of studies evaluating biochemical response to different kinds and doses of estrogens and progestins have been reported. There is an overall consistency, albeit fragmented, to suggest that estrogen stimulates proliferation of endometrial tissue and that progestins inhibit this stimulatory effect. The progestin exerts an antiestrogenic effect.

ESTROGEN RECEPTORS

In 1964 researchers demonstrated an active incorporation of estrogens into carcinomatous breast tissue. This was contrasted with benign adipose, muscle, and noncancerous breast tissue.[10] A search for estrogen receptors in uterine tissue showed elevated receptor concentration in carcinomatous samples compared with noncarcinomatous tissue. Buchi and Keller localized estrogen receptors in normal and myometrial tissue from different regions of the uterus. Levels were much lower in myometrium than in endometrium.[4] The myometrial receptors were not variable as a function of menstrual cycle time. The endometrial receptors were, which suggests that endometrial tissue is probably more responsive to hormonal variation than is myometrial tissue. Estrone receptors were searched for, and not found, in endometrial slices incubated with labelled estrone.[19] It therefore appeared that estradiol would have influential effects on endometrial tissue but that estrone, lacking suitable receptor complexes to bind to, would exert less of an effect on the tissue.[19]

Ochiai noted similar phenomena.[51] Figure 5-3 reveals the cyclic variation in endometrial receptor as well as the relative elevation in comparison with other uterine sites. It is surprising that the cervical tissue samples do not show a significant cyclic variation in receptor response. One wonders whether a cyclic variation could be better revealed if the endocervix were targetted specifically.

PROGESTERONE RECEPTORS

Studies of the ratio of progesterone receptor to estrogen content also showed that small myoma have a lower ratio than does normal myometrium.[51] This suggests that when the progesterone receptor gets too low in proportion to estrogen receptor, the likelihood of myoma may increase.[51]

Milgrom and co-workers demonstrated that progestins reduced the quantity of their own receptors in endometrium.[47] Progestins (Provera 60 mg per day) also reduced the 17-beta dehydrogenase, an enzyme that increases the conversion of 17-beta estrogen into estrone.[19] There is, therefore, a biochemical basis by which progesterone would remove E2 from endometrial media.[19]

Tseng and Gurpide concluded, in their studies of endometrial biopsy tissue, that progesterone acts to reduce the number of estrogen receptors rather than to compete directly with receptor sites.[61] Estrone and estradiol did not compete for the same binding sites.[61] Flickinger also has concluded that progestins reduce the endometrial receptors for estradiol and for progesterone as shown in a variety of ways in humans and monkeys.[12]

The preceding studies of receptor content suggest a powerful biochemical mechanism by which steroids (estrogen and/or progesterone) interact with each other to stimulate or inhibit the production of tissue. Although there are positive effects of estrogen with reversal on progestin, carcinoma itself is not defined by the quantity of estrogen receptor.[12,13] There appears to be much overlapping in the system. Nonetheless, studies of endometrial response to the different hormones have yielded important information.

RELATIVE POTENCY OF DIFFERENT ESTROGENS

Since the studies taken together could not be used to identify nuclear binding of estrone in human endometrial tissue, it was suggested that estradiol was the critical risk factor in endometrial hyperplasia.[18] Metabolic studies on the uptake of estrogens and

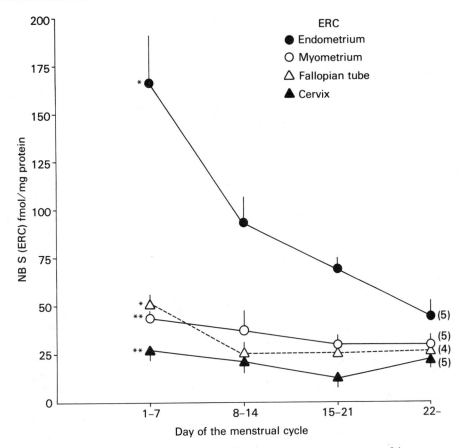

FIG. 5-3. Variation in the concentration of cytosol estrogen receptor of human uterus throughout the menstrual cycle; *values are significantly higher than those of second half of proliferative phase (p<0.02); **mean values of proliferative phase of myometrium and cervix are higher than those of secretory phase (p<0.05); (Ochiaik, 1980, Acta Obstet Gynaec Jpn 32:945-952)

progesterone by human endometrium provided some confirmatory evidence. Although most of the estrone and estradiol that enter tissue is released into the medium as estrone, and approximately the same proportion of perfused estrone and estradiol enters the endometrium from buffer, endometrial adenocarcinoma appears to retain estradiol and release estrone.[62] The demonstration, after incubation of tissue slices with labelled estrone, that there were no chromatin-bound estrone receptor complexes in human endometrium further implicates the other principal estrogen—estradiol.[19] Estriol, the presumed weakest of the three estrogens, is a short-acting steroid.[11] Daily repetitive (more than once a day, generally 2 or 3 times) oral administration of estriol is able to induce estrogenic activity in the endometrium just as estradiol can.[11] If it is orally administered in repetitive doses that result in prolonged elevation of the blood levels and continuous stimulation of the estrogen receptors, estriol can have profound influences on endometrial slices. It was noted, however, that estriol administration at a lower frequency (once a day) is usually effective in relieving menopausal symptoms and safe with respect to endometrial stimulation.[11] Thus the classification of estriol as a weak hormone was considered to be "probably" valid when estriol was administered once a day. Englund concluded that when estriol was administered in a way that yields prolonged elevation of the blood levels, as is the case in frequent daily administration, it produces the same effect on the endometrium as estradiol.

Studies of the endometrial response to 2 doses of Premarin (0.625 or 1.25), 3 weeks on, 1 week off, combined with progestin have shown that either dose has potent estrogenic effects.[38] An increase in the nuclear estrogen and progesterone receptors to levels that are equivalent to premenopausal proliferative levels was noted. Norethisterone, in doses ranging from 2.5 to 5 mg., did not affect the amount of estrogen entering the nucleus. It did temporarily suppress the biological activity of endometrium as measured by the number of estrogen and progestin receptors. This temporary effect is considered to last about 1 week.[38] Women without progesterone treatment have higher levels of cytoplasmic receptor for progesterone and from these data it was concluded that progesterone leads to a reduction in the number of progesterone receptors. One final measurement indicated that progesterone administration induced estradiol dehydrogenase, the enzyme that converts estradiol to estrone, thereby reducing the estrogenic effect. Because there was a small sample size (7), the results in this study were considered tentative.[38]

Ludwig, in 1982, reported the morphological response of the human endometrium to long-term treatment with progestational agents.[40] The endometria of 12 women were examined, 11 on a long-term, low-dose regimen of progestogens for contraception, and 1 on a short-term, high-dose regimen of injectable progestogen for adjuvant therapy of breast carcinoma. Endometrial examination, using the criteria of Noyes, indicated that the response, though variable, did have some clear effects. The authors concluded, "short term, high dose administration of progestogens produces a completely different endometrial pattern than long term, low dose treatment." The low-dose effects included a profound reduction of gland mitoses, tortuosity of glands, basal vacuolization, signs of secretion, and predecidual reaction.

An additional piece of evidence confirming the influence of estradiol on endometrial tissue was provided by Hughes and colleagues.[29] In their study of postmenopausal women with excessive uterine bleeding, histologic findings showed either a continuous proliferative phase endometrium, endometrial hyperplasia, or adenocarcinoma of the endometrium. The addition of estradiol to an organ culture that contained normal and abnormal endometrial tissue increased the cellular proliferation; the addition of progesterone increased the synthesis of glycogen from glucose in significant amounts. This glycogen response was interpreted as cellular evidence that progesterone prevents the development of overproliferation of endometrium. A breakdown of glycogen occurred, as is the case during the luteal phase.[29]

UTERINE STUDIES *IN VIVO*

The question of effective and appropriate progestin dosing has recently received significant attention in the literature. Because high doses of progestin have had adverse effects on plasma lipid status (see Chapter 6), and because high doses of progestin have been associated with unpleasant side-effects such as uterine cramping and a loss of general feeling of well-being, there is much interest in reducing the dose of progestin. In fact, recent studies have suggested that the original doses were unnecessarily high and that correct doses can be adjusted down to about one-fifth of the level commonly described in 1980, 1981, and 1982 publications. In the studies of Vanderick, the dose of progestin was found to be irrelevant in adequately protecting the endometrium; in the 1300 endometrial biopsies studied,[64] one sees the inefficacy of short-term, high-dose progestin. Whitehead and co-workers attempted to determine the time course and minimum effective daily dose of progestin because it was already known that duration of progestin use was far more important than dose of progestin.[71] When Whitehead and colleagues began their study, it was clear that prolonged duration was much better in preventing endometrial hyperplasia than short duration. They measured suppression of DNA synthesis and reduction in estradiol receptors as evidence of an antiestrogenic effect. They also looked for an increase in activity of the progestin-sensitive enzymes, estradiol dehydrogenase and isocitric dehydrogenase. As a control, they used endometria of premenopausal women in the proliferative and secretory phases.[71] The results indicated that a low dose of progestin was equally as, or more effective, in opposing the estrogen influence than a high dose of progestin when both doses were given for long duration (last 7 days of each month).

Whitehead and co-workers further evaluated the actions of progestins on the morphology and biochemistry of the endometrium of postmenopausal women receiving low-dose estrogen therapy.[72] Thirty-three women on 0.625 mg conjugated equine estrogen were evaluated for the endometrial response to different doses of progestins. The lowest doses of progestin produced as, or more effective, an inhibition of proliferation (as measured by morphological appearance, DNA synthesis). Lowest doses of progestin produced as great an increase in isocitric dehydrogenase activity as the currently prescribed higher doses. The authors suspected that even lower doses of progestin might be fully adequate. One mg norethindrone or 75 μg D/L-norgestrel for 13 days was, therefore, recommended as the appropriate dosage for opposing the 0.625 mg of conjugated equine estrogen.[72]

A year later, the same group, reviewing the literature and exploring their own studies, concluded:[73]

1. Medroxyprogesterone acetate can be lowered from the old doses in line with the new studies on 1-norethindrone and D/L-norgestrel.
2. Reducing norethindrone from 10 to 1 mg a day is associated with a lowering of the adverse effect on lipid status that had been reported by other groups.
3. These lower doses yielded less premenstrual tension, a common problem to perimenopausal women taking high doses of progestin.

The question to the clinician becomes one of determining when and for how long progestin is advisable to promote endometrial protection. Gambrell has offered The Progestin Challenge Test as one effective way of determining when progestin is needed to prevent endometrial hyperplasia.[16] The Progestin Challenge Test, as originally conceived, is a 10-day trial of progestin (norlutate 5 mg or Provera 10 mg was originally used) to each woman with an intact uterus. The progestin is continued each month for as long as withdrawal bleeding continues. When data from close to 3000 patients, collected during the period from 1975 to 1978, were combined, it was shown that malignancy declined each year in all groups. The Progestin Challenge Test was able to distinguish those at risk sufficiently that all treatments produced equally low rates of malignancy *if* The Progestin Challenge Test was used to define which treatment to give. The carcinoma incidence was initially higher in estrogen users, but started to decline significantly once The Progestin Challenge Test was started.[16] Elsewhere, women taking a total of 25 mg of norethisterone during a 5-day span were not as well protected from hyperplasia as those taking 15 mg over 13 days with a constant estrogen treatment (Menophase).[60]

Because these studies have indicated that lower doses of progestin appear to be even more effective than high doses, it remains for future investigators to define what level of progestin is most appropriate to provide an adequate challenge.

Although this chapter has emphasized the role of estrogen replacement therapy in the incidence of endometrial carcinoma, it is important to realize that estrogen replacement therapy is just one of a number of identified "risk-factors" for carcinoma—not even the major one. The others are considered next.

RISK FACTORS FOR ENDOMETRIAL CARCINOMA OTHER THAN ESTROGEN

Postmenopausal bleeding is the keynote heralder of hyperplasia or adenocarcinoma. Figure 5–4 shows the pathology of postmenopausal bleeding among women not taking exogenous estrogens and compares these data with those of women who were taking estrogen.[14] Evaluation of the endometrium in postmenopausal bleeders can disclose hyperplasia but it can just as likely yield a proliferative or an atrophic state. With increasing age, the probability of encountering a malignancy among the postmenopausal bleeders increases from about 20% to a maximum reported rate of about 40% of

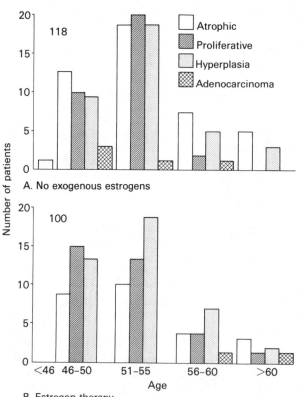

FIG. 5-4. (*A,B*) Pathology of postmenopausal bleeding (Gambrell RD, 1977, Clin Obstet Gynaecol 4:1)

cases.[36,42,53] Figure 5–2 demonstrates this relationship. In the population described in Figure 5–2, a group of Greek women, estrogen replacement therapy was extremely rare. In the population described in Figure 5–4, the Gambrell study, one part of that diagram reflects estrogen therapy users. The incidence of malignancy does not appear to be greater in postmenopausal bleeders that are on estrogen than in those who are not, although definitive studies remain to be carried out.

Although postmenopausal bleeding can reflect endometrial disease, endometrial disease can also occur in silent form. In the studies of Horwitz described previously, necropsy data indicated a high proportion (at least half of all cases) of silent cases of endometrial malignancies. Sturdee and co-workers, in their screening studies, found that 6% of those without unscheduled bleeding were also abnormal.[60] There does appear to be a large variation in the literature in reports of the incidence of silent pathologic conditions.

According to Kierse, malignancy was more common in those postmenopausal bleeding cases with profuse bleeding than in those with scanty bleeding,[36] but it should be noted that such results are not universal. Questions about the amount of bleeding as a reflection of the likelihood of pathology are addressed in detail in Chapter 8.

OBESITY

Several researchers have attempted to quantify the relative risks of obesity and other conditions in contributing to endometrial carcinoma through their epidemiologic association incidence. MacMahon showed that women with obesity are at high risk. Little risk difference was observed between those at normal weight and those who are very slender.[41] He also noted a markedly lower incidence for the parous than the nulliparous women, even when the first birth occurred after age 30. McDonald and co-workers found that the greatest risk factors in endometrial carcinoma were obesity (which increased the jeopardy to 3.5) and nulliparity (which increased the likelihood to 1.8).[44] These risk factors are much higher than the risk factor for estrogen therapy. Estrogen therapy was shown to have about one-third the influence that obesity had in predicting endometrial carcinoma over a 30-year-period in an entire county of Minnesota.[44] Many others have confirmed the influence of obesity. For example, in one study of 229 cases of adenocarcinoma of the endometrium in the United States, 64% of the women were obese.[46] Similar findings (51%) were reported by Ng and colleagues.[49] Gusberg summarized the literature and concluded that obesity carried a three- to nine-fold increased incidence of endometrial carcinoma.[20] Figure 5–5 illustrates the relative incidence of endometrial carcinoma as a function of height and weight in a patient population of younger women, aged 25 to 29. One notes an extremely high incidence of such pathology in tall, heavy young women.[75]

There is a clear consensus in the literature that obesity is a critical association of the development of endometrial carcinoma. Because of this, Lucas has suggested that obesity control may well be an excellent prophylactic.[39]

NULLIPARITY

Nulliparity, as well as delayed menopause, has been associated with increased incidence of endometrial carcinoma. According to McCall's study of 229 cases of adenocarcinoma, 66% of the women were of low parity.[46] McDonald computed an increased epidemiologic incidence of endometrial carcinoma for the nulliparous to be 1.8 times that of the parous woman.[44] Others have supported similar conclusions.[46,57,74]

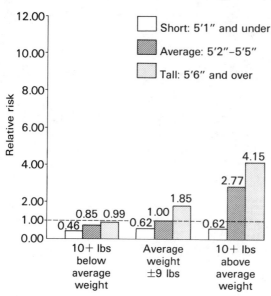

FIG. 5-5. Relative risk of endometrial cancer by height and weight at age 50 to 59, (Wynder EL, Escher GC, Mantel N, 1966, Cancer 19:489–520)

OTHER CONDITIONS

Hypertension has also been shown to be an associate of endometrial carcinoma.[49,57] Women with polycystic ovary syndrome—a disease characterized by excess production of androgens—also carry a similar propensity.[39]

CONCLUSIONS

The literature has provided a convincing case for the influence of unopposed high-dose estrogens on increasing the frequency of occurrence of endometrial carcinoma. An appropriate perspective, however, would be to keep in mind that other conditions have a greater influence on the potential for endometrial carcinoma. Obesity in particular has been shown to be a powerful risk factor for endometrial carcinoma. The use of progestins in opposition to estrogen therapies appears to offer a significant method of minimizing this carcinoma incidence. The use of the Progestin Challenge Test to define when progestins are useful is gaining wider acceptance. The reduction in progestin level to doses much lower than formerly considered appropriate is also likely to begin to gain acceptance as the molecular studies continue to demonstrate the efficacy.

Schiff and Ryan have addressed the question of appropriateness of hormonal replacement therapy in women at risk for endometrial carcinoma because of obesity or hypertension. They noted that these risks (obesity and so forth) did not increase the incidence of endometrial carcinoma with estrogen replacement therapy.[55] Such a statement offers hope for the obese women suffering from menopausal distress symptoms, but further documentation would be desirable.

REFERENCES

1. Abramson D, Driscoll SG (1966) Endometrial aspiration biopsy. *Obstet Gynecol* 27:381–391.

2. Andrews WC (1979) Estrogen and menopause. *Va Med* 106:517–521.

3. Aylward M, Maddock J, Parker A, Protherde DA, Ward A (1978) Endometrial factors under treatment with oestrogen and oestrogen/progestogen combinations. *Postgrad Med J* 54:2:74–81.

4. Buchi K, Keller PJ (1980) Estrogen receptors in normal and myomatous human uteri. *Gynecol Obstet Invest* 11:59–60.

5. Buchman MI, Kramer E, Feldman GB (1978) Aspiration curettage for asymptomatic patients receiving estrogen. *Obstet Gynecol* 51:339–341.

6. Calanog A, Sall S, Gordon G, Southren AL (1977) Androstenedione metabolism in patients with endometrial cancer. *Am J Obstet Gynecol* 129:553–556.

7. Callantine MR, Martin PL, Bolding OT, Warner PO, Greaney MO Jr. (1975) Micronized 17 Beta-estradiol for oral estrogen therapy in menopausal women. *Obstet Gynecol* 46:1:37–41.

8. Campbell S, Minardi J, McQueen J, Whitehead M (1978) Endometrial factors: the modifying effect of progestogen on the response of the post menopausal endometrium to exogenous estrogens. *Postgrad Med J* 54:59–64.

9. Carlstrom K, Damber M, Furuhjelm M, Joelsson I, Lunell N, von Schoultz B (1979) Serum levels of total dehydroepiandrosterone and total estrone in postmenopausal women with special regard to carcinoma of the uterine corpus. *Acta Obstet Gynecol Scand* 58:179–181.

10. Demetriou JA, Crowley LG, Kushinsky S, Donovan AJ, Kotin P, MacDonald I (1964) Radioactive estrogens in tissues of postmenopausal women with breast neoplasms. *Cancer Res* 24:926–934.

11. Englund DE, Johansson EDB (1980) Endometrial effect of oral estriol treatment in postmenopausal women. *Acta Obstet Gynecol Scand* 59:449–451.

12. Flickinger GL, Elsner C, Illingworth DV, Muechler EK, Mikhail G (1977) Estrogen and progesterone receptors in the female genital tract of humans and monkeys. *Ann NY Acad Sci* 286:180–189.

13. Galli MC DeGiovanni C, Nicoletti G, Grilli S, Nanni P, Prodi G, Gola G, Rocchetta R, Orlandi OC (1981) The occurrence of multiple steroid hormone receptors in disease-free and neoplastic human ovary. *Cancer* 47:6:1297–1302.

14. Gambrell RD, Jr. (1977) Postmenopausal bleeding in *Clinics Obstet Gynaecol* 4:1:129–143.

15. Gambrell RD Jr (1981) Preventing endometrial Ca with progestin. *Contemp Obstet Gynecol* 17:133–143.

16. Gambrell RD Jr, Massery FM, Castaneda TA, Ugenas AJ, Ricci CA, Wright JM (1980) Use of progestogen challenge test to reduce the risk of endometrial cancer. *Obstet Gynecol* 55:732–738.

17. Gordon J, Reagan JW, Finkle WD, Ziel HK (1977) Estrogen and endometrial carcinoma: an independent pathology review supporting original risk estimate. *N Engl J Med* 297:570–571.

18. Gurpide E (1978) Enzymatic modulation of hormonal action at the target tissue. *J Toxicol Environ Health* 4:249.

19. Gurpide E, Gusberg SB, Tseng L (1976) Oestradiol binding and metabolism in human endometrial hyperplasia and adenocarcinoma. *J Steroid Biochem* 7:891–896.

20. Gusberg SB (1975) A strategy for the control of endometrial cancer. *Proc R Soc Med* 68:163–168.

21. Gusberg SB (1976) The individual at high risk for endometrial carcinoma. *Am J Obstet Gynecol* 126:535–000.

22. Gusberg SB and Kaplan AL (1963) Adenomatous hyperplasia as Stage O carcinoma of the endometrium. *Am J Obstet Gynecol* 87:662–678.

23. Hammond CB (1980) Progestins with estrogen replacement curb Ca risk. *Obstet Gynecol News* 9/15/80:4–5.

24. Hammond CB, Jelovsek FR, Lee KL, Creasman WT, Parker RT (1979) Effects of long term estrogen replacement therapy. II Neoplasia. *Am J Obstet Gynecol* 133:537–547.

25. Hofmeister FJ (1974) Endometrial biopsy: another look. *Am J Obstet Gynecol* 119-773-777.

26. Hofmeister FJ, Barbo DM (1964) Cancer detection in private gynecologic practice: a concluding study. *Obstet Gynecol* 23:386–391.

27. Horwitz RI, Feinstein AR (1978) Alternative analytic methods for case control studies of estrogens and endometrial cancer. *N Engl J Med* 299:1089–1094.

28. Horwitz RI, Feinstein AR, Horwitz SM, Robboy SJ (1981) Necropsy diagnosis of endometrial cancer and detection-bias in case/control studies. *Lancet* July 11:66–67.

29. Hughes EC, Csermely TV, Jacobs RD, O'Hern PA (1974) Biochemical parameters of abnormal endometrium. *Gynecol Oncol* 2:205–220.

30. Hulka B (1980) Effect of exogenous estrogen on postmenopausal women: the epidemiologic evidence. *Obstet Gynecol Surv* 35:6:389–399.

31. Hutchison GB, Rothman KJ (1979) Correcting a bias? *N Engl J Med* 299:1129–1130.

32. Jick H, Watkins RN, Hunter JR, Dinan BJ, Madsen S, Rothman KJ, Walker AM (1979) Replacement estrogens and endometrial cancer. *N Engl J Med* 300:218–222.

33. Judd HL, Cleary RE, Creasman WT, Figge DC, Kase N, Rosenwaks Z, Tagatz GE (1981) Estrogen replacement therapy. *Obstet Gynecol* 3:267–275.

34. Judd HL, Davidson BJ, Frumar AM, Shamonki IM, Lagasse LD, Ballon SC (1980) Serum androgens and estrogens in postmenopausal women with and without endometrial cancer. *Am J Obstet Gynecol* 136:859–871.

35. Kay CR (1978) Logistics of study on hormone therapy in the climacteric. *Postgrad Med J* 54:2:92–94.

36. Keirse MJNC (1973) Aetiology of postmenopausal bleeding. *Postgrad Med J* 49:344–348.

37. Kelley RM, Baker WH (1961) Progestational agents in the treatment of carcinoma of the endometrium. *N Engl J Med* 264:216.

38. King RJ, Whitehead MI, Campbell S, Minardi J (1978) Biochemical studies of endometrium from postmenopausal women receiving hormone replacement therapy. *Postgrad Med J* 54:2:65–68.

39. Lucas WE (1974) Causal relationships between endocrine metabolic variables in patients with endometrial carcinoma. *Obstet Gynecol Surv* 29:507–528.

40. Ludwig H (1982) The morphologic response of the human endometrium to long-term treatment with progestational agents. *Am J Obstet Gynecol* 142:796–808.

41. MacMahon B (1974) Risk factors for endometrial cancer. *Gynecol Oncol* 2:122–129.

42. Mantalenakis SJ, Papapostolon MG (1977) Genital bleeding in females aged 50 and over. *Int Surg* 62:103–105.

43. McBride JM (1959) Premenopausal cystic glandular hyperplasia and endometrial carcinoma. *J Obstet Gynecol Br Commonwealth* 66:288–296.

44. McDonald TW, Annegers JF, O'Fallon WM (1977) Exogenous estrogen and endometrial carcinoma. *Am J Obstet Gynecol* 127:572–580.

45. Menczer J, Modan M, Ezra D, Serr DM (1980) Prognosis is pre- and postmenopausal patients with endometrial adenocarcinoma. *Maturitas* 2:37–44.

46. Mickal A, Torres J (1974) Adenocarcinoma of endometrium. In: *The Menopausal Syndrome*, pp 139–142. Greenblatt RB, Mahesh VB, McDonough PG (eds). New York, Medcom Press.

47. Milgrom E, Thi L, Atger M, Baulieu EE (1973) Mechanisms regulating the concentration and confirmation of progesterone receptor. *J Biol Chem* 248:6366–6374.

48. Nachtigall LE, Nachtigall RH, Nachtigall RD, Beckman EM (1979) Estrogen replacement therapy II: a prospective study in the relationship to carcinoma and cardiovascular and metabolic problems. *Obstet Gynecol* 54:74–79.

49. Ng ABP, Reagan JW, Storaasli JP, Wentz WB (1973) Mixed adenosquamous carcinoma of the endometrium. Am J Clin Pathol 59:765–781.

50. Ng ABP, Reagan JW (1970) Incidence and prognosis of endometrial carcinoma by histologic grade and extent. *Obstet Gynecol* 35:437–442.

51. Ochiai K (1980) Cyclic variation and distribution in the concentration of cytosol estrogen and progesterone receptors in the normal human uterus and myoma. *Acta Obstet Gynaecol Jpn* 32:945–952.

52. Paterson MEL, Wade-Evans T, Sturdee DW, Thom MH, Studd JWW (1980) Endometrial disease after treatment with oestrogens and progestogens in the climacteric. *Br Med J* 96:1–8.

53. Procope BJ (1971) Aetiology of postmenopausal bleeding. *Acta Obstet Gynecol Scand* 50:311–313.

54. Reagan JW, Ng ABP (1973) *The Cells of Uterine Carcinoma*, 2nd Edition. Basel, Kargers.

55. Schiff I, Ryan K (1980) Benefits of estrogen replacement. *Obstet Gynecol Surv* 35:400–411.

56. Shapiro S, Kaufman DW, Slone D, Rosenberg L, Miettinen OS, Stolley PD, Rosenshein NB, Watring WG, Leavitt T, Knapp RC (1980) Recent and past use of conjugated estrogens in relation to adenocarcinoma of the endometrium. *N Engl J Med* 303:485–489.

57. Smith DC, Prentice R, Thompson DJ, Herrmann WL (1975) Association of exogenous estrogen and endometrial carcinoma. *N Engl J Med* 293:1164–1167.
58. Stahl NL (1974) Hormones and cancer. In: *The Menopausal Syndrome.* Greenblatt RB, Mahesh VB, McDonough PG (eds). New York, Medcom Press.
59. Studd J, Thom M, White PJ (1978) Menopausal therapy and endometrial pathology. *Br Med J* 2:11/11:1369.
60. Sturdee DW, Wade-Evans T, Paterson ME, Thom M, Studd JW (1976) Relations between bleeding pattern, endometrial histology, and oestrogen treatment in menopausal women. *Br Med J* 1:6127:1575–1577.
61. Tseng L, Gurpide E (1973) Effect of estrone and progesterone on the nuclear uptake of estradiol by slices of endometrium. *Endocrinology* 93:245–248.
62. Tseng L, Stolee A, Gurpide E (1972) Quantitative studies on the uptake and metabolism of estrogens and progesterone by human endometrium. *Endocrinology* 90:390–404.
63. Van Campehout J, Choquette P, Vauclair P (1980) Endometrial pattern in patients with primary hypoestrogenic amenorrhea receiving estrogen replacement therapy. *Obstet Gynecol* 56:349–355.
64. Vanderick C, Beernaert J, De Muylder E (1975) Hormonal contraception. Sequential formulations and the endometrium. *Contraception* 12:655–665.
65. Van Keep PA, Ser DM, Greenblatt RB, Kopera H (1978) Effects, side effects, and dosage schemes of various sex hormones in the peri and postmenopause. Workshop Report in *Female and Male Climacteric: Current Opinion.* Baltimore, University Park Press.
66. Weiss NS (1975) Risks and benefits of estrogen use. *N Engl J Med* 293:1200–1202.
67. Weiss NS, Sayvetz TA (1980) Incidence of endometrial cancer in relation to the use of oral contraceptives. *N Engl J Med* 302:551–554.
68. Weiss NS, Szekely DR, Austin DF (1976) Increasing incidence of endometrial cancer in the United States. *N Engl J Med* 294:1259–1262.
69. Weiss NS, Szekely DR, English DR, Schweid AI (1979) Endometrial cancer in relation to patterns of menopausal estrogen use. *JAMA* 242:3:261–264.
70. Wentz WB (1974) Progestin therapy in endometrial hyperplasia. *Gynecol Oncol* 2:363–367.
71. Whitehead MI, Townsend PT, Pryse-Davies J, Ryder TA, King RJB (1981) Effects of estrogens and progestins on the biochemistry and morphology of the postmenopausal endometrium. *N Engl J Med* 305: 1599–1605.
72. Whitehead MI, Townsend PT, Pryse-Davies J, Ryder T, Lane G, Siddle N, King RJB (1982) Actions of progestins on the morphology and biochemistry of the endometrium of postmenopausal women receiving low-dose estrogen therapy. *Am J Obstet Gynecol* 142:791–795.
73. Whitehead MI, Townsend PT, Pryse-Davies J, Ryder T, Lane G, Siddle NC, King RJB (1982) Effects of various dosages of progestogens on the postmenopausal endometrium. *J Reprod Med* 27:8:539–548.
74. Woll EA, Hertig AT, Smith GV, Johnson LC (1948) The ovary in endometrial carcinoma with notes on the morphological history of the aging ovary. *Am J Obstet Gynecol* 56:617–633.
75. Wynder EL, Escher GC, Mantel N (1966) An epidemiological investigation of cancer of the endometrium. *Cancer* 19:489–520.
76. Ziel HK, Finkle WD (1975) Increased risk of endometrial carcinoma among users of conjugated estrogens. *N Engl J Med* 293:1167–1170.

6

Hormone Replacement Therapy and Coronary Heart Disease

Because of the risk association between oral contraceptives and circulatory diseases,[40,50,91,92] a great deal of attention has been focused on a similar question for menopausal hormone use. In fact, in most circumstances, judicious use of hormone replacement therapy appears to reduce the risks of coronary heart disease. It is necessary, however, to be alert to the particular subgroups of individuals who appear to be at increased risk. Almost paradoxically, hysterectomy, with or without ovariectomy, has been associated with an elevated risk of coronary heart disease. The use of synthetic estrogens has also consistently been the major associate of potentially deleterious lipid alterations for estrogen replacement therapy users. Details of these studies are reviewed in this chapter.

Moreover, oral contraceptives and thromboembolic events have recently been more extensively reviewed.[60] It is now well supported that a greater association of pill use and increased risk of circulatory disease exists among older women who smoke. Figure 6–1 shows the data that demonstrate the association between age, oral contraceptive use, smoking, and death from circulatory system disease.[59] One notes the significantly increased death rate among women over 45 years of age who both smoke and use oral contraceptives. One can also see an increased incidence with combined hormone use and smoking, even in the 35- to 44-year-old age group.

COHORT STUDIES

Cohort studies have limitations. While often useful in suggesting a new and important line of medical research, they are inherently imperfect. For example, Wiseman and Macrae have described a decline in mortality figures in the United Kingdom that has occurred simultaneously with an increased use of oral contraceptives.[93] This finding would support a protective effect of oral contraceptives on coronary heart disease, a conclusion opposite to that generally appreciated. Broader perspectives are needed. These authors suggested that when mortality trends are opposed to the results of a case-control study or cohort study, one should doubt the conclusions about causal relationships in the cohort studies.[93] Such has been the case with certain cohort studies and oral contraceptive use. Nonetheless, they do have value because, by suggesting trends, they focus attention on and facilitate isolation of particular subgroups or treatments of potential risk, despite not proving a cause and effect.

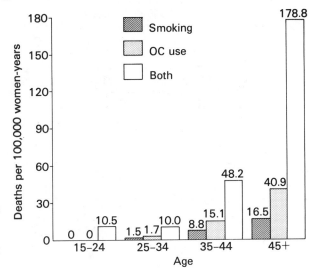

FIG. 6-1. Rates of excess circulatory system mortality as a function of age, smoking, and contraceptive use (Population Reports, 1982, Oral Contraceptives in the 1980's. *Population Information Program*. Baltimore, The Johns Hopkins University, Series A, No. 6. A 189-A 122)

ATHEROSCLEROSIS

Atherosclerotic processes appear to undergo a predictable progression with age.[83] Arterial intimal smooth muscle proliferation occurs, followed by an increase in connective tissue matrix, then extracellular and intracellular lipid deposition, with subsequent endothelial damage initiated either by hyperlipidemia of blood factors, such as flow disturbances as in hypertension, or platelet adherence to vessel wall and platelet aggregation causing the release of platelet factor, which leads to the proliferation of smooth muscle. One notes the variety of expressions that atherosclerotic processes can produce: abdominal aortic aneurysm, myocardial infarct, cerebral infarct, and peripheral vascular infarct that may reach the level of gangrene of the extremity.[83]

Hyperlipidemia and damage to the arterial vessels, in combination, are responsible for arteriosclerosis.[78] The initial risk factors in the development of coronary heart disease have been elusive. Some consider it to start with faulty diet and unfortunate genetic tendencies, both of which lead to hyperlipidemia.[83] Others have attributed the origins of the progression to psychological and behavioral factors leading to blood pressure reactivity.[78] Obesity and diabetes mellitus, combined with hypertension, promote the progression from hyperlipidemia to atherosclerosis. Once individuals become atherosclerotic, the forces of stress, physical inactivity, and cigarette smoking combine to speed development of coronary heart disease.[83] The critical questions of this chapter, therefore, revolve around the potential roles of hormone replacement regimens in the alteration of these factors.

LIPIDS AND COAGULATION

CHARACTERIZATION OF LIPIDS

The lipoproteins circulating in the blood fall, principally, into four classes: the chylomicrons, the prebeta, the beta, and the alpha lipoproteins.[83] Table 6-1 shows the

TABLE 6-1. Characteristics of lipoproteins

Electrophoresis	Density (Preparative)	Lipoprotein	Composition (% of Mass)			
			Triglyc-eride	Choles-terol	Pro-tein	Phospho-lipid
Chylomicrons	0.95	Chylomicron derived from exogenous source dietary fat†	90	5	1	4
Prebeta (2)	0.95–1.006	Very-low density lipoprotein	65*	13	10	12
Beta	1.006–1.063	Low-density lipoprotein produced from liver and intestine‡	10	43*	25	22
Alpha (1)	1.063–1.21	High-density lipoprotein	2	18	50*	30

*Major component of lipoprotein
†Derived from exogenous source
‡Produced in Liver & Intestine
Reproduced with permission from Tsang R, Glueck CJ, Atherosclerosis: A Pediatric Perspective. *In* Gluck L, et al (eds): Copyright © 1979 by Year Book Medical Publishers, Inc., Chicago

composition of these different lipoproteins with respect to triglyceride, cholesterol, protein, and phospholipid content.

One should be aware of the heterogeneity of these fractions. High-density lipo-protein–cholesterol (HDL–Ch) for example, is a composite representing a heterogeneous class of particles that float in that density. The state of the art in lipid research is moving rapidly. New knowledge focusing on the protein component probably heralds the wave of the future.[10,17,58] Nonetheless, the studies that form the available pool of information do provide a basis for understanding critical relationships between atherosclerotic potential and hormone balance.

Triglycerides, cholesterol, phospholipids, and the apoprotein have been characterized in cycling women.[53] The very-low-density lipoproteins (VLDL) contain the greatest concentration of triglycerides, the low-density lipoproteins (LDL) carry the greatest concentrations of both cholesterol and apoprotein B (the atherogenic fraction), and the HDLs contain 50% apoprotein B and 20% cholesterol (the antiatherogenic fraction).[53]

The function of the very low density lipoprotein (VLDL-prebeta) is to carry triglycerides to body tissues where they are hydrolized by the enzyme lipoprotein lipase. The resultant fatty acids and glycerol are taken up by the tissues for energy.[37] The "remnant" left behind is cholesterol rich and, in excess, alters the composition of the remaining VLDL to make it relatively more cholesterol dominant.

Knopp and co-workers investigated the effects of oral contraceptives as well as menopausal hormone replacement therapy regimens on these various lipid fractions.[37] Estrogen use in postmenopausal women caused no changes in the VLDL cholesterol concentration. The LDL cholesterol concentrations were slightly reduced. The HDL cholesterols were significantly increased, and no significant change in the cholesterol/triglyceride ratio was noted for hormone replacement therapy regimens.[37] In contrast, oral contraceptives, composed of synthetic hormones, produced a number of changes, which included increases in total plasma triglyceride concentration and increased triglyceride content of the VLDL.[37]

LIPIDS AND CORONARY HEART DISEASE

Studies in men and studies in women have elucidated the relative associated factors for subsequent coronary heart disease.[13,35,56,57,83] There are slight differences between the sexes. In men who took part in a 14-year follow-up after myocardial infarction, associated factors for subsequent systemic heart disease were listed in relative order: age, systolic blood pressure, smoking, and high serum triglycerides, especially in younger men. The rate of infarcts rose with the number of factors from 15 per 1000 for subjects with none to 150 per 1000 in subjects with 4 or more.[13] In that study the cholesterol level was directly correlated to the triglyceride level. The authors discussed the difficulty of using measures of plasma cholesterol as potential risk factors because the cholesterol in the HDL is beneficial but gets "counted" into the overall risk equation as a negative.[13]

HDL–Ch appears to have a protective effect for atherosclerosis.[13,35,83] Increases in HDL–Ch correlated with a lower incidence of coronary occlusion.[14] Gordon and co-workers have also noted that as HDL levels increased, the rate of incidence of coronary heart disease decreased.[24] Confirmation was also provided by Miller. Those with coronary heart disease showed lower HDL-Ch than those who were disease-free.[46] The degree of disease was an inverse function of the HDL level, and the HDL content appeared to be a more powerful predictor than other lipid fractions and independent of the other lipid fractions in its predictive capacity.[46]

Sex differences are apparent in the concentration of HDL-Ch. In young children (6 to 11), there is little difference between boys and girls. At adolescence, the HDL-Ch falls in males and rises in females,[83] perhaps accounting for the significantly lower incidence of coronary heart disease in young women than in young men. Racial differences in HDL-Ch are apparent as well. Blacks have higher HDL levels than whites.

The VLDL-Ch fraction appears to be highly correlated with the incidence of coronary heart disease.[35] In older women, the VLDL-Ch fraction discriminated distinctly better than the cholesterol level in predicting the potential for coronary heart disease.[35] Close to 3000 women and 2300 men, initially free of coronary heart disease, were prospectively followed to yield these conclusions.

In summary, the LDL-Ch fraction appears to be the principal atherogenic factor, whereas HDL-Ch appears to be the antiatherogenic fraction. Moreover, simple measures of total cholesterol levels are less useful because cholesterol is found in all fractions. Triglyceride concentrations also carry little or no useful information when more sophisticated information is available. This is revealed in Figure 6–2, which shows the relationship between HDL-Ch and triglycerides to coronary heart disease in women.[24] One notes the several relationships just described. As the HDL-Ch level increases, the number of cases of coronary heart disease per 1000 decreases. The figure shows clearly that when individuals are separated on the basis of the HDL-Ch level, the additional information provided by triglyceride content is not useful in predicting who might or might not be susceptible to coronary heart disease.[24] This study followed approximately 1500 women and 1000 men aged 49 to 82 who provided plasma for lipid analysis. All the individuals were free of coronary heart disease at the start of the study and were followed prospectively for several years.

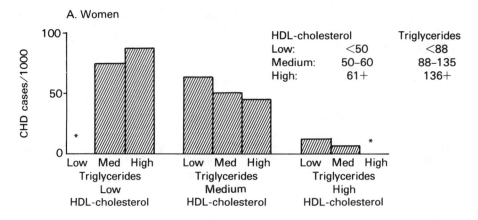

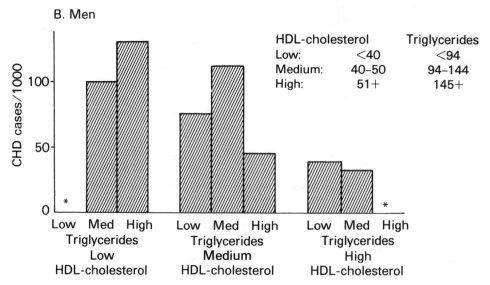

FIG. 6-2.   Incidence of coronary heart disease by level of HDL-cholesterol in the Framingham Study in (*A*) women and (*B*) men; *cells with fewer than 85 persons at risk (Grodan T, Castelli WP, Hjortland MP, Kannel WB et al, 1977, Am J Med 62:707–714)

CYCLIC VARIATION IN PLASMA LIPID LEVELS

A clear cyclic variation in plasma free and total cholesterol as well as plasma phospholipids exists.[52] The lipid levels are consistently lowest at those times of the cycle when estrogen levels are maximum, *i.e.,* the mid-cycle (presumed) ovulatory time and the mid-luteal phase.

HORMONE REPLACEMENT THERAPY AND LIPID CHANGES

A number of studies have been published evaluating the influence of hormone replacement therapy on levels of cholesterol, phospholipids, serum triglycerides, LDL-Ch, HDL-Ch, and beta/alpha lipid ratio. A review of these studies indicates an overall pattern of beneficial effects to users of natural estrogens and some potentially dangerous effects to users of some synthetic estrogens. Progestin use is also considered. The details follow.

PLASMA CHOLESTEROL

The influence of estrogen on plasma cholesterol has been found to be an inverse one. Reductions in plasma cholesterol after different forms of estrogen use have been consistently reported.[4,21,39,46,70] Equine estrogens were studied in 1500 women;[4] six forms of estrogen with and without progestogen were studied in other women;[39] and 0.5 mg stilbestrol administered on alternate days was evaluated in oophorectomized women.[21] All women consistently showed a reduction (varying degrees) in plasma cholesterol. Table 6–2 illustrates the cholesterol levels according to age and postmenopausal estrogen use among a large sample of women whose data were arrayed by different age groups.[4] One notes the consistently lower level of plasma cholesterol at each age for the users of, in this case, mostly conjugated equine estrogen. Table 6–3 assembles the serum levels of cholesterol, phospholipid, and other measures for several different groups of women: normal young women, normal postmenopausal women, women with coronary artery disease, and women with coronary artery disease treated with Premarin. This table will be referred to in sequence as appropriate.

The addition of progestin opposition to the estrogen regimen (in usual postmenopausal doses) appears to have little effect on the cholesterol response to estrogen. Monthly assays for plasma cholesterol in women taking norethisterone acetate (1 mg for 6 days) each cycle in opposition to continuous estrogens (4 mg estradiol, 2 mg estriol) yielded an approximate 15% drop in plasma cholesterol compared with pretreatment levels.[16] The phenomenon was consistently noted throughout a 24-month span. Ethinyl estradiol was reported to decrease cholesterol levels in six oophorecto-

TABLE 6-2. Cholesterol levels according to age and postmenopausal estrogen use*

Age, Yr	Cholesterol mg/dL	
	Users	Nonusers
55–59	219.6 ± 33.2	240.0 ± 38.7
60–64	223.0 ± 39.5	232.4 ± 39.3
65–69	221.5 ± 31.2	233.0 ± 39.0
70–74	215.8 ± 30.3	230.4 ± 38.3

*All data adjusted for obesity. Means and standard deviations are given. (Barrett-Conner E, Brown V, Turner J, et al, 1979 JAMA 20:2167–2169; Copyright 1966–79, 1981–82, American Medical Association.)

TABLE 6-3. Plasma levels of cholesterol, phospholipid, and beta/alpha in different groups of women

Group	Number of Women	Avg. Age	Cholesterol mg %	Phospholipids mg %	C/P Ratio	β/α Lipoprotein Cholesterol Ratio
Normal young women	22	20–30	189 ± 4.6	193 ± 6.1	0.99 ± 0.040	2.4 ± 0.3
Normal post-hysterectomized women	113	45–65	262 ± 4.1	226 ± 3.3	1.16 ± 0.015	3.4 ± 0.1
Women with coronary heart disease	58	55	270 ± 7.5	225 ± 5.6	1.20 ± 0.020	4.1 ± 0.1
Women with coronary heart disease after Premarin (5 or 10 mg/day)	30		238 ± 7.8	258 ± 6.6	0.92 ± 0.032	2.7 ± 0.1

Robinson RW, Cohen WD, Higano, N 1958, Ann Int Med 48:95–101

mized women, and the addition of norethisterone (a 21-day duration, 10-mg dose) was found to reverse the cholesterol-reducing effects of the ethinyl estradiol.[26] This was the only study of several that found a reversal of the cholesterol-reducing effect of estrogen in response to progestins. The other studies that added progestin opposition[31,39,46] did not use such excessive doses or durations and did not find a reversal of the estrogen effect.

The effect of hysterectomy with or without oophorectomy has also been studied. There is some ambiguity in the literature that may be due to age variation and concomitant steroid secreting capacity. Aitken has reported increased serum cholesterol levels after oophorectomy compared with hysterectomy without oophorectomy.[1] Serum cholesterol levels showed more pronounced increases in younger women, aged 36 to 45, presumably because the loss of their ovaries represented a greater steroid change than in older women. The older women, aged 46 to 55, did not show a significant increase in cholesterol levels in response to oophorectomy when compared with hysterectomy alone.[1] Utian has concluded that oophorectomy does not significantly increase serum cholesterol values; however, he used small groups whose age variation may have obscured an age-related variation.[84] Punnonen evaluated 25 castrated women (mean age = 48) and found little change in cholesterol level, either after bilateral oophorectomy or after subsequent estradiol valerate therapy (Fig. 6–3).[62] Here again, there is a small sampling with predominate skewing toward the age group of ovarian decline. One notes the 7-month duration of this study and the essential continuity of cholesterol level across time regardless of treatment or condition.[62]

The tendency for a moderately decreased plasma cholesterol level as a function of increased estrogen concentration is, therefore, generally confirmed.

PHOSPHOLIPIDS

Four major phospholipids—lysolecithin, sphingomyelin, lecithin, and ethanolamine phosphatide—were studied in 26 postmenopausal women before and 1 month after 2

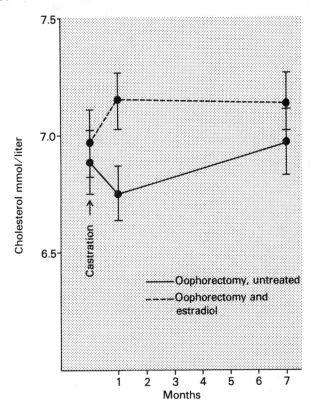

FIG. 6-3. Serum cholesterol levels after bilateral oophorectomy and after estradiol valerate therapy (Punnonen R, Rauramo L, 1976, Int J Gynaecol Obstet 14:13–16)

doses of conjugated equine estrogen (1.25 or 2.5 mg).[27] Of these four classes of phospholids, only one, lecithin, responded to estrogen replacement therapy. It increased by approximately 22%.[27] Punnonen also studied the issue of phospholipids with respect to bilateral oophorectomy and subsequent estrogen replacement therapy (2 mg a day peroral estradiol valerate).[62] Figure 6–4 shows these results. One notes the lack of effect of castration on serum phospholipids.[62] The subsequent estrogen replacement therapy did show significant effect. Phospholipids increased.

Phospholipid levels are lower in younger women (Table 6–3). Normal postmenopausal women and women with coronary heart disease do not show differences in phospholipid levels. The addition of high doses of conjugated equine estrogens (5 or 10 mg daily) has a tendency to increase the phospholipid level.[68] Lower doses of estrogen replacement therapy (estradiol valerate, 2 mg a day) also showed a tendency to increase phospholipid concentration in oophorectomized women—after 6 months of therapy.[63] Because phospholipids are detergents that act to reduce cholesterol plaques, one could speculate that the use of estrogen replacement therapy is acceptable with respect to the phospholipid effects.

SERUM TRIGLYCERIDES

Recalling Figure 6–2, which showed the incidence of coronary heart disease in relation to levels of HDL-Ch and triglycerides, one realizes that the triglyceride level itself has little

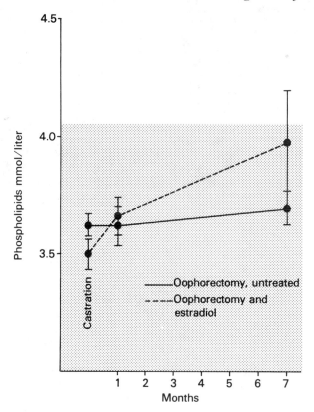

FIG. 6-4. The effect of bilateral oophorectomy and subsequent estradiol valerate therapy on serum phospholipids (Punnonen R, Rauramo L, 1976, Int J Gynaecol Obstet 14:13–16)

predictive value. Nonetheless, a great number of researchers have evaluated the influence of various estrogens and progestins on serum triglyceride levels. The results tend to be consistent. Natural estrogens have no negative effects on serum triglyerceride levels; progestins in hormone replacement therapy regimens tend to, if anything, reduce the triglycerides, and synthetic estrogens (ethinyl estradiol) tend to increase the serum triglyceride levels.

Figure 6-5 shows the triglyceride response to postmenopausal women treated with two different regimens of estrogen replacement therapy.[89] One can see the lack of triglyceride alteration in response to a 2-mg daily dose of estradiol valerate. In contrast, women taking ethinyl estradiol (0.05 mg daily) showed a marked increase in their serum triglyceride levels.[89] Others have reported similar phenomena. Synthetic hormones (ethinyl estradiol, 20 and 50 μg daily) were compared to Premarin (0.625 and 1.25 mg daily). There was a significant rise in serum triglyceride levels on both doses of ethinyl estradiol, but no significant change on either dose of Premarin.[5] This study was performed on 17 oophorectomized women in a crossover design. Pyorala confirms the phenomenon as well. Eight postmenopausal women, 41 to 53 years of age, were treated with estradiol valerate, 2 mg per day, 20 days of each 28-day cycle. After 3 to 4 months of treatment, the estradiol valerate had caused no significant changes in serum triglyceride levels, but the ethinyl estradiol dosage (25 μg) was reported to significantly increase the serum triglycerides.[60] Tikkanen has also noted that natural estrogens may have much less effect on triglyerceride metabolism.[80]

Wynn, in evaluating the effect of progestins in combined oral contraceptives, found a similar result and suggested that high doses of ethinyl estradiol with minimal progestin opposition affect mainly the increased triglyceride levels.[95] Oral contraceptives were also shown by Oster and co-workers to have a significant influence in increasing total plasma triglycerides in large samples of women aged 20 to 40.[53] The oral contraceptives were predominant synthetic estrogen-based and were taken in a much larger dose in comparison to hormonal replacement therapy.

In contrast to these potentially hypertriglyceridemic effects of ethinyl estradiol, the effects of the natural estrogens tend to be inconsequential in menopausal women.[6,22,39,48,62,63,74,90] Figure 6–6 shows the serum triglyceride response to oophorectomy and to subsequent estradiol valerate over the course of 7 months.[62] One notes the transient increase in the serum triglyceride level one month after castration and the overall lack of effect of estradiol valerate on the serum triglyceride level. There are, however, exceptions.[67]

Although serum triglycerides do not, by themselves, appear to have an atherogenic effect, the demonstration that natural estrogens appear not to influence the levels while synthetics do, should be borne in mind. Where there is a choice, it seems most conservative to prescribe the natural, as opposed to the synthetic, estrogens. Natural estrogens can be synthetically prepared but are identical with those produced by the body and are, in this context, considered "natural." Those synthetics that are prepared by altering the molecular configuration of the steroid could be the ones that are more likely to produce the potential adverse effects.

FIG. 6-5. Serum triglyceride response to estradiol valerate and ethinyl estradiol (Wallentin L, Larsson-Cohn U, 1977, Acta Endocrinol 86:597–607)

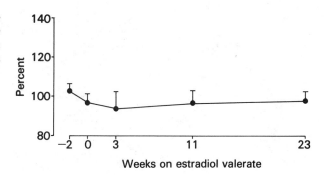

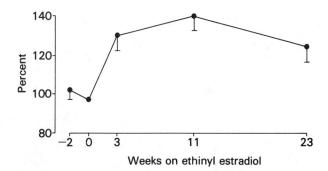

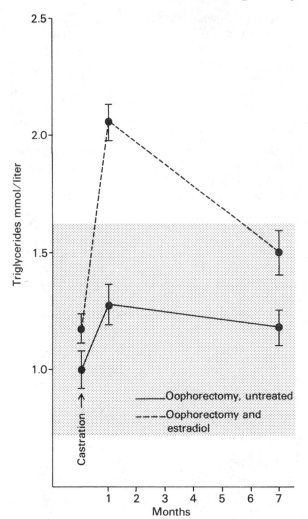

FIG. 6-6. Serum triglyceride response to oophorectomy and subsequent estradiol valerate (Punnonen R, Rauramo L, 1976, Int J Gynaecol Obstet 14:13–16)

LOW-DENSITY LIPOPROTEIN-CHOLESTEROL

The relationship between estrogen replacement therapy and LDL–Ch has been clear-cut; there is unanimity in the literature. Wallace and co-workers, in a large cross-sectional study that spanned 10 North American lipid research clinics, found significant reductions in the LDL-Ch among estrogen users at every age.[88] Robinson and Lebeau found that either of two doses of conjugated equine estrogens (0.625 mg or 1.25 mg per day) yielded a significant reduction in LDL–Ch levels among a group that was either naturally or surgically menopausal.[67] Gustafson, studying six oophorectomized women given ethinyl estradiol either alone or with 21 days norethisterone (10 mg), found that a 20-Lg dose of ethinyl estradiol significantly reduced the LDL–Ch levels.[26] Adding the high dose and duration of progestin reversed the changes produced by the estrogens.[26] More recently, Wahl and co-workers showed that norgestrel and norethindrone acetate in oral contraceptives yielded the highest LDL–Ch levels and cautioned against these progestins in oral contraceptives. Whether a lower dose of progestin would have so deleterious an effect is doubtful. The results are clear. Estrogen replacement treatment at menopause significantly lowers the LDL–Ch levels in plasma.

HIGH-DENSITY LIPOPROTEIN-CHOLESTEROL

With HDL–Ch being antiatherogenic, it becomes especially noteworthy that estrogen replacement therapy has been shown to significantly increase the level of this protective lipoprotein.[8,26,31,59,67,68] Bradley and co-workers evaluated serum HDL–Ch in women using oral contraceptives as well as menopausal estrogens and progestins.[8] A consistency was noted. All menopausal estrogens—conjugated equine estrogens (0.625 or 1.25 mg per day) and ethinyl estradiol (0.02 and 0.05 mg per day)—were associated with increased levels of HDL–Ch over nonuser levels. Norethindrone acetate (5.0 mg) had the reverse effect. It lowered the HDL–Ch level significantly.[8] Oral contraceptive users had mixed effects, which will not be reviewed here.[87] Gustafson, evaluating ethinyl estradiol alone (20 Lg per day) or with norethisterone (10 mg a day for 21 days) showed that the synthetic estrogen increased the HDL-Ch but that the addition of progestin reversed these effects.[26] Similar findings were reported by Hirvonen and co-workers.[31] For two consecutive cycles, constant estradiol valerate at 2 mg a day, combined with one of three different progestin regimens for the last 10 days of the cycle, was taken.[31] The progestin dose of 10 mg medroxyprogesterone acetate yielded no change in HDL-Ch; the other two progestin regimens (10 mg norethindrone acetate and 0.5 mg norgestrel) both reduced HDL-Ch by about 20%. All treatments led to a decrease in the total cholesterol level, which ranged from 10% to 18%: Medroxyprogesterone acetate had the most mild effect; norgestrel produced the greatest drop in total cholesterol.[31] The authors concluded that medroxyprogesterone acetate may have a limited advantage over the other two progestins for this reason. Conjugated equine estrogens alone (0.63 or 1.25) also were associated with an increase in HDL-Ch.[67]

The consistency with which the literature reports an increase in HDL-Ch after taking estrogen therapy coupled with the reports of the overall beneficial effects of increased levels of HDL-Ch, combine to show the value of hormone replacement therapy in enhancing this antiatherogenic factor.

BETA/ALPHA LIPID RATIOS

Recalling the earlier descriptions of beta lipoprotein and alpha lipoprotein, one remembers that beta lipoprotein represents the LDL-Ch (the atherogenic fraction) whereas the alpha represents the HDL-Ch (the antiatherogenic fraction). The ratio between these two figures, β/α, is a reflection of the relative balance. The higher the number, the greater is the atherogenicity. Higano and co-workers showed that the β/α lipoprotein level could be lowered by the ingestion of conjugated equine estrogens.[30] In contrast, short-term administration of three different androgens to men increased the serum β/α lipoprotein cholesterol in each group, mainly due to an increase in the β lipoprotein fraction.[30] Nachtigall and colleagues, in their 10-year, double-blind prospective study, evaluated 2.5 mg conjugated equine estrogen coupled with 10 mg medroxyprogesterone acetate (7 days per month).[47] Initially, 10 of the 84 patients had elevated β/α lipoprotein levels. All subjects on hormone replacement therapy showed a decreased level within the first 6 months. In comparison, the elevated controls did not show a similar decline with passage of time.[47] Table 6–3 shows the beneficial response to estrogens that women with coronary artery disease experience.[68]

There is, therefore a consistency in the literature with respect to the lowering of β/α lipoprotein ratios by estrogen replacement therapies. Thus, another aspect of the beneficial effects of estrogen replacement therapy on coronary risk factors is apparent.

HORMONE REPLACEMENT THERAPY AND BLOOD PRESSURE CHANGES

Hypertension has long been acknowledged as a risk factor for coronary heart disease.[73] Because of this, a number of researchers have evaluated whether hormone replacement therapy produces any alteration in either systolic or diastolic blood pressure. The overwhelming trend of the results is that hormone replacement at menopause does not influence blood pressure in any significantly negative way—with a few, rare exceptions. Oral contraceptives can carry a different prognosis and are not reviewed here.

Lind and colleagues, in a double-blind prospective study involving several treatment groups of six forms of hormone replacement therapy as well as a placebo group, found that both systolic and diastolic blood pressures are reduced a small but statistically significant degree in women on the various regimens of hormone replacement therapy.[39] Barrett-Conner and co-workers also investigated the incidence of heart disease and hormone use in a community study of a sample of 1500 older women in California.[4] They recorded the systolic and the diastolic blood pressures of age-matched users and nonusers, beginning with age 55 and moving up through age 74.[4] There was a consistently lower level of both systolic and diastolic blood pressure in every age group among hormone users, the differences varying between 1% and 10% lower. With one exception, these differences were not statistically significant, but the trend of consistently lower pressures at each age is noteworthy.

Although in general the tendency for a reduction in blood pressure is noted, several exceptions have occurred. These are considered first. Utian, in his study of 50 ovariectomized women, 45 to 55 years old, 1 to 2 years postovariectomy showed that two of the women showed a marked elevation of diastolic blood pressure after beginning estradiol valerate treatment.[85] Notelovitz noted a similar phenomenon to occur occasionally in his patients attending a climacteric clinic.[49] His patients were given 1.25 mg conjugated estrogens per day. In this population, a few postmenopausal women also were noted to have blood pressure elevations that, the author noted, occurred more commonly in older patients.[49] After the patients were taken off of hormones, the blood pressure (of those elevated cases) did fall, taking as long as 3 months to stabilize. In the same context, Crane and co-workers noted, in their study of 570 hypertensive patients, that 5 of them were postmenopausal women taking low doses of estrogens.[19] Each of the 5 became normotensive within 7 months after stopping estrogen treatment.

These several cases of hypertension in a few menopausal women who are taking estrogen therapy are rare exceptions and do not establish a role of estrogen in hypertension, but rather make clear that elevations in blood pressure can coexist with hormone replacement therapy. Therefore, blood pressure should be routinely monitored. Davis and co-workers, in their study of long-term estrogen substitution in atherosclerosis, compared menopausal women (stilbestrol, 5 mg every other day) to those who were not taking hormones.[21] After 10 years, estrogen replacement therapy users had a lower incidence of hypertension than untreated women.[21] Borglin and co-workers noted no blood pressure elevations in estrogen regimens with and without 10 days of progestin opposition each month.[6]

The search for a putative blood-borne agent responsible for hypertension led several investigators to evaluate the renin–aldosterone system in patients taking estrogen replacement therapy. Punnonen and colleagues studied 9 women, aged 48 to 52, after bilateral oophorectomy. Plasma renin activity and daily urinary excretion of aldosterone were evaluated. They found no activation of the renin–aldosterone system in patients taking estradiol valerate therapy (2 mg per day).[61] In contrast, Pallas and co-workers, studying the same question with respect to conjugated equine estrogen (neither dose nor duration was defined) reported an increased plasma renin activity in users of conjugated estrogens, but no effect on the renin concentration itself.[54] Furthermore, there was no effect of conjugated estrogen on blood pressure when hormone users were matched to controls and corrected for age and relative weight.[54]

These findings lend support to the conclusion that hormone replacement therapy does not tend to increase the risk of hypertension.

Von Eiff studied blood pressure and estrogens by injecting estradiol valerate and comparing diastolic and systolic blood pressures both before and after an "arithmetic stress test."[86] He reported that, under resting conditions, estrogen therapy was associated with a reduced pulse (by about 8 beats per minute) and reduced diastolic (by about 6 mm Hg) and systolic blood pressure.[86] Under the arithmetic test "stress," women who were taking estrogen showed a less pronounced systolic rise than women who were not taking estrogens. In reviewing the literature as well as his own study, Von Eiff concluded, "In our opinion, whenever hypertension appears under estrogen treatment, estrogen medication should *not* be stopped at once. Salt intake, however, should be reduced to a maximum of 3 g per day . . . should this prove to be insufficient, antihypertension drugs should be added to HRT. Whenever high estrogen doses are given, salt restriction becomes an important conjunct." Such a conclusion concurs wtih our own. The general tendency of the natural hormone therapies suggests a benefit rather than a risk to the cardiovascular health. Nonetheless, it is prudent to maintain an alert view for the occasional exceptions.

RISK FACTORS FOR CORONARY HEART DISEASE OTHER THAN LIPIDS

FAMILY HISTORY

Family history appears to play an important role in the potentiation of risk for coronary heart disease. Whether the family history is carrying a physiologic genetic trait or perhaps establishing a coronary prone behavior pattern is not clear. Von Eiff has pointed out that when family history is taken into account, he finds no effect of estrogen therapies. Whenever high doses of estrogen are given, salt restrictions are considered to be a critical safety factor.[86] Likewise, women who work excessively long hours have been identified as a population at great risk.[29] The only clearly higher incidence of coronary heart disease among women who work outside the home is in that group of working women who carry dual burdens and 80-hour workweeks. For example, those who hold full-time clerical positions and then come home to full-time housework and child-care responsibilities were found to be at excess risk for coronary heart disease.[29]

COAGULATION FACTORS

The question of whether alterations in coagulation factors increase the risk for intravascular clotting has been raised. The Boston Collaborative Drug Surveillance Program concluded that thromboembolic events are not influenced by estrogen replacement therapy.[6,7] Notelowitz has a similar view.[44] Studd and co-workers in prospective studies of five different replacement therapy regimens to hysterectomized women supported this, concluding: "This study does not reveal any change toward hypercoagulability in any of the . . . parameters with the treatment regimens studied."[79] They did emphasize that small sample sizes rendered their results tentative.

One exception is noted, however. Stangel and co-workers evaluated the effects of conjugated estrogens on coagulability in menopausal women.[77] The women were both naturally and surgically menopausal, ranging in age from 29 to 70. Conjugated equine estrogens (1.25 mg, 21 days on, 7-day, hormone-free period) were tested after more than one month of therapy. There was increased coagulability in some of these women.[77] The youngest women exhibited the greatest hypercoagulability; the effect may reflect a special propensity for young menopausal women who take estrogen or it may reflect that the young menopausal women had increased risks because of the hysterectomy itself.[15,20,25,65,69] However, the small sample size in each group of individuals, coupled with the short duration, made it impossible to check for subsequent readjustment to hormone therapy. Such tentative results demand replication before any final conclusion can be drawn.

Aylward prospectively studied 52 climacteric women complaining about menopausal distress symptoms.[2] He evaluated opposed versus unopposed estrogen treatment. The results suggest that progestin opposition did not alter the estrogen effect and that there were profound alterations for synthetic estrogen (ethinyl estradiol) that persisted for 9 months after the hormone had been stopped. In contrast, the "natural" estrogen tested (estrone piperazine sulfate) did not produce the alterations. The parameters tested included blood coagulation, prothrombin time, cephalin time, platelet aggregation time, and concentrations of factor VII and factor X.

In 1982, Mammen reviewed the literature on oral contraceptives and blood coagulation.[42] He noted that no test procedures that currently existed allowed plasma and serum levels of blood factors to predict who is at risk for thromoembolic episodes in association with hormone use.[42] He further noted that only a small number of women develop thrombosis in association with oral contraceptives and that absolute levels of proenzymes of cofactors (in reclotting) are not necessarily relevant in defining the state of the coagulation system. Abnormalities detected in the blood of the patient with a massive thromboembolic event may be the result of the event and not necessarily had led to it.

Until more definitive studies can be carried out, the clinician would appear to be most conservative who limits estrogen therapies to the natural estrogens. Ethinyl estradiol is the one synthetic product that has shown some potentially disturbing effects.

HYSTERECTOMY WITH OR WITHOUT OOPHORECTOMY

A growing number of reports are highlighting negative effects of hysterectomy and oophorectomy. The operations appear to increase the frequency of occurrence of coronary heart disease in women not given hormonal replacement therapy. Particularly at risk are young women. Johanson and co-workers evaluated late effects of bilateral oophorectomy in young women, 15 to 30 years old at surgery.[34] They noted increased morbidity and/or mortality in later years from coronary artery disease occurring in those women whose operations were performed when they were young. It was considered that changes in serum lipids that accompany the premature menopause were related to these effects, although mechanisms are not resolved from their work.

Centerwall, in a review of premenopausal oophorectomy and cardiovascular disease, concluded that among the many studies that have been published, there was a trend for a three- to five-fold increase in the incidence of coronary heart disease among hysterectomized young women.[15] He concluded that the relative odds ratio was the same whether or not the ovaries were removed. Despite this conclusion, until a systematic evaluation of age and ovarian status at time of hysterectomy is provided for critical viewing by readers, definitive conclusions cannot be drawn.[20]

Among the 2900 women who were followed up for 24 years in the Framingham study of menopause and coronary heart disease, no premenopausal woman ever developed a myocardial infarct or a documented case of coronary heart disease.[25] The latter were common among postmenopausal women dating from the time of the menopause. Removing either the uterus alone or the uterus and one or both ovaries increased the risk of coronary heart disease by an equal amount. The authors did not know how to explain this finding, but they suggested that alterations in lipids metabolism with the cessation of menses might partially account for the results.[25] Such a phenomenon may explain the apparently paradoxical report of Jick and co-workers.[33] They reported an increased risk of nonfatal myocardial infarctions among noncontraceptive estrogen users (hormone replacement therapy). It turns out that these estrogen users developing myocardial infarction are overwhelmingly disproportionately hysterectomized women. In fact, among the 14 women in their study that did develop myocardial infarction on estrogen, 12 had been hysterectomized before menopause.[32,33] This was the only report in the literature of increased risk of myocardial infarction among natural estrogen users, and it now appears that the confounding of estrogen use with a young hysterectomized population may have been responsible for the aberrant result.

Metabolic studies in oophorectomized women have shown that any of three different progestogens given to young oophorectomized women (under 45 years of age) induced two negative effects: large increases in LDL-Ch and decreases in HDL-Ch.[75] Differentiating the three different progestins revealed a difference between the 19-nortestosterone derivates (norethisterone acetate, 10 mg per day and D-norgestrel, 1.8 mg per day) and the progesterone derivative (medroxyprogesterone acetate, 10 mg per day). The former two caused decreases in the HDL-Ch levels whereas the latter did not produce such changes.[75] These dosages of progestins have been shown to be equipotent in postponement of menstruation assays, but apparently are not equipotent in their effects on lipid alterations. One notes that it is the 19-norethisterone derivatives that have the androgenlike influences on lipid metabolism in these oophorectomized women.

Other approaches yield similar conclusions.[11,12,28] Bain and co-workers evaluated the use of postmenopausal hormones and the risk of myocardial infarction through a mail survey response from over 120,000 registered nurses.[3] One hundred twenty-three of the women with prior menopause had been hospitalized for myocardial infarction in this sample. There was no association between hormone replacement therapy and myocardial infarction. Bilateral oophorectomy, however, was different. Bilateral oophorectomy increased the risk for myocardial infarction in this population.[3]

Using autopsy records, Rivin evaluated the incidence and severity of atherosclerosis in females with hypoestrogenic or hyperestrogenic state.[66] There was a significantly increased incidence of coronary artery atherosclerosis in untreated castrated females. There was, in contrast, a significant decrease below normal for atherosclerosis in patients who had conditions reflective of a hyperestrogenic state. These subjects were compared with normative age-matched populations from the work of others to draw these conclusions.[66] Wuest provided similar data.[94] The hearts of 49 bilaterally oophorectomized women were examined 2 to 42 years before death for the degree of coronary atherosclerosis. Oophorectomized women were consistently more atherosclerotic than normal women.[94] Subsequent autopsies of oophorectomized women showed more advanced atherosclerosis in those who had not had estrogen treatments as compared with those who had.[94] It was noted that the site of predilection for the development of severe atherosclerosis was in the anterior descending branch of the left coronary artery.

Atherosclerotic disease was also compared by Robinson and co-workers in age-matched castrates versus hysterectomized women with ovaries intact. The ovariectomized women fared worse. Atherosclerotic disease occurred in 22% of the castrates and in 9% of the noncastrated hysterectomized women. These women were in their 50s and 60s and had been hysterectomized before age 45.[69] Such a finding is not universal. Ritterband and colleagues in their attempt to separate oophorectomized from simply hysterectomized patients on the basis of atheroarteriosclerotic disease, found equal percentages (8%) for both groups of patients.[65] The incidence of coronary artery disease was significantly higher in the two surgical groups than in the general population of age-matched women. Wide variation in age clumping makes it probable that the difference in the level of ovarian activity at the time of hysterectomy could not be adequately evaluated in the two groups. This may explain why ovariectomy was equivalent to simple hysterectomy, thereby differing from the results of Robinson and co-workers.[69] Gordon and colleagues, in their review of the Framingham data, concluded that hysterectomized women show a three- to fivefold increased risk of coronary heart disease, with or without ovariectomy.

Hypertension was also shown to be more common among hysterectomized women than among nonhysterectomized controls.[76]

It is critically important that the clinician be aware of the consistency with which the literature shows the potentially deleterious effects of hysterectomy and oophorectomy on the cardiovascular physiology. Many hysterectomies are performed (see Chap. 8) and the alteration in cardiovascular health that may result from such surgery should certainly be part of the decision process before surgery. As described, hormone therapies for hysterectomized young patients may not offer the same protective effect against cardiovascular diseases that it does for the intact menopausal women. These issues are not yet resolved and require more detailed studies that will reflect the ovarian status at the time of hysterectomy.

SYNTHETIC ESTROGENS

A growing number of reports reveal profound differences between synthetic and natural estrogens and their effect on the cardiovascular system.[37,38,41,48,51,55,59,76,80,82,89] The natural estrogens (Premarin) have been compared to the synthetics (in oral contraceptives) to show the potential beneficial effect of conjugated equine estrogens in contrast to the synthetics, which potentially offer deleterious alterations in plasma triglyceride, VLDL, and HDL fractions.[37] Synthetic estrogens have been acknowledged to cause a rise in the triglyceride concentration in young subjects; this phenomenon has been contrasted with the fact that postmenopausal women treated with natural estrogens do not show these rises.[38] Maddock has demonstrated that administration of cyclic "natural estrogens" (Premarin, piparazine estrone sulfate, or estradiol valerate) are essentially beneficial.[41] Several investigators have shown that synthetic estrogens increase serum triglycerides in menopausal women whereas natural estrogens do not.[48,64,89] Blood pressure has been reported to increase more in response to ethinyl estradiol than to other estrogens among hysterectomized young women.[76]

The synthetic steroid component in the contraceptive steroids has been noted and contrasted with the predominantly "natural" estrogen component in the menopausal hormone prescriptions.[55,59] Although these differences are considered to be related to the increase in thromboembolic events in certain oral contraceptive users,[51] this still requires better documentation.

Because of the increasing incidence of reports that ethinyl estradiol has been associated with various cardiovascular physiologic phenomena that are not health promoting, a conservative view would suggest avoiding this particular class of hormone regimens for the time being. There are many others that do not carry such potentials.

CERTAIN PROGESTOGENS

The role of progestins in the hormone replacement therapy regimen has been well studied albeit not completely. Several issues need to be considered: the relative strength of the progestogen in question, the age of the woman who is ingesting it, her ovarian status (functioning or nonfunctioning), and the difference between the use of progestins in oral contraceptives as opposed to their use in hormone replacement therapy regimens. Each of these conditions carries with it a slightly different prognosis.

Brenner has characterized the pharmacology of progestogens by different animal assays. The androgenic potency of synthetic progestins can be measured by prostatic size or by steroid displacement.[9] Along the dimension of prostatic size, he notes the following relative androgenic potencies:

Relative Prostatic Weight Change

Levonorgestrel	9.4
d/l-Norgestrel	4.7
Norethindrone (reference standard)	1.0
Medroxyprogesterone acetate	0

In terms of its steroid displacement capacity, the relative ratios are somewhat different. If norethindrone again has a reference standard unit of 1, levonorgestrel is given an androgenic potency of 2.0 and medroxyprogesterone acetate corresponds to 1.0.[9] Another dimension by which the progestins can be measured is their "antiestrogenic potency." On such a scale, measured by the inhibition of keratinization of vaginal epithelium, progestins yield the following relative antiestrogenic potencies:

Antiestrogenic Potency

Progesterone	1
d/l-Norgestrel	74
Norethindrone	7.0
Medroxyprogesterone acetate	active

One sees that, depending upon which dimension of the progestin is measured, variations occur in the relative potency.[9]

The 19-norethisterone derivatives (norethisterone acetate and norethindrone) have androgenlike influences on lipid metabolism, whereas medroxyprogesterone acetate, being a 17-α-hydroxyprogesterone, causes much less change on lipid metabolism (there is no HDL-Ch change and a small LDL-Ch increase).[75] By 1967, it was clear that estrogen and androgens had opposite effects on serum lipids among users of certain hormones.[23] The HDL fraction was the lipid fraction most influenced by progestogens and then specifically by the 19-norethisterone derivatives.[75]

The dose of progestin appears to be critically relevant for its potential for lipid alterations. Low doses of norgestrel (0.5 mg) in the study of Nielsen significantly lowered the triglyceride level in women with hyper- and polymenorrhea 39 to 55.[48] In the Silfverstolpe study, the higher dose of norgestrel (1.8 mg/day) did not change serum triglyceride levels.[75]

The studies of oral contraceptives have shown a potential role for progestogens in the development of arterial diseases.[36,43,45,95] In 1982, Wynn noted that among oral contraceptive users taking ethinyl estradiol, those who would and who would not show an increased level of triglycerides varied according to the particular progestin.[95] The level increased by about 50% in the users of norethindrone acetate (1 mg plus 50 μg of ethinyl estradiol) and it increased by a lesser 20% in women who used 1 mg of norethindrone acetate coupled to a lower dose (20 μg) of ethinyl estradiol. The apparent difference was the dosage of synthetic estrogen, as described earlier.[95] Recent investigations by Meade, however, led him to conclude that the progestational component of oral contraceptives may contribute to the increased risk of stroke and ischemic heart disease in women, probably mediated in part by elevations in blood pressure.[45] He concluded that progestin did not appear to influence the risk of venous thromboembolism and suggested that heart disease risk would be reduced by the reduction in dose of both the estrogen and progestin components.[45] The conclusion of Mann, who evaluated progestin and cardiovascular disease by reviewing the epidemiologic data, was similar.[43] All death certificates for women aged 14 to 44 who died in England and Wales during 1978 that were coded for myocardial infarction were studied. He noted that "despite the very small numbers, there was a tendency within both groups (2 estrogens, low and high dose progestin) for the patients (myocardial infarct) to have received a higher daily dose of progestogen than was given to controls."[43]

Kaye, in 1982, evaluated progestogen and arterial disease using evidence from the Royal College of General Practitioners' Study. Cardiovascular disease noted over a 14-month period in the records of 1400 general practitioners was studied for dose of estrogen and progestin, as well as for recruited controls matched for age and other parameters.[36] There was a clear association between high rates of reporting of all three categories of arterial disease and larger doses of progestogens.[36]

In conclusion, it appears that progestin used in oral contraceptives is increasingly associated with an increased potential for pathologic factors as is the case with the synthetic estrogen (ethinyl estradiol) in both menopausal and oral contraceptive users. The effect of low-dose progestins, especially when the 19-nortestosterone derivatives are avoided, appears to be innocuous. The earlier demonstration (see Chap. 4) that even lower doses of progestins are protective of endometrial transformations is particularly comforting when considering the merits of these *low*-dose progestins in cardiovascular physiology.

PROTECTIVE FACTORS AGAINST CORONARY HEART DISEASE

In studies on hormone replacement therapy, a number of investigators concluded that certain hormone replacement therapy regimens are protective against coronary heart disease. Moreover, Rosenberg and co-workers concluded that there was no evidence for a synergistic effect of estrogen with the other predisposing factors for coronary heart disease.[71] Such a conclusion would, if replicated, have important clinical implications. It would suggest that a patient who is at risk for coronary heart disease has no reason to avoid hormone replacement therapy, if prescribed in appropriate doses. In the Rosenberg and co-workers study, 2.4% of the 336 myocardial infarction patients were regular estrogen users. In contrast, twice as many (4.9%) of the 6730 reference patients were regular estrogen users at the time of hospitalization.[71] Adjusting for confounding variables has led authors to conclude that there was a slight reduction in incidence of myocardial infarction for the estrogen users. The duration of use was not different in the two groups, and the dose was not known. Ross and colleagues concluded that there was evidence of a protective effect of menopausal estrogen therapy and protection from death from ischemic heart disease.[72] They studied a Los Angeles retirement community, evaluating records of 20,000 residents. Women dying from ischemic heart disease were compared to age-, race-, and socioeconomically matched controls. The women using conjugated estrogens had a markedly lowered incidence of ischemic heart disease than those with disease.[72] Heart disease victims, therefore, use fewer conjugated estrogens than healthy women do.

The moderate use of alcohol has also been considered to be a protective factor against coronary heart disease.[8,72] "Moderate" is defined as the consumption of two drinks, or less, each day. Seven ounces of wine, or its equivalent, probably constitutes the most beneficial "moderate" quantity.

ESTROGEN TREATMENT FOR LIPID PATHOLOGIES

Several investigators have shown that, appropriately used, certain estrogen replacement therapy regimens can reverse lipid excesses. Although men given high doses (5 mg conjugated equine estrogen per day) do increase their risk for cardiovascular pathology,[18] women do not. In 1958, Robinson and co-workers treated 58 women who had evidence of coronary heart disease with 5 or 10 mg of oral Premarin daily for an average of 14 months.[68] They compared pretreatment levels to post-treatment levels of cholesterol (C) (mg%), phospholipids (P) (mg%), C/P, and β/α lipoprotein cholesterol ratio. Table 6–3 shows the therapeutic results obtained with this dose of estrogen replacement therapy and compares these results to normative data from normal young women, normal postmenopausal women, women with coronary heart disease, and women with coronary heart disease after an average of 14 months of treatment. One notes the beneficial response in each of the parameters that are measured. The β/α lipoprotein cholesterol ratio, which was initially elevated, returned to levels that were equivalent to those in normal postmenopausal women. The other measures showed equivalent beneficial responses to estrogen therapy.

At about the same time, Marmorston and colleagues evaluated the effects of small doses of estrogen on serum lipids on female patients with myocardial infarction. Twenty-six postmenopausal women who had sustained a myocardial infarction were given ethinyl estradiol (10 μg per day) continuously. No negative side-effects were noted. Their results showed the following:[44]

- Serum cholesterol levels fell, phospholipid levels rose, and thus the cholesterol/phospholipid (C/P) ratio declined. This was a time-dependent response over the 6 months of this study.
- The magnitude of these changes was equal to that of the Robinson study just mentioned in which massive doses of estrogen were given.

• The magnitude of the effect, here, depended on the pretreatment level. If it was initially normal, the change was small; if it was initially high, the change was larger, suggesting the homeostatic influence of estrogen on serum lipids.

Further support for the therapeutic value of estrogen followed. In 1978 and then 1979, Tikkanen and colleagues evaluated the influences of natural estrogen as an effective treatment for postmenopausal hypercholesteremia.[80,81] In the first study, serum LDL–Ch concentration decreased in 16 or 17 postmenopausal women with elevated serum total and LDL–Ch; this beneficial response was evident after 6 months of estradiol valerianate treatment (Fig. 6–7).[80] One notes the changes in LDL–Ch level as a function of the initial LDL–Ch level after 3 months of treatment with estradiol valerianate (2 mg daily). Data of 17 hypercholesterolemic and 22 normocholesterolemic postmenopausal women are shown. Those with the highest initial levels showed the greatest LDL–Ch reducing effects. Simultaneously with these results, they also noted two beneficial results: Both major risk factors for coronary heart disease—the elevated LDL–Ch levels and reduced HDL–Ch levels—were changed in the direction of increased cardiovascular health.[81] The authors also noted that a modest VLDL triglyceride-increasing effect was limited to those women whose initial levels were within the normal ranges. Such a small effect would not seem to be harmful.

FIG. 6-7. Treatment response of hyperlipidemic women to estradiol valerianate therapy (Tikkanen MJ, Nikkila EA, 1978, Lancet Sept 2:490–501)

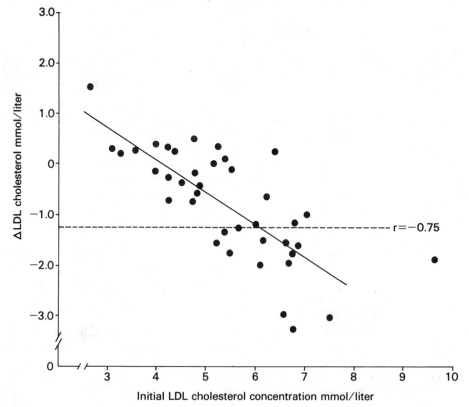

CONCLUSIONS

The overall consistency in the reports in the literature tends to support the relative protective effect of estrogen replacement therapy for postmenopausal women. Cardiovascular physiology does not seem to be at risk of detrimental effects of natural estrogens or to low doses of the 17α progestins. One should be cautioned, however, that individuals at especially high risk for cardiovascular disease should be identified and treated accordingly as part of their routine workup for their menopausal care. Each of the defined elements in cardiovascular physiology (especially LDL-Ch and HDL-Ch) seems to benefit from rational hormone replacement therapy regimens. Synthetic estrogens should be avoided in any conservative hormone replacement therapy program. Progestogen prescriptions should be maintained at relatively low dose levels.

REFERENCES

1. Aitken JM, Lorimer AR, Hart DM, Lawrie TDV, Smith DA (1971) The effects of oophorectomy and long term mestranol therapy on the serum lipids of middle aged women. *Clin Sci* 41:597–603.
2. Aylward M (1978) Coagulation factors in opposed and unopposed oestrogen treatment at the climacteric. *Postgrad Med J* 54:2:31–37.
3. Bain C, Willett W, Hennekens CH, Rosner B, Belanger C, Speizer FE (1981) Use of postmenopausal hormones and risk of myocardial infarction. *Circulation* 64:1:42–46.
4. Barrett-Conner E, Brown V, Turner J, et al (1979) Heart disease risk factors and hormone use in postmenopausal women. *JAMA* 20:2167–2169.
5. Bolton CH, Ellwood M, Hartog M, Martin R, Rowe AS, Wensley RT (1975) Comparison of the effects of ethinyl oestradiol and conjugated equine oestrogens in oophorectomized women. *Clin Endocrinol (Oxf)* 4:2:131–138.
6. Borglin NE, Staland B (1975) Oral treatment of menopausal symptoms with natural oestrogens. *Acta Obstet Gynecol Scand* 43:3–11.
7. Boston Collaborative Drug Surveillance Program (1974) Surgically confirmed gallbladder disease, venous thromboembolism, and breast tumors in relation to postmenopausal estrogen therapy. *N Engl J Med* 290:15–19.
8. Bradley DD, Wingerd J, Petitti DB (1978) Serum high density lipoprotein cholesterol in women using oral contraceptives, estrogens and progestins. *N Engl J Med* 299:17–20.
9. Brenner PF (1982) The pharmacology of progestogens. *J Reprod Med* 27:8(supp)490–497.
10. Brown MS, Goldstein J (1983) Lipoprotein receptors in the liver. Control signals for plasma cholesterol traffic. J Clin Invest 72:743–747.
11. Burch JC, Byrd BF, Vaughn WK (1975) The effects of long-term estrogen administration to women following hysterectomy. *Front Horm Res* 3:208–214.
12. Byrd BF, Burch JC, Vaughn WK (1977) The impact of long-term estrogen support after hysterectomy. A report of 1016 cases. *Ann Surg* 185:5:574–580.
13. Carlson LA, Bottiger LE, Ahfeldt, PE (1979) Risk factors for myocardial infarction in the Stockholm prospective study. *Acta Med Scand* 206:351–360.
14. Castelli WP, Doyle JT, Gordon T (1977) HDL cholesterol and other lipids in coronary heart disease. *Circulation* 55:767–772.
15. Centerwall BS (1981) Premenopausal hysterectomy and cardiovascular disease. *Am J Obstet Gynecol* 139:58–61.
16. Christiansen C, Christensen MS, Hagen C, Stocklund KE, Transbol I (1981) Effects of natural estrogen/gestagen and thiazide on coronary risk factors in normal postmenopausal women. *Acta Obstet Gynecol Scand* 60:407–412.
17. Cooper RA, Strauss JF (1984) Regulation of cell membrane cholesterol. In: *Physiology of Membrane Fluidity* Boca Raton, CRC Press.
18. The Coronary Drug Project Research Group (1970) The coronary drug project: initial findings leading to modifications of its research protocol. *JAMA* 214:1303–1313.
19. Crane MG, Harris JJ, Winsor WIII (1971) Hypertension, oral contraceptive agents and conjugated estrogens. *Ann Intern Med* 74:13–21.

20. Cutler W (1980) Premenopausal hysterectomy and cardiovascular disease. *Am J Obstet Gynecol* 141:849.

21. Davis ME, Jones RJ, Jarolim C (1961) Long-term estrogen substitution and atherosclerosis. *Am J Obstet Gynecol* 82:1003-1018.

22. Fedor-Freybergh P (1977) The influence of estrogens on the well-being and mental performance in climacteric and postmenopausal women. *Acta Obstet Gynecol Scand* 64:1-66.

23. Furman RH, Alaupovic P, Howard RP (1967) Effects of androgens and oestrogens on serum lipids and the composition and concentration of serum lipoproteins in normolipemic and hyperlipidemic states. *Prog Biochem Pharmacol* 2:215-249.

24. Gordon T, Castelli WP, Hjortland MP, Kannel WB, Dawber TR (1977) The Framingham Study. High density lipoprotein as a protective factor against coronary heart disease. *Am J Med* 62:707-714.

25. Gordon T, Kanel W, Hjortland M, McNamara P (1978) Menopause and coronary heart disease: the Framingham Study. *Ann Intern Med* 89:157-161.

26. Gustafson A, Svanborg A (1972) Gonadal steroid effects on plasma lipoproteins and individual phospholipids. *J Clin Endocrinol Metab* 35:203-207.

27. Hagopian M, Robinson RW (1965) Estrogen effect on human serum levels of the major phospholipids. *J Clin Endocrinol Metab* 25:283-285.

28. Hammond CB, Jelovsek FR, Lee KL, Creasman WT, Parker RT (1979) Effect of long-term estrogen replacement therapy. I. Metabolic. *Am J Obstet Gynecol* 133:525-536.

29. Haynes SG, Feinleib M (1982) Women, work and coronary heart disease: Results from the Framingham 10-year follow up study. In *Women: A Developmental Perspective*. Berman PW, Ramey ER (eds). US Dept Health and Human Services, NIH Publication No. 82-2298.

30. Higano N, Cohen WD, Robinson RW (1959) Effects of sex steroids on lipids. *Ann NY Acad Sci* 72:970-979.

31. Hirvonen E, Malkonen M, Manninen V (1980) Effects of different progestogens on lipoproteins during postmenopausal replacement therapy. *N Engl J Med* 304:560-563.

32. Jick H, Dinan B, Herman R, Rothman K (1978) Myocardial infarction and other vascular diseases in young women. *JAMA* 240:2548-2552.

33. Jick H, Dinan B, Rothman K (1978) Noncontraceptive estrogens and non fatal myocardial infarctions. *JAMA* 239:1407-1408.

34. Johansson BW, Jaij L, Kullander S, Lenner HC, Svanberg L, Astedt B (1975) On some late effects of bilateral oophorectomy in the age range of 15-30 years. *Acta Obstet Gynecol Scand* 54:449-461.

35. Kannel WB, Castelli WP, Gordon T, McNamara P (1971) Serum cholesterol, lipoproteins, and the risk of coronary heart disease. *Ann Intern Med* 174:1-12.

36. Kay CR (1982) Progestogens and arterial disease—evidence from the Royal College of General Practitioners' study. *Am J Obstet Gynecol* 142:762-765.

37. Knopp RH, Walden CE, Wahl PW, Hoover JJ (1982) Effects of oral contraceptives on lipoprotein triglycerides and cholesterol: relationships to estrogen and progestin potency. *Am J Obstet Gynecol* 142:725-731.

38. Lebech PE, Broggaard B (1974) Serum lipid and antithrombin-III changes effected by synthetic and natural estrogen therapy. In *The Menopausal Syndrome*. Greenblatt RB, Mahesh VB, McDonough PG (eds). New York, Medcom Press.

39. Lind T, Cameron EC, Hunter WM, Leon C, Moran PF, Oxley A, Gerrard J, Lind UOG (1979) A prospective controlled trial of six forms of hormone replacement therapy given to postmenopausal women. *Br J Obstet Gynaecol* 86:3:1-29.

40. MacMahon B (1978) Cardiovascular disease and non-contraceptive oestrogen therapy. In *Coronary Heart Disease in Young Women*, pp 197-207. Edinburgh, Churchill Livingstone.

41. Maddock J (1978) Effects of progestogens on serum lipids in the post-menopause. *Postgrad Med J* 54:2:38-41.

42. Mammen EF (1982) Oral contraceptives and blood coagulation: a critical review. *Am J Obstet Gynecol* 142:781-790.

43. Mann JI (1982) Progestins in cardiovascular disease: an introduction to the epidemiologic data. *Am J Obstet Gynecol* 142:752-757.

44. Marmorston J, Madgson O, Lewis JJ, Mehl J, Moore FJ, Bernstein J (1958) Effect of small doses of estrogen on serum lipids in female patients with myocardial infarction. *N Engl J Med* 258:583-586.

45. Meade TW (1982) Effects of progestogens on the cardiovascular system. *Am J Obstet Gynecol* 142:776-780.

46. Miller NE (1979) The evidence for the antiatherogenecity of high density lipoprotein in man. *Lipids* 13:914-919.

47. Nachtigall LE, Nachtigall RH, Nachtigall RD, Beckman EM (1979) Estrogen replacement therapy II: a prospective study in the relationship to carcinoma and cardiovascular and metabolic problems. *Obstet Gynecol* 54:74–79.

48. Nielsen FH, Honore E, Kristoffersen K, Secher NJ, Pedersen GT (1977) Changes in serum lipids during treatment with norgestrel, oestradiol-valerate and cycloprogynon. *Acta Obstet Gynecol Scand* 56:4:367–370.

49. Notelovitz M (1975) Effect of natural oestrogens on blood pressure and weight in postmenopausal women. *S Afr Med J* 49:2251–2254.

50. Notelovitz M (1977) Coagulation, oestrogen and the menopause. *Clin Obstet Gynaecol* 4:107–128.

51. Notelovitz M, Southwood B (1974) Metabolic effect of conjugated oestrogens (USP) on lipids and lipoproteins. *S Afr Med J* 48:2552–2556.

52. Oliver MF, Boyd GS (1953) Changes in plasma lipids during the menstrual cycle. *Clin Sci* 12:217–222.

53. Oster P, Arab L, Kohlmeier M, Mordasini R, Schellenberg B, Schlierf G (1982) Effects of estrogens and progestogens on lipid metabolism. *Am J Obstet Gynecol* 142:773–775.

54. Pallas KG, Holzwarth GJ, Stern MP, Lucas CP (1977) The effect of conjugated estrogens on the renin-angiotensin system. *J Clin Endocrinol Metab* 44:1061–1068.

55. Pasquale SA, Murphy RJ, Norwood PK, McBride LC (1982) Results of a study to determine the effects of three oral contraceptives on serum lipoprotein levels. *Fertil Steril* 38:559–563.

56. Pfeffer RI, Whipple GH, Kurosaki TT, Chapman JM (1978) Coronary risk and estrogen use in postmenopausal women. *Am J Epidemiol* 107:479–487.

57. Pfeffer RI, Van Den Noort S (1976) Estrogen use and stroke risk in postmenopausal women. *Am J Epidemiol* 103:445–456.

58. Phillips NR, Havel RJ, Kane JP (1983) Sex related differences in the concentration of apolipoprotein E in human blood plasma and plasma lipoproteins. *J Lipid Res* 24:1525–1535.

59. Plunkett ER (1982) Contraceptive steroids, age, and the cardiovascular system. *Am J Obstet Gynecol* 142:747–751.

60. Population Reports (1982) Oral contraceptives in the 1980's *Population Information Program*, The Johns Hopkins University, Hampton House, Maryland. Series A, Number 6, May-June, pp. A189–A222.

61. Punnonen R, Lammintausta R, Erkkola R, Rauramo L (1980) Estradiol valerate therapy and the renin-aldosterone system in castrated women. *Maturitas* 2:91–94.

62. Punnonen R, Rauramo L (1976) Effect of bilateral oophorectomy and peroral estradiol valerate therapy on serum lipids. *Int J Gynaecol Obstet* 14:13–16.

63. Punnonen R, Rauramo L (1976) The effect of castration and oral estrogen therapy on serum lipids. In *Consensus on Menopause Research.* van Keep PA, Greenblatt RBV, Albeaux-Fernet M (eds). Proc First International Congress on the Menopause Help in France, Baltimore, University Park Press.

64. Pyorala T (1976) The effect of synthetic and natural estrogens on glucose tolerance, plasma insulin and lipid metabolism in postmenopausal women. In *The Management of the Menopause and Postmenopausal Years* Campbell S (ed). Lancaster, England, MTP Press, pp 195–210.

65. Ritterband AB, Jaffe IA, Densen PM, Magagna JF, Reed E (1963) Gonadal function and the development of coronary heart disease. *Circulation* 27:237–251.

66. Rivin AU, Dimitroff SP (1954) The incidence and severity of atherosclerosis in estrogen-treated males and in females with a hypoestrogenic or hyperestrogenic state. *Circulation* 9:533–539.

67. Robinson RW, Lebeau RJ (1965) Effect of conjugated equine estrogens on serum lipids and the clotting mechanism. *J Atheroscler Res* 5:120–124.

68. Robinson RW, Cohen WD, Higano N (1958) Estrogen replacement therapy in women with coronary artherosclerosis. *Ann Intern Med* 48:95–101.

69. Robinson RW, Higano N, Cohen WD (1959) Increased incidence of coronary heart disease in women castrated prior to menopause. *Arch Intern Med* 104:908–913.

70. Robinson RW, Higano N, Cohen W (1960) Effects of long-term administration of estrogens on serum lipids of postmenopausal women. *N Engl J Med* 263:828–831.

71. Rosenberg L, Armstrong B, Jick H (1976) Myocardial infarction and estrogen therapy in postmenopausal women. *N Engl J Med* 294:1256–1259.

72. Ross RK, Paganini-Hill A, Mack TM, Arthur M, Henderson B (1981) Menopausal estrogen therapy and protection from death from ischaemic heart disease. *Lancet* 1:858–860.

73. Rowe JW (1983) Systolic hypertension in the elderly. *N Engl J Med* 309:1246–1247.

74. Saunders DM, Hunter JC, Shutt DA, O'Neill BJ (1978) The effect of oestradiol valerate therapy on coagulation factors and lipid and oestrogen levels in oophorectomized women. *Aust NZ J Obstet Gynaecol* 18:3:198–201.

75. Silfverstolpe G, Gustafson A, Samsioe G, Svanborg A (1979) Lipid metabolic studies in oophorectomized women. Effects of three different progestogens. *Acta Obstet Gynecol Scand* 88:89–95.

76. Spellacy WN, Birk SA (1972) The effect of intrauterine devices, oral contraceptives, estrogens and progestogens on blood pressure. *Am J Obstet Gynecol* 112:912–919.

77. Stangel JJ, Innerfield I, Reyniak JV (1976) The effects of conjugated estrogens on coagulability in menopausal women. *Obstet Gynecol* 49:314–316.

78. Sterling P, Eyer J (1981) Biological Basis of stress-related mortality. *Soc Sci Med* 15E:3–42.

79. Studd J, Dubiel M, Kakkar VV, Thom M, White PJ (1978) The effect of hormone replacement therapy on glucose tolerance, clotting factors, fibrinolysis and platelet behaviour in post-menopausal women. In: *The Role of Estrogen/Progestogen in the Management of the Menopause*, pp 41–60. Cooke ID (ed) Baltimore, University Park Press.

80. Tikkanen MJ, Nikkila EA (1978) Natural oestrogen as an effective treatment for Type-II hyperlipo-proteinaemia in postmenopausal women. *Lancet* September 2:490–501.

81. Tikkanen MJ, Kuusi T, Vartianien E, Nikkila EA (1979) Treatment of post-menopausal hyper-cholesterolaemia with estradiol. *Acta Obstet Scand (Suppl)* 88:83–88.

82. Toy JL, Davies JA, McNicol GP (1978) The effects of long-term therapy with oestriol succinate on the haemostatic mechanism in postmenopausal women. *Br J Obstet Gynaecol* 85:5:363–366.

83. Tsang R, Glueck CJ (1979) Atherosclerosis, a pediatric perspective. *Curr Probl Pediatr* 9:3:3–11.

84. Utian WH (1972) Effects of oophorectomy and estrogen therapy on serum cholesterol. *Int J Gynecol Obstet* 10:95–101.

85. Utian WH (1978) Effect of postmenopausal estrogen therapy on diastolic blood pressure and bodyweight. *Maturitas* 1:3–8.

86. Von Eiff AW (1975) Blood pressure and estrogens. *Front Horm Res* 3:177–184.

87. Wahl P, Walden C, Knopp R, Hoover J, Wallace R, Heiss G, Rafkind B (1983) Effect of estrogen/progestin potency on lipid/lipoprotein cholesterol *N Engl J Med* 308:862–867.

88. Wallace RB, Hoover J, Barrett-Conner E, et al (1979) Altered plasma lipid and lipo-protein levels associated with oral contraceptive and oestrogen use. *Lancet* ii:112–114.

89. Wallentin L, Larsson-Cohn U (1977) Metabolic and hormonal effects of post-menopausal oestrogen replacement treatment. *Acta Endocrinol* 86:597–607.

90. Walter S, Jensen HK (1977) The effect of treatment with oestradiol and oestriol on fasting serum cholesterol and triglyceride levels in postmenopausal women. *Br J Obstet Gynaecol* 84:11:869–872.

91. Weir RJ, Briggs, E, Mack A, Taylor L, et al (1971) Blood pressure in women after one year of oral contraception. *Lancet* 1:467–471.

92. Weir RJ, Buggs E, Mack A (1974) Blood pressure in women taking oral contraceptives. *Br Med J* 1:533–535.

93. Wiseman RA, MacRae KD (1981) Oral contraceptives and the decline in mortality from circulatory disease. *Fertil Steril* 35:277–283.

94. Wuest JH, Dry TJ, Edwards JE (1953) The degree of atherosclerosis in bilaterally oophorectomized women. *Circulation* 7:801–809.

95. Wynn V, Niththyananthan R (1982) The effect of progestins in combined oral contraceptives on serum lipids with special reference to high-density lipoproteins. *Am J Obstet Gynecol* 142:766–772.

7

Hormone Replacement Therapy: Dosing

INITIAL CONSIDERATIONS

Hormone replacement therapy regimens for the perimenopausal and menopausal woman have had to be empirically defined because available dosing data are incomplete. Nonetheless, an analysis of about 100 recent studies does permit some preliminary conclusions. Firstly, it becomes clear that low doses of estrogen as well as progestin—started early in the perimenopausal period—provide adequate hormonal support to prevent osteoporosis for most women, if adequate calcium is provided from the diet. Moreover, contrary to some beliefs, it is never too late.[3] Whenever estrogen supplementation is started, the rate of bone degeneration seems to decline (Fig. 7-1). Women entered this study at different intervals after bilateral oophorectomy. Some were treated with placebo, others with mestranol replacement therapy. Data were obtained at varying intervals after inception of therapy. The data in this study support the fact that, even 6 years after oophorectomy, the initiation of estrogen replacement therapy has merit, even though only after 3 years of estrogen therapy was there a consistent halt to further bone loss.[3] More recent observations show a dose–response relationship in which lower levels of ethinyl estradiol were inadequate to fully prevent the loss of bone and in which the highest doses yielded a net increase in bone mass.[39] For details, see Chapter 2.

The benefits of progestin opposition to estrogen have recently been revealed; unopposed progestin has also been studied.[25,50] Its beneficial effect on the bone remodeling cycle was discussed in Chapter 2. Its role in preventing and reversing endometrial hyperplasias was described in Chapter 5. Its potential for reducing breast cancer incidence was also discussed.[32] The question of whether to prescribe hormones in cyclic or continual regimens has not been well studied but the absence of adverse effects from continuous estrogens has been recently shown.[12,15,35] The protective value of using unopposed progestin has also been studied.

Whereas originally estrogen doses were far too high and were subsequently reduced, progestin opposition to the estrogen has also followed a similar pattern. Original progestin doses tended to be too high and of too short a duration to promote maximal effectiveness. Recent studies have provided strong support for prescribing progestin, where it is appropriate to do so, in very low doses for a long (10 to 13 days) duration each month.

Other relevant estrogen and progestin dose considerations include assessing the height of the patient as well as her relative stature. Thus, for those patients who are appropriate candidates for hormone replacement therapy (see Chapter 1 for discussion of appropriateness), a recent body of information has accumulated for preliminary

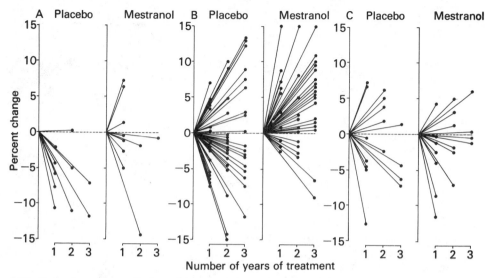

FIG. 7-1. Percentage change of metacarpal mineral content after oophorectomy: effect of mestranol and placebo (*A*) within 2 months of oophorectomy; (*B*) within 3 years after; (*C*) within 6 years after (Aitken JM, Hart DM, Lindsay R, 1976, Postgrad Med J (suppl) 6:18–25)

suggestions of optimal doses. The clinician should be alert to new information in this field. Hopefully, studies published in the next 3 or 4 years should add a great deal of sophistication to our ability to establish the most effective and safe dose.

ESTROGEN THERAPIES AND PLASMA HORMONE LEVELS

ESTRADIOL CREAMS

There are differences in absorption and metabolism relating to the route and form of hormones administered. For example, vaginal creams appear more likely than oral tablets to increase the 17β-estradiol level at similar doses.[96] Estradiol cream, 2 mg per day, or 1.25 mg a day of conjugated equine estrogens are reasonably optimal doses for achieving plasma estrogen concentrations that are equivalent to premenopausal early follicular phase.[54,71]

Figure 7–2 shows the plasma estrone and estradiol levels in response to Premarin cream therapy before treatment, during the 4 weeks of therapy, and during the followup.[96] One notes the apparent decline in each estrogen during the fourth week of therapy that the authors have suggested might reflect decreased patient compliance. Nonetheless, lacking more accurate information, they concluded the decline might also be due to a refractory phase in steroid metabolism. Short-term studies have confirmed the rapid absorption and plasma response of conjugated vaginal cream therapies. Whitehead and colleagues have suggested that the vaginal epithelium cleaves the sulfate radical from estrone more effectively.[96] Figure 7–3 shows the preferential increase of the particular estrogen dominant in the cream. When 0.05 mg estrone is delivered vaginally (Fig. 7–3A), the estrone levels show excessive increases whereas the estradiol levels are moderately elevated.[79] One notes in contrast that within 60 minutes of applying 0.5 mg of

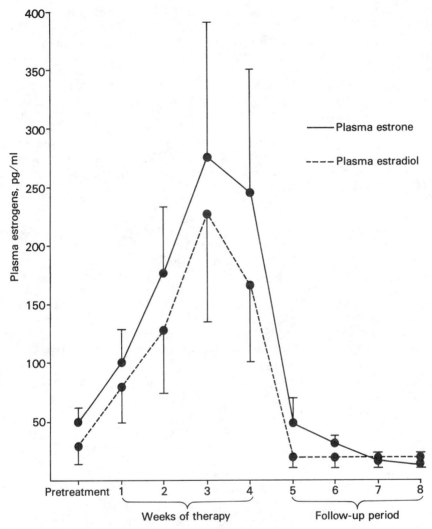

FIG. 7-2. Vaginal Premarin therapy (1.25 mg/day): effect on plasma estrogens (Whitehead MI, Minardi J, Kitchin Y, Sharples MJ, 1978, In: *The Role of Estrogen/Progestogen in the Management of Menopause.* Baltimore, Univ. Park Press, 63–72)

micronized estradiol per vagina (Fig. 7-3B), the plasma estradiol levels reach excessive concentrations. The estrone levels, while rising, do not show as drastic an increase. Thus the vaginal application of an estrogen cream is reflected in increases in both E1 and E2; however, the major estrogen increase is defined by the specific estrogen in the cream. Further refinements in dose have followed. Vaginal estradiol (estrace) of 0.2 mg a day for women with vaginal atrophy yielded plasma levels that appeared more physiologic. Within 12 hours, E2 levels had increased from 18.1 ± 1.2 pg/ml to 62.6 ± 18 pg/ml, a level maintained 15 days later for women who continued to use the creams.[54] Premarin cream (1.25 mg a day) yielded somewhat lower plasma 17β-estradiol levels but much higher estrone levels. The estrone level had increased from baseline levels of approximately 21.6 ± 3.0 pg/ml to about 80 pg/ml within 12 hours. This was approximately double the estrone level achieved with the Estrace cream. Premarin contains 10 different estrogens, the largest component (48%) being estrone sulfate.[100] Indeed, all preparations were very effective in relieving symptoms of atrophic vaginitis and hot flashes. Premarin has the widest and longest clinical use experience.

Vaginal administration of 0.5 mg of estriol cream has also been evaluated.[80] Estriol, 0.5 mg, yielded LH suppression to about 84% of baseline within 2 hours and a significant suppression of FSH by 5 hours. The maximal estriol response in plasma was achieved in 2 hours as well. Although oral doses of estriol suffer from rapid conversion into the conjugated state, thereby rendering the steroid less effective, vaginal administration of estriol appears to avoid this and has, therefore, been recommended.[80]

CREAMS COMPARED WITH OTHER ROUTES

The degrees of systemic absorption of vaginally and of orally administered estrogens at different dose levels in postmenopausal women have been compared.[22] Relief of vaginal symptoms and a change from atrophic to greater than 70% superficial cell count has been achieved with every level of vaginal cream (0.3 mg a day and higher.)[22] Moreover, at minimum effective doses, the creams consistently provided lower blood levels of estrogen to achieve symptom relief than the oral route did. Figure 7–4 compares the blood estrogen levels after 1 week of oral versus 1 week of vaginal therapy for each of 3 doses of conjugated equine estrogens. One notes the lower blood estrogen levels achieved by the vaginal estrogen creams. Because it seems best to prescribe the lowest

FIG. 7-3. Effect of vaginal estrogen therapy, (*A*) estrone (0.05 mg/day) and (*B*) micronized estradiol (0.5 mg/day) on plasma estrogens and gonadotropins (Schiff I, Tulchinsky D, Ryan KJ, 1977, Fertil Steril 23:1063–1066)

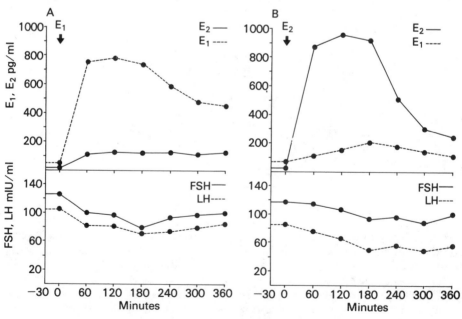

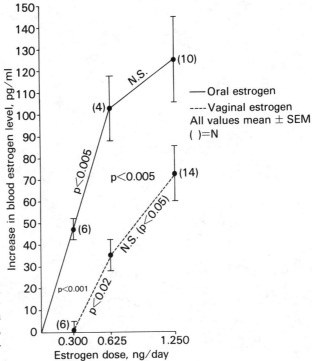

FIG. 7-4. Oral and vaginal estrogen therapy: effect of different doses on plasma estrogen level (Deutsch S, Ossowski R, Benjamin I, 1981, Am J. Obstet. Gynecol. 139:967–968)

adequate dose for symptom relief, the vaginal route would appear to be safest, particularly since it avoids the hepatic circulation in the main. Figure 7–5 compares three different dose cream regimens. Plasma responses of estradiol and estrone vary with dose administered.[71] Although other vaginal creams are available, their use is less well defined.[23] Percutaneous oestradiol cream (3 mg) estradiol 17β has been studied for its influence on plasma levels of parathyroid hormone and calcitonin.[87] Plasma estrogen response to transdermal estradiol cream was not reported in this study; however, a more recent report did provide some initial data.[46]

ESTROGEN IN ORAL FORM

Pharmacologic Properties of Various Estrogen Formulations

One of the difficulties of determining appropriate hormone doses for the specific estrogen lies in the variation in the response of these in the different target-tissue systems of the body.

The commercially available synthetic estrogens have been listed by Deghenghi:

Ethynyl estradiol (EE) (oral tablets or capsules)
Mestranol
Quinestrol
Diethylstilbestrol (DES)
Chlorotrianisene (TACE)
Clomiphene

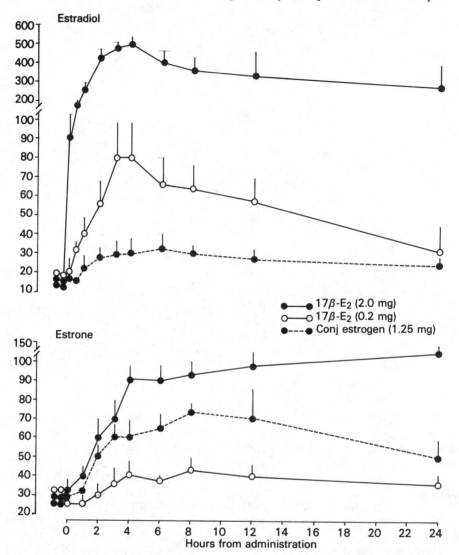

FIG. 7-5. Vaginal estrogens: differential plasma estrogen response to different therapies (Rigg IA, Herman H, Yen SSC, 1977, reprinted by permission of the New England Journal of Medicine 298:195–197)

He considers the following to be included among the natural estrogens:

17β-Estradiol
17β-Estradiol benzoate
17β-Estradiol cyclopentylpropionate
17β-Estradiol dipropionate
17β-Estradiol valerate*

Estriol
Conjugated estrogens (equine)
Estrone
Piperazine estrone sulfate
Zeranol

Some of the hormones that are considered natural by some are considered synthetic by others.[18] Most consider E1, E2, E3 and the conjugated estrogens to be natural. The others described as natural by Deghengi may undergo a systemic conversion from the esterified state to the natural estrogen. Zeranol, in particular, should not be considered a natural estrogen since it is not even a steroid.

Mashchak and co-workers evaluated the human pharmacodynamic properties of various estrogen formulations, comparing varied doses of piperazine estrone sulfate, micronized estradiol, estrace, Premarin, ethinyl estradiol, and DES (Table 7–1).[55] The relative potency for a number of systems was determined by parallel line analysis for each response (Table 7–2). Table 7–1 shows these data. One notes that the relative strengths are not consistent across the systems. Thus, for example, DES has more pronounced influences on changes in sex hormone binding globulin whereas conjugated equine estrogens have more profound influences on angiotensinogen levels.[55] In general, however, the hepatic measures were exaggerated three- to ten-fold by oral Premarin with

TABLE 7-1. Pharmacodynamics of various estrogen preparations

Estrogen Preparation	Δ SHBG-BC (nM) (mean ± SEM)	Δ CBG-BC (μg/dl) (mean ± SEM)	Angiotensinogen (ng/ml) (mean ± SEM)	FSH Suppression (%) (mean ± SEM)
Piperazine estrone sulfate (mg)				
0.3	−5.7 ± 2.8	1.0 ± 1.2	QNS	6.3 ± 10.7
0.6	3.0 ± 2.3	−2.4 ± 0.4	QNS	27.8 ± 5.2
1.25	10.3 ± 7.0	−0.3 ± 0.5	4,600 ± 1,500	29.3 ± 7.3
2.5	46.7 ± 18.4	2.7 ± 2.6	6,000 ± 1,400	51.0 ± 13.3
5.0	65.3 ± 23.9	6.5 ± 2.2	9,500 ± 1,200	62.9 ± 3.4
Conjugated estrogens (mg)				
0.3	6.7 ± 3.8	−2.6 ± 0.3	QNS	19.9 ± 6.8
0.625	38.0 ± 20.0	0.6 ± 0.3	6,100 ± 0	18.6 ± 20.6
1.25	54.0 ± 16.0	3.3 ± 0.4	10,000 ± 900	55.0 ± 9.8
2.5	104.3 ± 26.8	8.6 ± 1.6	11,300 ± 400	51.5 ± 7.9
Micronized estradiol (mg)				
1.0	15.7 ± 8.1	0.7 ± 1.6	2,900 ± 500	34.7 ± 8.4
2.0	62.7 ± 25.4	5.0 ± 1.4	6,400 ± 200	54.0 ± 10.7
10.0	90.0 ± 7.0	18.2 ± 1.1	8,400 ± 3,300	77.0 ± 5.5
Diethylstilbestrol (mg)				
0.1	45.7 ± 11.6	8.1 ± 1.1	7,700 ± 2,600	23.7 ± 2.0
0.5	109.7 ± 23.1	20.3 ± 1.2	9,100 ± 1,800	38.7 ± 9.9
Ethinyl estradiol (mg)				
0.01	71.3 ± 11.8	12.3 ± 1.8	7,500 ± 900	42.6 ± 10.4
0.02	110.7 ± 29.8	12.5 ± 3.4	9,200 ± 3,900	41.8 ± 5.3

QNS, Quantity not sufficient.
Mashchak CA, Lobo RA, Dozono-Takano R et al, 1982, Am J Obstet Gynecol 144:511–518.

TABLE 7-2.   Relative potency estimated according to four specific parameters of estrogenicity

Estrogen Preparation	Serum FSH	Serum CBG-BC	Serum SHBG-BC	Serum Angiotensinogen
Piperazine estrone sulfate	1.1	1.0	1.0	1.0
Micronized estradiol	1.3	1.9	1.0	0.7
Conjugated estrogens	1.4	2.5	3.2	3.5
DES	3.8	70	28	13
Ethinyl estradiol	(80–200)*	(1,000)*	614	232

*Estimate in the absence of parallelism.
Mashchak CA, Lobo RA, Dozono-Takano R et al, 1982, Am J Obstet Gynecol 144:511–518

much greater excesses produced by the synthetic estrogens (ethinyl estradiol and DES). For angiotensinogen response, micronized estradiol and piperazine estrone sulfate were equally potent: Premarin was 3.5-fold greater; DES was 13-fold greater; and ethinyl estradiol was 232-fold more potent than the piperazine estrone sulfate. The persistent parallelism strongly suggested that the five preparations were all subsets of one estrogen family in which each estrogen affects target tissues in a qualitatively similar manner.[55] General support for the liver effect (excess binding globulin production) of oral estrogen has been well documented in the literature.[33,76] Although the role of estrone is not biologically clear and needs study,[42] there have been several reports indicating a relative constancy of the E2/E1 ratio when estrogens are taken orally—regardless of whether estrone or estradiol is prescribed.[43] Individual estrogens, specifically Premarin, estradiol valerate, micronized estradiol, piperazine estrone sulfate, ethinyl estradiol and mestranol, have each been evaluated for estrogen and gonadotropin plasma response to varying doses of the replacement hormone. Each of the estrogens does show dose–response tendencies that are positive for steroid response and inverse for gonadotropins.

Conjugated Equine Estrogens

Conjugated equine estrogens have been well characterized.[6,11,22,30,31,47,49,55,60,72,76,77,82,83,86,88,89,91,93,94,101] The measurement of equilin in human plasma has shown that women who ingest conjugated equine estrogens circulate large quantities of equilin.[100,101] The biological effects of these large quantities are currently unclear, but conjugated equine estrogens contain approximately 30%, or more, equilin or equilin derivatives.[100] Figure 7-6A shows the plasma FSH response to administration of increasing doses of conjugated equine estrogen interspersed with weeks during which hormones were not given. Figure 7-6B shows the plasma estradiol response to the same dose regimen. One notes the rapid and graded response to conjugated equine estrogen in both systems.[94] Figure 7-4 illustrates equivalent dose–response tendencies.

The general dose of conjugated equine estrogens found in the literature ranges from 0.3 mg per day to 1.25 mg or more.[23] The relative doses of conjugated equine estrogens necessary to produce relief of distress have been studied. Hot flashes are generally relieved with either a 0.625 mg per day dose or 1.25 mg dose.[6,47,88] Sleep quality has been reported to be improved at doses as low as 0.625 mg.[77] Vaginal atrophy appears to require a higher dose once the atrophy is well underway and a 1.25 mg dose appears to be

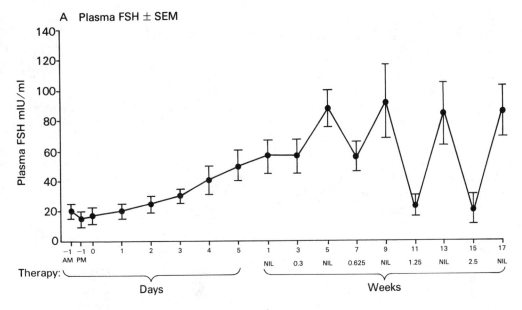

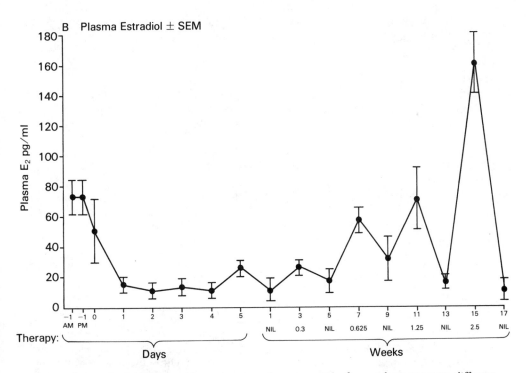

FIG. 7-6. Oral conjugated equine estrogens: dose response after oophorectomy to different doses interspersed with placebo; (*A*) plasma FSH: (*B*) plasma E2 (Utian W, Katz M, Davey D, Carr P, 1978, Am J Obstet Gynecol 132:297–302)

sufficient.[82,88] High doses, 5 mg a day, were reported to yield improved well-being in contrast with placebo.[93] Withdrawal bleeding is more likely when doses are higher—1.25 vs. 0.625 was tested.[47] No harmful effects for the blood lipid factors, as described earlier, were noted at doses as high as 1.25 mg per day.[7,8] For details, see Chapter 6. At doses as high as 1.25 mg there was no influence on osteoarthrosis.[21] Studies of calcium/creatinine ratio, renin substrate, thyroxine-binding globulin, sex hormone-binding globulin, and corticosteroid-binding globulin have shown positive dose-dependent responses from conjugated equine estrogen beginning with doses as low as 0.15 through 0.3, 0.625 and 1.25 mg.[31,34,55,76] The use of conjugated equine estrogens for osteoporotic individuals appears to require a somewhat higher than normal symptom-relief dose, reported at about 2.5 mg in one study.[72] No impairment of glucose tolerance was reported at doses as high as 1.25 mg.[86,89,91] The propensity for cystic glandular hyperplasia is dose-dependent, as described earlier; at doses of 0.625 or less, it rarely poses a problem.[60] Doses of 0.625 mg or less per day occupy the "low-dose" end of a prescribing continuum.

Estradiol Valerate

Estradiol valerate equilibrates rapidly, reaching plasma levels within one day of hormone ingestion that are equal to those found on the fifth day.[69] Estradiol valerate has been studied at its common dose of 2 mg a day.[16,24,45,67] At this level, in women who were in early postmenopause, estradiol levels went from pretreatment averages of 15.6 +/− 7.8 pg/ml to approximately 52 pg/ml by day 21 of the first cycle, reaching 57 pg/ml in the third cycle and 64 pg/ml by the sixth cycle of hormone therapy.[45] Estrone levels showed much larger increases—from basal levels of 3 pg/ml to 218, 263, and 259 pg/ml in the first, third, and sixth cycles respectively.[45] Although estrone levels were always considerably greater than estradiol levels during estradiol valerate therapy, the ratio itself appeared to be stable within each woman.[24]

Estradiol valerate use has been reported in doses ranging from 1 mg (low dose) through 2 mg per day (high dose) and in one study to 4 mg a day (very high dose).[93] At the 2-mg dose, glucose tolerance was shown to be normal.[89,91] Cystic glandular hyperplasia incidence was dose-related, as described in Chapter 5.[47,60] Low doses, 1 mg, vs. higher doses, 2 mg, yield a lower incidence of either withdrawal or breakthrough bleeding as well as a lower incidence of flush relief.[6,47] At very high doses, 4 mg, improved well-being (over placebo) was reported.[93] At the 2-mg dose, there were no changes observed in serum triglyceride levels and there were slight increases in cholesterol levels, yielding an overall neutral or beneficial response to the lipid factors.[58,66,67,74] Plasma renin activity was not altered at the 2-mg dose.[65] Skin thickness was reduced with the 2-mg dose, indicating that it may be too strong an estrogen for this system.[64]

Micronized Estradiol

Micronized estradiol is readily absorbed and also undergoes significant conversion to estrone.[104] Figure 7–7 shows the response to a 2-mg dose of oral micronized estradiol over the 24 hours following administration. One notes the much larger response of estrone and the rapid achievement of high plasma levels within the first several hours after ingestion of a single tablet.[104]

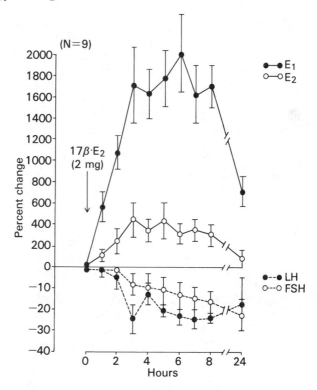

FIG. 7-7. Oral micronized estrogen: Plasma estrogens and gonadotropins; response to a single 2-mg tablet (Yen SS, Martin PL, Burnier AM, Czekala NM et al, 1975, J Clin Endocrinol Metab 40(3):518–521)

TABLE 7-3. Effects of piperazine oestrone sulphate 1.5 and 3.0 daily on mean serum levels of LH, FSH, oestrone, and oestradiol in eight subjects

Dose (mg)	LH (u/l)	FSH (u/l)	Oestrone (pg/ml)	Oestradiol (pg/ml)
Basal	60.9	25.2	58	10
1.5	50.3	17.7	410	72
3.0	47.2	11.9	931	148

Differences between LH levels not significant. All other differences significant. Basal levels of FSH, oestrone, and oestradiol significantly different from all levels on treatment ($p < 0.001$). Levels on 1.5 mg and 3.0 mg significantly different for FSH ($p = 0.023$), oestrone ($p = 0.003$) and oestradiol ($p = 0.003$).

Isaacs AJ, Havard CW, 1978. Clin Endocrinol (Oxf) 9:4:297–302.

Piperazine Oestrone Sulfate

Piperazine oestrone sulfate in two different cyclic doses (1.5 or 3.0 mg) also yields dose-dependent increases in estrone and estradiol with a much greater response for the estrone. Table 7-3 shows these data for 33 postmenopausal women. Gonadotropin showed similar responses to this estrogen as to the others arrayed elsewhere.[41]

Ethinyl Estradiol

Ethinyl estradiol, although less satisfactory for heart health parameters,[8] appears to have been commonly prescribed in dosages ranging from 20 to 50 μg a day.[23,29] At 50 μg per day, estrone levels showed rapid increases that approximately doubled from baseline.[45] Gonadotropins both dropped approximately 25% at this dose.[45] Elsewhere, at 15 μg per day, the dose was initially sufficient to suppress gonadotropins to premenopausal levels, but a subsequent "escape" to the menopausal elevation levels followed.[102] With a 200-μg dose, adrenal influences have been reported.[49] Increases in corticosteroids among eight ovariectomized women were demonstrated with a subsequent return to baseline after withdrawal from the hormone.[52] Liver effects, as already described, were shown to be dose-dependent.[58,76] Glucose tolerance was unaffected by either 50- or 500-μg doses given to hysterectomized women.[86] Twenty-microgram doses did produce significant increases in midday calcitonin concentrations.[87]

Mestranol

Mestranol at 25 μg a day in five oophorectomized women also yielded rapid elevations in both estrone and estradiol levels that were greater for the former.[53]

Although 20 μg has been suggested as the optimal daily dose, it has also been mentioned that individual variation in 9 AM fasting cortisol concentration should facilitate adjusting the dosage.[3] If the cortisol level is high (more than 1.2 mmol/liter), the woman should probably be given a higher dose of mestranol, if that is the hormone of choice. At 20 to 40 μg a day, no adverse effects on serum lipids were revealed.[4] However, even at 80 μg per day, no changes in glucose tolerance test results could be found.[86]

Estriol

Estriol has also been studied at 2 mg per day,[68,92] as well as at high doses of 4, 6, and 8 mg per day. While it did not induce endometrial proliferation at any dose, it did improve vaginal maturation.[92] It also retarded the loss of epidermal thickness during one 3-year course.[68]

Thus all forms of oral estrogens show consistent plasma response that is dose dependent—positive for the estrogens and inverse for the gonadotropins.

SUBLINGUAL TABLETS

Burnier and colleagues have reported the time-course in a minimal dose of sublingual micronized estradiol.[10] Estrace, in a 1-mg tablet broken in half (*i.e.*, 0.5 mg) was either taken once a day or on alternate days for a month. At this low dose, vaginal atrophy was relieved with complete reversal of the maturation index, yielding an estrogenized pattern. Since this route bypassed the liver and was preferable for those patients who were annoyed by the messiness of the vaginal cream, the report was particularly noteworthy.[10] The authors noted a good deal of conversion of the estrogen from E2 to E1, which takes about 4 hours to start and is similar to the oral administration results described previously. See Figure 7–8. This finding therefore suggests that another major pathway for the conversion of estradiol to estrone (besides the small bowel) does exist. The authors suggested that it is possibly due to the reticuloendothelial system since the region of the neck is rich in lymphatic channels and tissue. With vaginal administration the conversion to estrone did not take place in such great magnitude.[10] Burnier and

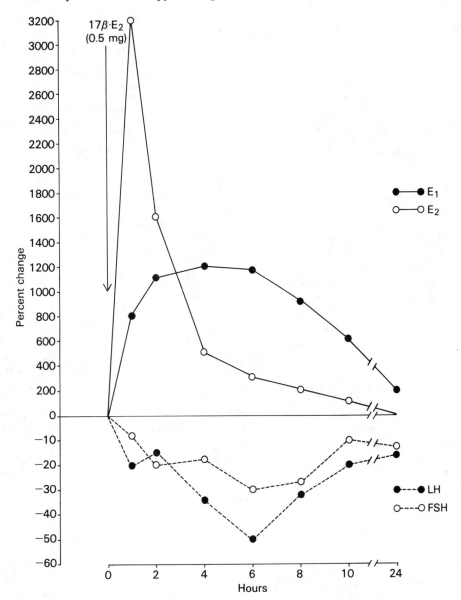

FIG. 7-8. Sublingual 17β-estradiol (0.5 mg) yields rapid plasma estrogen and gonadotropin response (Burnier AM, Martin PL, Yen SSC, Brooks P, 1981, Am J Obstet Gynecol 140:146–150)

co-workers concluded that the most physiologic way of administering estrogen is vaginally and is acceptable to at least 75% of the patients. They considered the sublingual route to be the next most physiologic method with a much lower effective dose necessary to achieve satisfactory results than through the oral route.[10] Estrogen, either transdermal or vaginal, provides an effective way to accomplish estrogen replacement therapy. Although patient compliance can be achieved, there is a reluctance on the part of most. The dose as well as the estrogen being supplied will determine the blood levels. While alternate days of administration have been suggested, a smaller dose, used daily, should provide a more consistent blood level and thus a better therapeutic effect.

ESTROGEN IMPLANTS

Estrogen delivered by implant has been utilized but is felt to be a less desirable route because of the repeated interventions necessary. Nonetheless, they appear to yield effects similar to those of the other routes described.[40,51,85] Particularly in obese women, estradiol implants have been noted to yield excess levels of androgens circulating in plasma.[51] This was noted in the presence of normal (equivalent to premenopausal women) serum estrogen levels. A 100-mg dose, by an estrogen implant, has been effective in relieving symptoms and yielding plasma responses that are equivalent to the studies described earlier.[40]

Once implanted, even as silicone implants, there is less recourse to altering doses. Retrieving may also pose some difficulties. Nonetheless, some find this approach functional when other methods fail. In contrast, the transdermal approach, recently explored by Laufer and colleagues, shows potential as a new and effective method of hormonal delivery.[46] The skin does absorb estrogen rapidly. What remains to be determined is a full panoply of dose–response evaluations.

CONCLUSIONS—ESTROGEN THERAPIES

Because of the obvious disparities in different response measures for varying doses of different estrogens, the clinician is presented with a problem in dosing. There is no universal response to different hormones and we are left with the essential question, How does one achieve the greatest benefit with the lowest dose? For the present, the oral route, in yielding increased stimulation of the liver, would appear to be less desirable and offer less of an advantage to the patient who is comfortable with the use of a vaginal cream or sublingual tablet. The oral route is still the most popular but may be losing its lead as the prime route of administration. The lowest doses of transmucosal estrogens have been sufficient to prevent osteoporosis as well as to relieve other menopausal symptoms. However, if treatment begins later in the degeneration sequence, higher doses, at least initially, appear desirable. Particularly worthy of caution is the indiscriminate use of the synthetic estrogens, ethinyl estradiol and diethylstilbestrol, because of their potential for the heart health risks described in Chapter 6.

HOW MUCH PROGESTIN?

RELATIVE PROGESTIN STRENGTHS

The practice of using progestin in opposition to estrogen therapy in menopausal hormone replacement therapy regimens has recently begun to gain more widespread acceptance. As described previously (see Chapters 4–6), recent evidence supports the value of progesterone in a menopausal therapy plan. Utian has outlined the most well known of the orally active progestational compounds.[95] He lists three principal classes:

1. *Progesterone derivatives*
   didrogesterone (6-dehydroretroprogesterone)

2. *Acetoxyprogesterone derivatives*
   medroxyprogesterone acetate
   megestrol acetate
3. *19-Nortestosterone derivatives and relatives*
   chlormadinone acetate
   ethynodiol diacetate
   lynestrenol (3-desoxonorethindrone)
   norethindrone (norethisterone)
   norethindrone acetate (norethisterone acetate)
   norethinodrel
   norgestrel
   norgestrienone

Of these compounds, many of which are available only in oral contraceptive formulations, several could be used in menopausal regimens as well. Figure 7–9 reviews the metabolic pathway of the principal relevant progestins.

Rozenbaum has described the relationship between chemical structure and biological properties of the progestogens.[73] Progestogens are classified in three ways that are mutually not interconnected: by isomeric configurations, by biologic activity, and by their affinity for hormone receptors.[73] Potency varies greatly from one to another. Norethindrone acetate is considered more potent than norethindrone because the added acetyl grouping decreases the binding affinity but increases the progestational activity, probably because of its delayed catabolism. Norgestrel is one of the most potent progestogens now in use due to the substitution of a 13β methyl group by an ethyl group—a phenomenon that produces increased progestational activity. At doses of norethindrone acetate approaching 30 mg per day, increased serum renin substrate is produced, but, the clinician should note that this is 30 times the dose currently being recommended for this hormone at menopause. Therefore, such a problem is not likely to occur at currently recommended menopausal doses of progestin.

The most widely studied compounds include norethindrone (norethisterone) norethindrone acetate (norethisterone acetate), megestrol acetate, medroxyprogesterone acetate, and norgestrel.

PROGESTIN IN OPPOSITION TO ESTROGEN

The studies are incomplete and cannot answer, properly, the urgent questions of how much progestin to prescribe for what duration in what opposition to particular doses of estrogen. Nonetheless, some evidence is available and the trend of information is becoming clearer. Particularly clear is the need for at least 10 days of progestin in order to induce endometrial shedding.[47]

Original menopausal replacement therapy regimens appear to have contained progestin doses that were approximately 5 to 10 times too high. The more recent studies of endometrial response to lower-dose, long-duration progestins clearly show maximal benefits to be derived from the lowest possible doses for the longest duration (see Chap. 5).[57,60,61] Studies of the effect of progestins on carbohydrate metabolism also support the value of the lower progestin doses.[12,89,91,103] In addition, studies of lipid response to different doses of progestin also support the beneficial value of the lower doses.[14,34,38,58,61] Particularly noteworthy were indications of a reversal of the beneficial effects of estrogen on lipid factors when high doses of progestin for long duration were given;[34] however, such potentially deleterious effects were not evident when low doses of progestin were

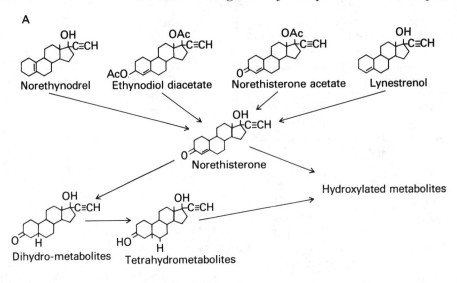

FIG. 7-9. Metabolism of synthetic progestogens related to (*A*) 17α-ethyl-19-nortestosterone and (*B*) 17α-acetoxyprogesterone (adapted from Fotherby K, 1974, Acta Endocrinol 185(suppl): 119-147)

taken for a long time.[14] There appears to be a lower risk of lipid imbalance when the progestin selected is a progesterone derivative such as medroxyprogesterone acetate rather than one of the 19-nortestosterone derivatives such as norgestrel. However, the particular effect noted, *i.e.*, the alteration in the total cholesterol level, which was described earlier, is probably not a particularly critical factor in defining risks since total cholesterol contains both beneficial and deleterious fractions.[38] For greater detail on the influences of progestin opposition on the coronary heart disease risk factors, the reader is referred to Chapter 6.

The influences of progestin opposition to estrogen on the osteoporotic process are currently unresolved. However, the several studies in which one or another form of progestin was added to different estrogen replacement therapy regimens appeared comforting. The beneficial effects in bone response when progestins were involved were equivalent to results when they were not involved.[13,15,70] Norethisterone acetate (1 mg 10 days per month) and methyltestosterone (5 mg per day 21 days per month) have each been evaluated in opposition to estrogen therapies. In all cases the response to hormones was decidedly better than the response to placebo. It therefore appears that progestin by itself is effective in providing benefits to bone, and in opposition to estrogen it may be even better. The reader is referred to Chapter 2.

PLASMA HORMONE RESPONSE TO PROGESTIN OPPOSITION

A few reports reveal the plasma responses to different doses of progestin,[35,49,69,101] but the paucity of studies makes any firm conclusions untenable. Nonetheless, some information can be gleaned. Progestin appears to be equilibrated rapidly within the system. One day appears to be all it takes.[69] Pharmacokinetic studies and pharmacodynamic studies of estradiol valerianate opposed with 0.5 mg D/L norgestrel have been clear in showing a rapid equilibration.[24] Figure 7–10 provides an example in one woman, although other women showed similar patterns.

When norethisterone acetate (5 mg, 7 days each cycle) was given in opposition to conjugated equine estrogens (1.25 mg) cyclic with a 7-day, hormone-free period each cycle, the addition of norethisterone tended to increase serum equilin and to depress by about 15% the levels of E2 and E1.[10]

In general, high doses of estrogen are opposed with high doses of progestin, and low doses of one permit low doses of the other. Aylward and co-workers combined norethisterone 5 mg with ethinyl oestradiol 30 μg, Premarin 1.25 mg, oestrone piperazine sulfate 3.0 mg daily, or oestradiol valerate 2.0 mg daily.[6] Lower doses of

FIG. 7-10. Pharmacodynamic response to 17β-estradiol (2 mg) opposed by 0.5 mg DL/norgestrel in one woman (Englund DE, Johnson EDB, 1977, Acta Obstet Gynecol Scand 65:27–31)

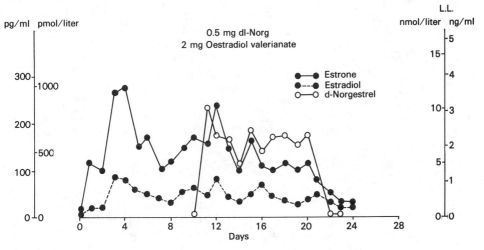

norethisterone (2.5 mg) were opposed to lower doses of estrogen (half of each of the foregoing). All regimens showed satisfactory endometrial effects. In the Aylward study, one hormone-free week per cycle was prescribed, as was 6 days of progestin with 21 days of estrogen therapy.

Prolactin response to progestin appears to be initially minimal.[35,49,105] Short-term studies indicate no change.[49] Longer-term studies indicated that prolactin was consistently increased in plasma in all women who had taken progestin opposition to estrogen for more than 12 months.[35] The elevation was statistically significant but the magnitude was too slight to be of concern. It was not related to the dose of estrogen involved in one study of low-dose progestin (1 mg norethisterone acetate 10 days each cycle) opposed to different strengths of estradiol 17β (both cyclic and continuous). Not only does progestin therapy have a protective effect on the endometrium but it is complementary to the estrogen in these other factors—provided that the doses of estrogen and progestin are balanced with each other.

PROGESTIN INFLUENCE ON AFFECT

There has been some suggestion in the literature that progestin has a pharmacologic effect on mood in the higher doses that were prescribed originally. For example, Dennerstein and co-workers, in opposing 50 μg per day of ethinyl estradiol with 250 μg of levonorgestrel, showed that anxiety, irritability, and insomnia were less well relieved on progestin-opposed estrogens than on estrogen alone.[20] In time, this changed and by the third therapy month, some kind of accommodation was apparent.[20] Women taking progestin with their estrogen did report comfort. In contrast, the study of Fedor-Freybergh described in earlier chapters reported no difficulties with the progestin opposition they used.[26] However, they had prescribed a 30-μg dose of D-norgestrel —considerably less than in the Dennerstein study. Dennerstein had also shown differences in flush response to estrogen alone (excellent) versus estrogen combined with progestin for a sequence each month (less good at first).[19] These issues remain unresolved but the antiestrogenic effect of the progestogen is apparent.

CURRENT DOSING RECOMMENDATIONS

Recent data support the value of a low-dose, long-duration progestin regimen each month. The low-dose quantity for norethisterone acetate is 1 to 1.5 mg/day; for medroxyprogesterone acetate it is likely to be 2.5 mg/day; doses for others are discussed in sequence below. Long duration means more than 9 days.

Norethindrone (Norethisterone)

Norethindrone (norethisterone) has been studied in several doses, generally from 2.5 mg to 5 mg per day, usually for 5 to 13 days per cycle.[6,34,60,91,97-99,101] Endometrial response to different doses of the progestins has indicated that whereas the high doses of progestins opposed to estrogens given for long durations (see Chap. 5) are also fully adequate for protection,[6,60] the newer, low doses of norethindrone are fully able to suppress DNA synthesis and nuclear estradiol receptor in endometrial tissue.[97-99] The fully effective norethindrone dose appears to be 1 mg per day for 10 days.[97,99]

Studies of the response of lipoproteins to equivalent doses of norethisterone indicate that the higher doses sometimes produce marginally adverse effects.[34] One can refer to Chapter 6 for details. Norethisterone in doses of 10 mg for 3 full weeks coordinated with simultaneous ingestion of 20 μg per day of ethinyl estradiol did show some tendency to adversely affect the lipoprotein response.[34] The addition of norethisterone tended to reverse the beneficial effects on lipids of ethinyl estradiol. However, the fact that progestin was administered over such a long period (21 days) and at such a high dose (10 mg) renders the normal physiological response to lower doses undefined.

Norethindrone Acetate (Norethisterone Acetate)

One of the most beautifully characterized progestin/estrogen combination studies has been carried out by the Scandinavian group. Figure 7–11A–D shows the different combinations of estradiol, estriol, and norethisterone acetate with protocols involved.[12] One notes that the high-dose and medium-dose estrogen therapies were continuous, that is, they contained no hormone-free days. The low-dose regimen included a 6-day, hormone-free interval each cycle. In Figure 7–11B, the Kupperman index indicates the dose response for the three different doses compared with placebo. Figure 7–11C shows that women with high-dose continuous therapy had the greatest incidence of regular bleeding. Regular bleeding was defined as a bleed beginning between days 19 and 22, shortly after the initiation of the progestogen opposition. This occurred in every one of the 12 cycles studied for 80% of the women in the high-dose group. This is especially noteworthy because it occurred in the face of continuous therapy with no hormone-free days. Figure 7–11D indicates the percent suppression of serum FSH calculated during the 12 months of treatment. This dose, 1 mg of progestin, is much lower than the 10-mg dose described in other recent research studies.[38] If a low dose of progestin can effectively induce endometrial shedding, one can avoid the problems (lipid alterations, affective symptoms) of the higher doses.

More recently, 1.5-mg norethisterone acetate opposition to 1.5 mg estrone did significantly reduce serum HDL-Ch.[105] The effects of various doses of progestins on glucose tolerance have not been systematically studied, although the finding that even on high doses of progestin all women were within normal limits rendered the carbohydrate metabolism system less likely to be a critical one for potential adverse effects.[91]

D-Norgestrel, L-Norgestrel, D/L-Norgestrel

A number of reports have evaluated different doses of norgestrel with respect to endometrial response and lipid factors. Affect and symptom response have also been evaluated with this hormone. Dose ranges have been wide, ranging from 37.5 μg per day[61] to 75 μg per day[97] and up to as much as 500 μg per day.[24,38,58,60] In addition, Fedor-Freyburgh studied D-norgestrel at doses of 30 μg.[26] Duration of progestin administration, each cycle, ranged from 5 to 21 days, opposed to 21 to 28 days per cycle of estrogen. The lowest doses tested are fully effective at relieving the risk of endometrial hyperplasia. Although high doses consistently are effective, the low doses are at least as effective.[6,97–99]

Medroxyprogesterone Acetate

Probably because medroxyprogesterone acetate is not an androgenic derivative, it has enjoyed the greatest popularity in hormone replacement therapy regimens. Rightly so. Although 10-mg doses for 10 to 13 days had been the recommended level,[38,57] the more recent discoveries of endometrial response at much lower doses of the 19-

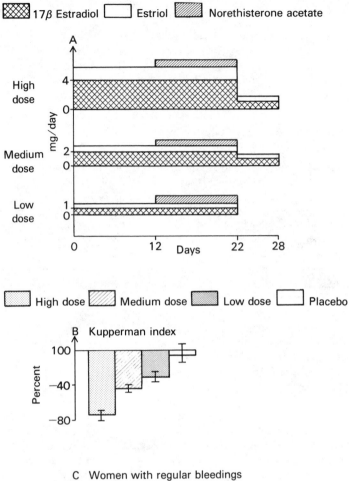

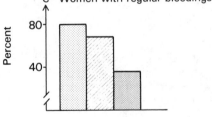

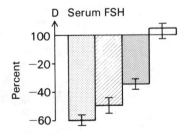

FIG. 7-11. Oestrogen/progestin variations: dose response results with 1 mg norethisterone acetate in three different regimens, contrasted with placebo (Christensen C, Hagen C, Christiasen C, Transbol I, 1982, Am J Obstet Gynecol 144:873–879

nortestosterone derivatives leads to the likelihood, currently untested however, that adequate doses of medroxyprogesterone acetate will prove to be much lower than those currently in use.

Megestrol Acetate

Two reports of sequential ethinyl estradiol 100 μg coupled to 1 mg megestrol acetate for 5 days in each cycle were published.[89,91] At these dosages, all were within normal limits on glucose tolerance tests and there was no change toward hypercoagulability in any of the measures evaluated: platelet aggregation, fibrinolysis, and platelet count.[89] Moreover, these ethinyl estradiol and progestin doses exceed current recommendations.

More recently, 5 mg megestrol acetate for 10 days each month was coupled with 1.5 mg sodium estrone sulfate (21 days each month).[105] Symptom relief was excellent with no changes in the serum triglycerides; fasting blood glucose levels were unaffected as well.

PROGESTINS UNOPPOSED TO ESTROGENS

For the patient who should not be taking estrogens, there has been some question about the value of unopposed progestin therapy. A number of investigations of different progestins have been reported using oral medroxyprogesterone acetate, norgestrel, norethindrone acetate (norethisterone acetate), norethindrone (norethisterone), and ethinyl diacetate. Unfortunately, only one or two studies per hormone have been reported, and they have not necessarily evaluated the same dimension.

Several studies on oral medroxyprogesterone acetate have been reported. The dosages ranged from 10 mg a day to 20 mg per day;[5,78] in one study, 50-, 100-, and 150-mg/day dosages were used.[56] At 20 mg per day, hot flushes responded significantly better to progestin than to placebo.[5,78] At the higher dosages, given by injection, all were fully effective at relieving hot flashes.[56] The 10-mg a day dose increased LDL-Ch (harmful) but caused no change in the (beneficial) HDL-Ch concentration.[84]

Ethinyl-diol-diacetate at 0.05 mg per day yielded no abnormal glucose tolerance in postmenopausal women.[91] Norethisterone in doses of 5 mg per day showed an effect on calcium metabolism that was similar to that of estrogens.[30] Although there was no consistent change in plasma calcium, there was a clear decline in the amount of calcium excreted in urine.

Norgestrel, at a 1-mg a day dose for a year, yielded no change in androstenedione but did reduce gonadotropins in one study of 36 ovariectomized women.[83] Elsewhere, 1.8 mg per day resulted in a 36% increase in the level of serum triglycerides.[84] In the studies of Nielsen, a dosage of 0.5 mg per day for 10 days out of every month yielded a decline in triglycerides of about 10% with no change in cholesterol level.[58]

Norethindrone acetate at a dosage of 5 mg per day given to 12 women yielded a decline in serum HDL-Ch—the beneficial lipid.[8] In one study using 10 mg per day, norethisterone acetate, also produced a decline in HDL-Ch.[84]

It therefore appears that there is a dose-dependent difference in the triglyceride, HDL-Ch, and LDL-Ch responses. The potential tendency of unopposed progestin at high doses to adversely alter lipid metabolism is real. It also appears that such effects do not occur at the new lower doses currently being tested. Progestin is also being studied in repository, injection, and suppository form. In one study, five subjects were provided with vaginal suppositories created specially for that study; one of three different media was used in combination with 25 mg of progestin per suppository.[63] All three forms, glycerinated gelatin, cocoa butter, and polyethylene glycol, were effective vehicles for carrying the progestin, and plasma levels were similarly elevated by all three.[63]

Depot medroxyprogesterone acetate has been studied in doses ranging from 10-mg injections to 150-mg injections in normal postmenopausal patients[9,59] as well as in cancer patients at much higher doses of 400, 700, and 1200 mg.[37] Whereas at the high doses the adrenals were suppressed,[37] at the lower 10-mg or 100-mg doses plasma progestin increases were noted. At the lowest dose of progestin injections (10 mg) an LH surge followed, but at the higher dosage (100 mg) no LH response was noted.[59] At a dosage of 150 mg per month, there was effective relief of hot flashes but no change in the vaginal physiology.[9]

It therefore becomes apparent that unopposed progestin has limited benefit in a menopausal hormone replacement therapy regimen. Although it is effective at relieving hot flashes, its potential deleterious effects on lipid metabolism, gonadotropins and adrenal activity, renders unopposed progestin a less worthy choice for menopausal management.

CYCLIC VERSUS CONTINUOUS: WHICH IS BEST?

Although there are researchers who feel that one or the other of the two methods is preferable, no real conclusion is justifiable from the data at hand. The work of the Scandinavian group (Fig. 7–11) shows that, contrary to the impression of some, women on continuous hormone replacement therapy do show regular bleeding as a dose-dependent response. If one considers the increased comfort obtained by continuous hormone therapy and the failure to show any true benefit of taking a withdrawal period, the issue becomes moot. Perhaps future studies will reveal more information on this issue. For now, there is no obvious answer.

OTHER ENDOCRINE RELATIONSHIPS

CATECHOLESTROGENS

Catecholestrogens are formed in the liver and central nervous system through hydroxylation at the C-2 carbon.[28] A high binding affinity to uterine estradiol receptors has been noted for catecholestrogens.[28] Therefore, catecholestrogens, in certain systems, are antiestrogenic because they have less than 0.1% of the uterotrophic activity but occupy the receptors. In an early report of the human biological activity of catecholestrogens, Adashi and co-workers showed that with prior estrogen priming (ethinyl estradiol) but not without, 2-hydroxyestrone produced effects.[1] After a 5-day course of treatment, progressive decrements in the release of both gonadotropins were observed for 18 hours. The prolactin levels remained unaltered, which suggested to the authors that 2-hydroxyestrone does not interact with the dopaminergic receptors. Adashi and colleagues concluded that catecholestrogen inhibits the release of gonadotropins and may be involved in the feedback regulation of gonadotropin secretion.[1]

In a study of postmenopausal women, a 4-hour infusion of the catecholestrogen, 2-hydroxyestrone, was evaluated.[8] Among women taking Premarin, powerful prolactin suppression was noted. Among women taking no hormones (unprimed), no effect on prolactin or gonadotropins was observed.[81] It does therefore appear that catecholestrogens play a significant role in the suppression of gonadotropin.

THE INFLUENCE OF THYROID HORMONE LEVELS

The effect of altering thyroid hormone concentrations on plasma gonadotropins in postmenopausal women has been studied.[90] Taylor and co-workers showed an inverse relationship between thyroid hormone and the concentration of FSH in hyperthyroid patients that responded to carbimazole by a reduction of T4, an increase of TSH, and an increase of FSH. In the untreated, thyrotoxic (high T4) state, abnormalities in LH-FSH ratios were noted.[90] The LH did not change but the FSH did, yielding a higher LH to FSH concentration when the drug lowered the T4. Others have shown that in thyrotoxicosis a decrease in metabolic clearance rate of 17β-estradiol and testosterone occurs that is due to an increase in the sex hormone-binding globulins (SHBC). During thyrotoxicosis therapy, a decrease in SHBG occurs with a subsequent increase in metabolic clearance rate for the 17β-estradiol. This finding of an inverse relationship between FSH and T4 suggested to Taylor and co-workers that thyroid concentrations have a significant effect on the feedback control of FSH—either by changes in steroid metabolism or by feedback alterations at the hypothalamic level.

Five postmenopausal women were given TRH, and hormone response was measured.[48] All showed significant T4 response with no changes noted for either gonadotropin or the steroids, estrogens, and progesterone. Thus, TRH, while elevating the T4, did not produce the clinical thyrotoxic response.[48]

HUMAN GROWTH HORMONE

Human growth hormone (HGH) appears to be affected by estrogen in both men and women.[27] There is a striking sex difference in ambulatory state growth hormone levels in plasma, although basal levels, within the first 2 minutes of first awakening in the morning, are not considerably different between men and women.[27] Ambulatory levels of human growth hormone in men remain at about the same levels as basal levels, but ambulatory levels in women show a striking cyclic effect that almost identically parallels the rise and fall of estrogen levels through the menstrual cycle. At menopause, this ambulatory elevation is lost and ambulatory levels appear, on the basis of small sample size, to match those of men. Menopausal women and normal men treated with diethylstilbestrol show striking elevations of ambulatory growth hormone without any appreciable elevation of basal levels.[27]

CORTICOSTEROIDS

Corticosteroids produce marked reductions in plasma levels of estrone, androstenedione, and testosterone in menopausal women.[17] The details of these data are provided in Figures 2–20, 2–21, and 2–22. Because of the adverse effect of corticosteroids on gonadal steroid levels, Crilly has suggested that corticosteroid-treated women be prophylactically treated with dehydroepiandrosterone, a precursor of androstenedione. In his initial trials, 10 mg b.i.d. provided an effective dosage for increasing androstenedione, oestrone, and testosterone to more appropriate physiologic levels.[17] The clinician should be alerted that corticosteroids have a profound influence on promoting osteoporosis that can be modified by estrogen therapy.

HUMAN CHORIONIC GONADOTROPIN

Although it is no longer in use, it is relevant to note the effect of human chorionic gonadotropin (HCG) in postmenopausal women. Dynamic tests in which the ovaries were stimulated by gonadotropins yielded estrogens produced by nonovulable postmenopausal follicles. This was observed when 50,000 IU of HCG was given, resulting in an estrogen type vaginal maturation index and an increase in estrogen in the urinary assays.[62]

NEED FOR VITAMIN B₆ ON ESTROGEN REPLACEMENT THERAPY

As described earlier, vitamin B_6 is suggested as an adjunct to estrogen therapy since xanthurenic acid secretion is abnormally high after L-tryptophan challenge in estrogen users. This high excretion, or L-tryptophan depletion, is associated with depression in women taking oral contraceptives, though not necessarily in menopausal estrogen users.[36] Currently, the recommended dosage of vitamin B_6 is 100 mg per day. One should be cautioned, however, that persistent high dosages of vitamin B_6 (2 to 6 g/day) may have adverse effects.[75]

GONADOTROPIN RESPONSE TO HORMONE REPLACEMENT THERAPY

The gonadotropin response to various doses of estrogen with or without progestins was described elsewhere in this chapter. In summary, there is a clear tendency for a dose-related decline in gonadotropins when hormone therapies are given. Particularly noteworthy is the failure to achieve premenopausal levels even though high doses of estrogen may be given. Such results caused some investigators to postulate an ovarian inhibin to account for the reduction in gonadotropin in women with younger ovaries. Because the catechoestrogens, in the estrogen-primed woman, further reduce gonadotropin levels, these may act as an inhibin. The issue remains unresolved.

A WOMAN'S PHYSICAL STATURE AND HORMONE DOSING

Slender women taking estrogen replacement therapy and obese women seem to be at highest risk for endometrial cancer.[44] Judd and co-workers have suggested that slender women may have more symptoms due to lower endogenous estrogen production, which causes them to seek therapy, and that the estrogen is overdosed in thin women because the size of the woman is generally not counted as relevant in defining appropriate doses. Nonetheless, given a lower body mass, there is a strong likelihood of a lower ability to metabolize equivalent quantities of hormone. Since continued unopposed estrogen appears to increase the likelihood of malignant transformation, it is important that the clinician attempt to titrate the doses to the size of the women as well as to the specific agent, because some estrogens are reposited in the fatty stores to a greater extent than others. No definitive studies have yet appeared to guide with numbers.

CONCLUSIONS

Replacement hormone therapy is of inestimable value to the perimenopausal and postmenopausal woman provided that it is prescribed judiciously. In general, it is apparent that this replacement therapy should be provided with a sensitivity to the specific needs of the individual woman. Progestin opposition is proving its value as well. The lowest doses of progestin as well as estrogen (if adequate calcium is ingested) will relieve the symptoms. Moreover, it also prevents or corrects osteoporosis and minimizes the risks of coronary heart disease. Furthermore, it probably represses the carcinogenic transformation of the endometrium and the breast. Continuous daily ingestion of a natural form of estrogen supported by some 10 to 13 days of a low-dose progestogen (preferably not a nortestosterone) each month appears to be optimal.

Sublingual or vaginal estrogen, at the appropriate dose, may be an acceptable route of administration. Presently, only Premarin is available as a vaginal cream in appropriate doses. If micronized estradiol is given by the sublingual route, one-half a tablet on alternate days is necessary to achieve an acceptable blood level.

REFERENCES

1. Adashi EY, Rakoff J, Divers W, Fishman J, Yen SSC (1979) The effect of acutely administered 2-hydroxyestrone on the release of gonadotropins and prolactin before and after estrogen priming in hypogonadal women. *Life Sci* 25:2051–2055.

2. Aitken JM, Hart DM, Lindsay R (1973) Oestrogen replacement therapy for prevention of osteoporosis after oophorectomy. *Br Med J* 3:515–518.

3. Aitken JM, Hart DM, Lindsay R (1976) Long term oestrogens for the prevention of postmenopausal osteoporosis. *Postgrad Med J* 6:18–25.

4. Aitken JM, Lorimer AR, Hart DM, Lawrie TDV, Smith DA (1971) The effects of oophorectomy and long term mestranol therapy on the serum lipids of middle aged women. *Clin Sci* 41:597–603.

5. Albrecht BH, Schiff I, Tulchinsky D, Ryan K (1981) Objective evidence that placebo and oral medroxyprogesterone acetate therapy diminish menopausal vasomotor flushes. *Am J Obstet Gynecol* 139:631–635.

6. Aylward M, Maddock J, Parker RJ, Protherde DA, Ward A (1978) Endometrial factors under treatment with oestrogen and oestrogen/progestogen combinations. *Postgrad Med J* 54:74–81.

7. Bolton CH, Ellwood M, Hartog M, Martin R, Rowe AS, Wensley RT (1975) Comparison of the effects of ethinyl oestradiol and conjugated equine oestrogens in oophorectomized women. *Clin Endocrinol (Oxf)* 4:2:131–138.

8. Bradley DD, Wingerd J, Petitti DB (1978) Serum high density lipoprotein cholesterol in women using oral contraceptives, estrogens and progestins. *N Engl J Med* 299:17–20.

9. Bullock JL, Massey FM, Gambrell RD Jr. (1975) Use of medroxyprogesterone acetate to prevent menopausal symptoms. *Obstet Gynecol* 46:2:165–168.

10. Burnier AM, Martin PL, Yen SSC, Brooks P (1981) Sublingual absorption of micronized 17β-estradiol. *Am J Obstet Gynecol* 140:146–150.

11. Campbell S, Whitehead M (1977) Oestrogen therapy and the menopausal syndrome. *Clin Obstet Gynaecol* 4:1:31–47.

12. Christensen MS, Hagen C, Christiansen C, Transbol I (1982) Dose response evaluation of cyclic estrogen/gestagen in postmenopausal women. *Am J Obstet Gynecol* 144:873–879.

13. Christiansen C, Christensen MS (1981) Bone mass in postmenopausal women after withdrawal of oestrogen/gestagen replacement therapy. *Lancet* 28:459–461.

14. Christiansen C, Christensen MS, Hagen C, Stocklund KE, Transbol I (1981) Effects of natural estrogen/gestagen and thiazide on coronary risk factors in normal postmenopausal women. *Acta Obstet Gynecol Scand* 60:407–412.

15. Christiansen C, Christensen MS, Larsen NE, Transbol I (1982) Pathophysiological mechanisms of estrogen effect on bone metabolism. *J Clin Endocrinol Metab* 55:1124–1130.

16. Cooke ID, Anderton KJ, Lenton E, Burton M (1976) Hormone patterns at the climacteric. *Postgrad Med J* 52:6:12–16.

17. Crilly RG, Horsman A, Marshall DH, Nordin BEC (1978) Post-menopausal and corticosteroid-induced osteoporosis. *Front Horm Res* 5:53–75.

18. Deghenghi R (1980) Chemistry and biochemistry of natural estrogens. In: *The Menopause and Postmenopause: Proceedings of an International Symposium Held in Rome, June, 1979*, pp 3–16. Pasetto N, Paoletti R, Ambrus JL (eds). Lancaster, MTP Press.

19. Dennerstein L, Burrows G, Hyman G (1978) Menopausal hot flushes: a double blind comparison of placebo, ethinyl oestradiol and norgestrel. *Br J Obstet Gynaecol* 85:852–856.

20. Dennerstein L, Burrows GD, Hyman G (1979) Hormone therapy and affect. *Maturitas* 1:247–259.

21. Dequeker J, de Proft G, Ferin J (1978) The effect of long-term oestrogen treatment on the development of osteoarthrosis at the small hand joints. *Maturitas* 1:27–30.

22. Deutch S, Ossowski R, Benjamin I (1981) Comparison between degree of systemic absorption of vaginally and orally administered estrogens at different dose levels in postmenopausal women. *Am J Obstet Gynecol* 139:967–968.

23. Edgren RA (1981) Pharmacology of hormonal therapeutic agents. In: *Menopause: Comprehensive Management.* Eskin BA (ed). New York, Masson.

24. Englund DE, Johansson EDB (1977) Pharmacokinetic and pharmacodynamic studies on estradiol valerianate administered orally to postmenopausal women. *Acta Obstet Gynecol Scand* 65:27–31.

25. Erlik Y, Meldrum DR, Lagasse LD, Judd HL (1981) Effect of megestrolacetate on flushing and bone metabolism in postmenopausal women. *Maturitas* 3:167–171.

26. Fedor-Freybergh P (1977) The influence of estrogens on the well-being and mental performance in climacteric and postmenopausal women. *Acta Obstet Gynecol Scand* 64:1–66.

27. Frantz AG, Rabkin MT (1965) Effects of estrogen and sex difference on human growth hormone. *JCEM* 25:1470–1490.

28. Gahwyler (1978) Introduction. In: *The Role of Estrogen/progestogen in the Management of the Menopause,* pp 1–8. Cooke ID (ed). Baltimore, University Park Press.

29. Gallagher JC, Aaron J, Horsman A, Marshall DH, Wilkinson R, Nordin BEC (1973) The crush fracture syndrome in postmenopausal women. *Clin Endocrinol Metab* 2:293–315.

30. Gallagher J, Nordin BEC (1975) Effects of oestrogen and progestogen therapy on calcium metabolisms in post-menopausal women. *Front Horm Res* 3:150–176.

31. Gambrell RD, Castaneda TA, Ricci CA (1978) Management of postmenopausal bleeding to prevent endometrial cancer. *Maturitas* 1:99–106.

32. Gambrell RD, Maier RC, Sanders BI (1983) Decreased incidence of breast cancer in postmenopausal estrogen-progestogen users. *Obstet Gynecol* 62:435–443.

33. Geola F, Frumar AN, Tataryn I, Lu K, Hershman J, Eggena P, Sambhi M, Judd H (1980) Biological effects of various doses of conjugated equine estrogens in postmenopausal women. *J Clin Endocrinol Metab* 51:620–625.

34. Gustafson A, Svanborg A (1972) Gonadal steroid effects on plasma lipoproteins and individual phospholipids. *J Clin Endocrinol Metab* 35:203–207.

35. Hagen C, Christiansen C, Christensen MS, Transbol I (1982) Long term effect of oestrogens in combination with gestagens on plasma prolactin and FSH levels in postmenopausal women. *Acta Endocrinol* 100:486–491.

36. Haspels AA, Bennink HJ, Van Keep PA, Schreurs WH (1975) Estrogens and Vitamin B6. *Front Horm Res* 3:199–207.

37. Hellman L, Yoshida K, Zumoff B (1976) The effect of medroxyprogesterone acetate on the pituitary adrenal axis. *J Clin Endocrinol Metab* 42:912–917.

38. Hirvonen E, Malkonen M, Nanninen V (1980) Effects of different progestogens on lipoproteins during postmenopausal replacement therapy. *N Engl J Med* 304:560–563.

39. Horsman A, Jones M, Francis R, Nordin C (1983) The effect of estrogen done on postmenopausal bone loss. *N Engl J Med* 309:1405–1407.

40. Hunter DJ, Julier D, Franklin M, Green E (1977) Plasma levels of estrogen, luteinizing hormone, and follicle-stimulating hormone following castration and estradiol implant. *Obstet Gynecol* 49:2:180–185.

41. Isaacs AJ, Havard CW (1978) Effect of piperazine oestrone sulphate on serum oestrogen and gonadotropin levels in postmenopausal women. *Clin Endocrinol (Oxf)* 9:4:297–302.

42. Jacobs HS, Hutton JD, James VHT (1981) Hormonal changes after the menopause and during hormone replacement therapy. In *Functional Morphology of the Human Ovary.* Coutts JRT (ed). Baltimore, University Park Press.

43. Jacobs HS, Hutton JD, Murray MAF, James VHT (1977) Plasma hormone profiles in post-menopausal women before and during oestrogen therapy. *Br J Obstet Gynaecol* 84:314.

44. Judd HL, Davidson BJ, Frumar AM, Shamonki IM, Lagasse LD, Ballon SC (1980) Serum androgens and estrogens in postmenopausal women with and without endometrial cancer. *Am J Obstet Gynecol* 136:859–871.

45. Larsson-Cohn U, Johansson ED, Kagedal B, Wallentin L (1977) Serum FSH, LH and oestrone levels in postmenopausal patients on oestrogen therapy. *Br J Obstet Gynaecol* 85:5:367–372.

46. Laufer L, De Fazio J, Lu J, Meldrum D, Eggen P, Sambhi M, Hershman J, Judd H (1983) Estrogen replacement therapy by transdermal estradiol administration. *Am J Obstet Gynecol* 146:533–540.
47. Lauritzen C (1973) The management of the premenopausal and the postmenopausal patient. *Front Horm Res* 2:2–21.
48. Lee SG, Lundy LE, Kashef M, Dorn J (1975) Influence of thyrotropin-releasing hormone on the postmenopausal female. *Obstet Gynecol* 45:1:25–26.
49. Lind T, Cameron EH, Hunter WM (1978) Serum prolactin, gonadotropin and oestrogen levels in women receiving hormone replacement therapy. *Br J Obstet Gynaecol* 85:2:138–141.
50. Lindsay R, Hart DM, Purdie D (1978) Comparative effects of oestrogen and progestogen on bone loss in postmenopausal women. *Clin Sci Mol Med* 54:193–195.
51. Lobo RA (1982) The modulating role of obesity and 17β-estradiol (E2) on bound and unbound E2 and adrenal androgens in oophorectomized women. *J Clin Endocrinol Metab* 54:320–324.
52. Mahajan DK, Billiar RB, Jassani M, Little AB (1978) Ethinyl estradiol administration and plasma steroid concentrations in ovariectomized women. *Am J Obstet Gynecol* 130:4:398–402.
53. Manolagas SC, Anderson DC, Lindsay R (1979) Adrenal steroids and the development of osteoporosis in oophorectomized women. *Lancet* 2:597–600.
54. Martin P, Yen SSC, Burnier AM, Hermann H (1979) Systemic absorption and sustained effects of vaginal estrogen creams. *JAMA* 242:2699–2700.
55. Mashchak CA, Lobo RA, Dozono-Takano R, Eggena P, Nakamura RM, Brenner PF, Mishell DR (1982) Comparison of pharmacodynamic properties of various estrogen formulations. *Am J Obstet Gynecol* 144:511–518.
56. Morrison JC, Martin DC, Blair RA, et al (1980) The use of medroxyprogesterone acetate (DepoProvera) for relief of climacteric symptoms. *Am J Obstet Gynecol* 138:99–104.
57. Nachtigall LE, Nachtigall RH, Nachtigall RD, Beckman EM (1979) Estrogen replacement therapy II: a prospective study in the relationship to carcinoma and cardiovascular and metabolic problems. *Obstet Gynecol* 54:74–79.
58. Nielsen FH, Honore E, Kristoffersen K, Secher NJ, Pedersen GT (1977) Changes in serum lipids during treatment with norgestrel, oestradiol-valerate and cycloprogynon. *Acta Obstet Gynecol Scand* 56:4:367–370.
59. Nilius SJ, Wide L (1971) Effects of progesterone on the serum levels of FSH and LH in postmenopausal women treated with oestrogen. *J Clin Endocrinol Metab* 42:362–370.
60. Paterson MEL, Wade-Evans T, Sturdee DW, Thom MH, Studd JWW (1980) Endometrial disease after treatment with oestrogens and progestogens in the climacteric. *Br Med J* 96:1–8.
61. Plunket ER (1982) Contraceptive steroids, age, and the cardiovascular system. *Am J Obstet Gynecol* 142:747–751.
62. Poliak A, Seegar-Jones G, Goldberg IB (1968) Effect of human chorionic gonadotropin on postmenopausal women. *Am J Obstet Gynecol* 101:731–739.
63. Price JH, Ismail H, Gorwill RH, Sarda IR (1983) Effect of the suppository base on progesterone delivery from the vagina. *Fertil Steril* 39:4:490–493.
64. Punnonen R (1972) Effect of castration and peroral estrogen therapy on the skin. *Acta Obstet Gynecol Scand* 21:1–44.
65. Punnonen R, Lammintausta R, Erkkola R, Rauramo L (1980) Estradiol valerate therapy and the renin-aldosterone system in castrated women. *Maturitas* 2:91–94.
66. Punnonen R, Rauramo L (1976) Effect of bilateral oophorectomy and peroral estradiol valerate therapy on serum lipids. *Int J Gynaecol Obstet* 14:13–16.
67. Punnonen R, Rauramo L (1976) The effect of castration and oral estrogen therapy on serum lipids. In *Concensus on Menopause Research* Van Keep PA, Greenblatt RB, Albeaux-Fernet M (eds). Proc First International Congress on the Menopause Help in France. . .1976. Baltimore, University Park Press.
68. Punnonen R, Rauramo L (1977) The effect of long-term oral oestriol succinate therapy on the skin of castrated women. *Ann Chir Gynaecol* 66:4:214–215.
69. Rauramo L, Punnonen R, Gronroos M (1979) Serum estrone estradiol and estriol concentrations during oral hormone therapy after oophorectomy. *Int J Gynecol Obstet* 16:348–350.
70. Recker RR, Saville PC, Heaney RP (1977) Effect of estrogens and calcium carbonate on bone loss in postmenopausal women. *Ann Intern Med* 87:6:649–655.
71. Rigg LA, Hermann H, Yen SSC (1977) Absorption of estrogens from vaginal creams. *N Engl J Med* 298:195–197.

72. Riggs BL, Jowsey J, Goldsmith RS, Kelly PJ, Hoffman DL, Arnaud CD (1972) Short and long-term effects of estrogen and synthetic anabolic hormone in postmenopausal osteoporosis. *J Clin Invest* 51:1659–1663.

73. Rozenbaum H (1982) Relationship between chemical structure and biological properties of progestogens. *Am J Obstet Gynecol* 142:7719–724.

74. Saunders DM, Hunter JC, Shutt DA, O'Neill BJ (1978) The effect of oestradiol valerate therapy on coagulation factors and lipid and oestrogen levels in oophorectomized women. *Aust NZ J Obstet Gynaecol* 18:3:198–201.

75. Schaumberg H, Kaplan J, Windebank A, Vick H, Rasmus S, Pleasure D, Brown M (1983) Sensory neuropathy from pyridoxine abuse: a megavitamin syndrome. *N Engl J Med* 309:445–448.

76. Schiff I, Ryan K (1980) Benefits of estrogen replacement. *Obstet Gynecol Surv* 35:400–411.

77. Schiff I, Regestein Q, Tulchinsky D, Ryan KJ (1979) Effects of estrogens on psychological state of hypogonadal women. *JAMA* 242:2405–2407.

78. Schiff I, Tulchinsky D, Cramer D (1980) Oral medroxyprogesterone in the treatment of postmenopausal symptoms. *JAMA* 244:1443–1445.

79. Schiff I, Tulchinsky D, Ryan KJ (1977) Vaginal absorption of estrone and 17β estradiol. *Fertil Steril* 23:1063–1066.

80. Schiff I, Wentworth B, Koos B, Ryan KJ, Tulchinsky D (1978) Effect of estriol administration on the hypogonadal woman. *Fertil Steril* 30:278–282.

81. Schinfeld JS, Tulchinsky D, Schiff I, Fishman J (1980) Suppression of prolactin and gonadotropin secretion in post-menopausal women by 2-hydroxyestrone. *J Clin Endocrinol Metab* 50:2:408–410.

82. Semmens JP, Wagner G (1982) Estrogen deprivation and vaginal function on postmenopausal women. *JAMA* 248:445–448.

83. Sexton L, Anderton KJ, Lenton EA, Brooke LM, Cooke ID (1978) The effects of premarin and norgestrel on plasma FSH, LH and androstenedione in post-menopausal women. *Postgrad Med J* 54:2:42–46.

84. Silfverstolpe G, Gustafson A, Samsioe G, Svanborg A (1979) Lipid metabolic studies in oophorectomized women. Effects of three different progestogens. *Acta Obstet Gynecol Scand* 88:89–95.

85. Simon JA, diZerega GS (1982) Physiologic estradiol replacement following oophorectomy: failure to maintain pre-castration gonadotropin levels. *Obstet Gynecol* 59:511–513.

86. Spellacy WN, Buhi WC, Birk SA (1972) The effect of estrogens on carbohydrate metabolism: glucose, insulin, and growth hormone studies on one hundred and seventy-one women ingesting Premarin, mestranol, and ethinyl estradiol for six months. *Am J Obstet Gynecol* 114:378–392.

87. Stevenson JC, Hillyard CJ, Abeyasekara G, Phang KG, MacIntyre I, Campbell S, Young O, Townsend PT, Whitehead MI (1981) Calcitonin and the calcium-regulating hormones in postmenopausal women: effect of estrogens. *Lancet* 693–695.

88. Stone SC, Mickal A, Rye PH (1975) Post-menopausal symptomatology, maturation index, and plasma estrogen levels. *Obstet Gynecol* 45:6:625–627.

89. Studd J, Dubiel M, Kakkar VV, Thom M, White PJ (1978) The effect of hormone replacement therapy on glucose tolerance, clotting factors, fibrinolysis and platelet behaviour in post-menopausal women. In: *The Role of Estrogen/progestogen in the Management of the Menopause,* pp 41–60. Cooke ID (ed). Baltimore, University Park Press.

90. Taylor MA, Chapman C, Hayter CJ (1977) The effect of altering thyroid hormone concentrations on plasma gonadotropins in postmenopausal women. *Br J Obstet Gynaecol* 84:4:254–257.

91. Thom M, Chakravarti S, Oram DH, Studd JWW (1976) Effect of hormone replacement therapy on glucose tolerance in postmenopausal women. *Br J Obstet Gynaecol* 84:776–783.

92. Tzingounis V, Aksu M, Greenblatt R (1978) Estriol in the management of the menopause. *JAMA* 239:1638–1641.

93. Utian WH (1972) The mental tonic effect of oestrogens administered to oophorectomized females. *S Afr Med J* 46:1079–1082.

94. Utian WH, Katz M, Davey D, Carr P (1978) Effect of premenopausal castration and incremental dosages of conjugated equine estrogens on plasma follicle-stimulating hormone, luteinizing hormone and estradiol. *Am J Obstet Gynecol* 132:297–302.

95. Utian WH (1980) *Menopause in Modern Perspective: A Guide to Clinical Practice* New York, Appleton-Century-Crofts.

96. Whitehead MI, Minardi J, Kitchin Y, Sharples MJ (1978) Systemic absorption from Premarin in vaginal cream. In: *The Role of Estrogen/Progestogen in the Management of the Menopause,* pp 63–72. Cooke ID (ed). Baltimore, University Park Press.

97. Whitehead MI, Townsend PT, Pryse-Davies J, Ryder TA, King RJB (1981) Effects of estrogens and progestins on the biochemistry and morphology of the postmenopausal endometrium. *N Engl J Med* 305:1599–1605.

98. Whitehead MI, Townsend PT, Pryse-Davies J, Ryder T, Lane G, Siddle N, King RJB (1982) Actions of progestins on the morphology and biochemistry of the endometrium of postmenopausal women receiving low-dose estrogen therapy. *Am J Obstet Gynecol* 142:791–795.

99. Whitehead MI, Townsend PT, Pryse-Davies J, Ryder T, Lane G, Siddle NC, King RJB (1982) Effects of various dosages of progestogens on the postmenopausal endometrium. *J Reprod Med* 27:8:539–548.

100. Whittaker PG, Dean PDG (1978) The measurement of equilin in human plasma. In *The Role of Estrogen/progestogen in the Management of the Menopause*, pp 101–109. Cooke ID (ed) Baltimore, University Park Press.

101. Whittaker PG, Morgan MRA, Cameron EHD, et al (1980) Serum equilin, estrone, and estradiol levels in postmenopausal women receiving conjugated equine estrogens ("Premarin"). *Lancet* 1:14–16.

102. Wise AJ, Gross MA, Schalch DA (1973) Quantitative relationships of the pituitary gonadal axis in post-menopausal women. *J Lab Clin Med* 81:28–36.

103. Wynn V (1982) Effect of duration of low dose oral contraceptive administration on carbohydrate metabolism. *Am J Obstet Gynecol* 142:739–746.

104. Yen SS, Martin PL, Burnier AM, Czekala NM, Greaney MO Jr., Callantine MR (1975) Circulating estradiol, estrone and gonadotropin levels following the administration of orally active 17beta-estradiol in postmenopausal women. *J Clin Endocrinol Metab* 40:3:518–521.

105. Ylostalo P, Kauppila A, Kivinen S, Tuimala R, Vihko R (1983) Endocrine and metabolic effects of low dose estrogen progestin treatment in climacteric women. *Obstet Gynecol* 62:682–686.

8

Perimenopausal Bleeding and Hysterectomy

The problems of unexplained vaginal bleeding are perhaps the most troublesome of the clinical menopausal picture. A vigorous approach to diagnosis and treatment is mandatory. First, one must distinguish normal from abnormal vaginal bleeding. In Chapter 1, a detailed description of the menstrual habit at the perimenopause showed an enormous range of normal variation in menstrual cycle length and flow pattern. It is particularly difficult to gauge abnormality from the simple self-report of a perimenopausal woman. Most clinicians first presume an abnormality when unscheduled or unexpected bleeding occurs. Such a cautious attitude has value. Nonetheless, without individualization, too often, invasive studies are relied upon. With an objective, perceptive mind, one can reflect and select the studies that will best define the cause of bleeding described by the patient. The length, timing, the amount, and the quality in context with the history from the patient can be helpful guides. Broadly speaking, the etiology of abnormal bleeding can be either gynecologic or medical. Some may be variations of the norm.

NONGYNECOLOGIC MEDICAL CAUSES OF ABNORMAL BLEEDING

Constitutional diseases such as hypothyroidism and cirrhosis of the liver and chronic anemia, leukemia, and other hematologic malfunctions should all be considered in the diagnostic evaluation of abnormal uterine bleeding.[118] Any one of these may promote a uterine bleeding secondary to the effects of the pathologic conditions reflected.

Hypertension and cardiovascular disease are, perhaps, the most common causes of systemic disease-induced excessive uterine bleeding. Hypothyroidism is the most common metabolic disease provoking hypermenorrhea. Hematologic causes such as platelet diseases, iron deficiency, and anemia appear to promote alterations in mucous membranes as well as in the endometrium that often lead to excess uterine bleeding. Cirrhosis of the liver can also lead to persistent and excessive uterine blood losses. Proper management of the underlying medical problems should stem the bleeding. Detailed management of medical complications are best reviewed in a monograph of internal medicine. It should be noted that, while infrequent in occurrence, these etiologic medical problems should always enter into our diagnostic review.

GYNECOLOGIC PATHOLOGY

The more commonly encountered causes of aberrant uterine bleeding are secondary to gynecologic pathologic conditions. Having said this, we should remember that not all aberrant bleeding is necessarily pathological.[15,107,115,156] Nonetheless it should be part of the differential diagnosis until proven otherwise. The variation and frequency of pathologies are, in the main, ovarian or uterine and vary by age, obesity status, and use of unopposed high-dose estrogen replacement regimens for long durations.[15,25,90,119,174] Fortunately fewer than 15% of women who present with postmenopausal bleeding are found to have endometrial carcinoma, and the incidence of any malignant disease has rarely been found to be higher than 25% of all cases presented.[107] A perspective on the particular pathological conditions found together with the frequency with which they occur offers a realistic view of the problem.

INCIDENCE

There is a paucity of information detailing the incidence of different forms of gynecological pathology associated with uterine bleeding. Several lines of available data suggest disparate results concerning the clinical pictures.

Detection is either heralded with bleeding, pain, or some other condition that forces the patient to seek medical help or is picked up at a general screening, as is sometimes common before starting hormone replacement therapy. Incidence rates vary according to the approach.[112] Less than half of postmenopausal endometria show the atrophic changes of senile tissue. Many are in the proliferative stages even many years after menopause.[14]

Cystic hyperplasia and adenomatous hyperplasia were reported in about 3% of patients in a 1966 large-scale study.[1] However, the detection rate of endometrial cancer at necropsy was 4 to 6 times greater than the detection rate during life. Aspiration curettage of asymptomatic patients receiving estrogen yielded a 16% rate of women who showed either focal adenomatous hyperplasia or a more severe lesion in one sample for which no pretreatment biopsy data had been obtained.[15] About 60% of cervical malignancies are asymptomatic at routine screenings.[73] Ovarian cancer is also silent until well-advanced, with more than half the patients having tumors that extend beyond the confines of the pelvis when first seen and most occurring without any tell-tale postmenopausal bleeding.[156] It would thus appear that a great deal of gynecologic pathology is silent.

Among the most common uterine pathologic conditions that present as a variant function of age are polyps, uterine fibroids, endocrine dysfunction, and malignancy.[118] The fibroids were said to result from the same endocrine dysfunction that created or stimulated the bleeding.[118]

Procope analyzed the etiology of postmenopausal bleeding by reviewing a series of 1100 women over age 45:[124]

Atrophic endometrium, 28%
Hormonal overstimulation, 19%
Malignant conditions, 28%
Polyps, either endometrial or cervical, 17%

Merrill reviewed the causes of postmenopausal bleeding to determine the relative incidence of malignancy (cervix and/or endometrium), endometrial hyperplasia, and atrophic or inadequate endometria.[107] In review of studies from 1930 through 1980, he noted a wide variation in relative rates of malignancy (7% to 63% as the cause for postmenopausal bleeding) as well as in rates of hyperplasia (2% to 46% of cases) and atrophic or inadequate endometrium (3% to 71% of the cases).[107] Other data support these large variations.[31,46,85,99,157,163] It is obvious that there is no consistency.

Some suggest that the rise of unopposed high-dose estrogen replacement therapy in the 1960s and early 1970s accounted for this shift in percentages, but true documentation has not appeared. Nonetheless, it is well accepted that unopposed high doses of estrogen therapies given for long duration do affect the rates of cystic glandular hyperplasia and probably of adenomatous hyperplasia.[59,119]

The relative rates of particular malignancies vary by ethnic pattern also. Jewish females with postmenopausal bleeding have many fewer cases of cervical malignancy[24] whereas those in India have excessively high rates, approaching 50% of all postmenopausal bleeding.[117] The uterine cancer rates in England show equivalent rates of cervical and uterine body disease.[156] The US population may be similar. In 1980, in the United States, invasive cancer of the endometrium accounted for half of all new genital cancers in women.[98] In a 1973 survey of 1600 consecutive primary uterine neoplasms detected over a 30-year period, it was reported that the cervical cancer rate had been declining while the endometrial cancer rate was increasing.[113] The phenomenon was attributed largely to adenosquamous carcinoma. Five-year survival rates were less than 20%, and exogenous estrogens were used by fewer than 20% of these cancer patients. The incidence of endometrial malignancy for all ages in the United States has been reported to be somewhere between slightly less than 1% to figures one-fifth that size.[74,91] Hofmeister reported that 60% of the cervical malignancies were asymptomatic.[73] The data of Horwitz, which suggested asymptomatic rates of endometrial cancer, appear much higher than this.

One is thus left with the obvious dilemma: On the one hand, there may be asymptomatic gynecologic pathology; on the other hand, there may be abnormal bleeding that carries no pathology. Moreover, even this seeming "abnormal" bleeding often is merely a variance of normal. The critical skills of the clinician must be sufficiently sensitive to provide optimal health care for this very difficult problem[135] while not overlooking the underlying pathology.

The Role of Obesity in Gynecologic Pathology

Endometrial cancer is closely associated with height and weight.[174] Heavy women and those of at least average height or taller had a disproportionately large relative incidence of endometrial cancer (see Fig. 5–5). This is presumably due to the increased endometrial stimulation secondary to excess fat conversion of androstenedione into estrogen. Thus, the clinician should counsel obese patients to diet and should also schedule follow-ups more frequently.

Age has also been associated with increased incidence of endometrial cancer (see Fig. 5–1). After age 50, malignancies increase sharply in number.[174] Table 8–1 provides demographic data by country and age for several reproductive pathologies.[123] Parsons and Sommers also observed the age-related increasing vulnerabilities to gynecologic pathology after the age of 40.[118]

THE ETIOLOGY OF ABERRANT BLEEDING

Hypermenorrhea is generally diagnosed unscientifically without any accurate measure of blood loss. Greenberg noted that heavy bleeders are commonly depressed and that depressed patients frequently have hypochondriacal symptoms.[63] The implication is serious—that depression may stimulate false estimates of blood flow. Parsons and Sommers also drew attention to the need for a very patiently taken history in which

TABLE 8-1. Rates of death from selected neoplasms among women age 25 to 34, 35 to 44, and 45 to 54 in selected countries (in deaths per 100,000 women per year)

Place and Year	Age 25-34			Age 35-44			Age 45-54		
	Breast Cancer	Cervical Cancer	Cancer of Corpus Uteri*	Breast Cancer	Cervical Cancer	Cancer of Corpus Uteri*	Breast Cancer	Cervical Cancer	Cancer of Corpus Uteri*
Developing Areas									
Chile 1976	0.8	4.1	0.8	9.0	16.5	2.7	29.8	35.9	7.5
Costa Rica 1976	—	5.7	—	7.6	9.8	4.4	21.9	28.2	6.3
Egypt 1974	1.1	0.1	0.5	4.0	0.2	1.8	7.7	0.8	4.1
Hong Kong 1977	1.0	1.4	—	11.3	4.7	1.4	18.3	17.8	1.7
Mauritius 1977	—	1.6	1.6	12.3	4.9	—	20.1	20.1	11.5
Philippines 1975†	1.5	0.4	1.3	6.9	1.5	4.6	12.3	3.6	8.7
Thailand 1977†	0.2	0.1	1.1	1.3	0.7	4.7	2.6	2.1	7.4
Developed Areas									
England & Wales 1977	4.0	2.1	0.1	22.2	6.0	0.5	64.4	13.6	4.0
Japan 1977	1.5	0.3	0.6	6.5	1.6	2.8	14.2	6.0	9.3
United States 1976	3.2	1.5	0.2	17.3	4.9	1.2	51.1	9.2	3.8

*Includes malignant neoplasms of endometrium, myometrium, body and fundus of uterus, and epithelium of chorionic villi; also unspecified uterine cancer
†Civil registration data considered incomplete and therefore unreliable
—Nil or negligible
Population Reports, 1982, Oral contraceptives in the 1980's. Series A, No. 6 *Population Information Program.* Johns Hopkins University, Baltimore, from World Health Statistical Annual 1979—Vital Statistics and Causes of Death, Geneva.

careful assessment was attempted regarding the amount of bleeding.[118] The problem is a difficult one because the loss of blood is rarely quantified and one must rely on one's own perceptual process in teasing out the information from a potentially stressed patient whose judgment may be skewed.

In general, the quality and the quantity of flow, the time since menopause, and the fact that the bleeding may not necessarily reflect the character of the pathologic condition means that all factors need to be considered.[14,74,107,164] For example, the patient with a submucous fibroid that is located contiguous with the endometrium presents a thinned-out endometrium overlying the tumor. This tumor potentially interferes with the local constrictive effect of the uterine musculature, thereby disrupting the vascular control of bleeding. This does not occur only with submucous fibroids, albeit they are most commonly associated with heavy bleeding; it also occurs with the presence of intramural fibroids, presumably producing vascular backflow. However, a fibroid may not be the sole source of postmenopausal bleeding since, frequently, another condition may also be present.[118,157] Such confusion is more likely in the perimenopausal phases.

Duration of aberrant uterine bleeding has ranged from 1 day to 17 years in one report of 514 cases studied. No relationship between duration and pathology could be obtained. Likewise, the type of bleeding, varying from profuse hemorrhage to spotting, also bore no significant relationship to pathology.[31] Some studies confirmed this absence of a relationship,[14] whereas others have shown that malignancy was more common in those with profuse postmenopausal bleeding than in those with scanty postmenopausal bleeding.[85] The rapid growth of a myomatous uterus in the postmenopausal patient should be considered highly suspicious of malignancy.[102]

Likewise, pain may or may not reflect the degree of pathology.[74,118] For example, a polyp extruding through the uterine cervix can, by its growth and loss of blood supply, produce constrictions that yield pain although the polyps themselves have a generally benign course.[118] Nonetheless, with increasing time since the onset of the menopause, the presence of bleeding increasingly reflects a greater danger (see Fig. 5-2).

In Endometrial Cancer

Investigation of aberrant uterine bleeding will frequently reveal endometrial pathologies. The presence of cystic glandular hyperplasia does not carry a particularly alarming prognosis.[145] Fewer than 1% of patients with cystic glandular hyperplasia will subsequently develop endometrial carcinoma.[104,118] However, adenomatous hyperplasia carries a more serious implication. Among patients not treated, 30% will subsequently develop endometrial carcinoma within 10 years.[66,68] Survival rates vary inversely with age.[106] Moreover, the presence of adenomatous hyperplasia (see Chap. 5) that overgrows and invaginates into the stroma bears careful watching but is not in itself considered appropriate indication for hysterectomy.[118] The diagnosis of atypical hyperplasia, where the individual cells show microscopic abnormalities with great variation from one cell to the next, often seen with cancer may not by itself justify a hysterectomy. However, in concert with other pathologic conditions, atypical hyperplasia may well warrant consideration of hysterectomy. Moreover, confirmation of carcinoma in situ requires a microscopic diagnosis. This carcinoma is slow-growing and appears to take 5 years before placing the patient at risk for invasive cancer. Nonetheless this form, the only of the above described, has been considered irreversible. Adenocarcinoma of the endometrium generally presents with abnormal bleeding. Unfortunately this implies erosion into the vascular bed.

There does appear to be some overlap in the incidence of various pathologic conditions. For example, when Sharma and colleagues evaluated fibroid tumors, the most common finding was cystic glandular hyperplasia, which in the majority of cases occurred at the edge of the tumor.[144] Other common changes included adenomyosis with its separation of glands by muscle fibers from the basal layer of endometrium with distortion and elongation and dilatation of glands.[144] Those authors concluded that the findings of mixed changes in endometrial curettings are common.

In Cervical Cancer

Cervical cancer will also, at times, stimulate bleeding; squamous carcinoma occurs in 95% of cases and adenocarcinoma, in 5%.[82] Herpesvirus may have some responsibility for this cancer, and it is suggested by Jordan that sexually active patients be advised to use occlusive contraceptive therapy. However, cervical cancer does not positively correlate with the number of sexual partners. Nonetheless, it is particularly prevalent among promiscuous or the partners of promiscuous males.[156]

The mean age of the cervical cancer patient at diagnosis is about 51 years for localized cases and 56 years for more diffuse spreading cases.[69] Hakama noted that the stage at diagnosis is an indication of the rate of growth. Furthermore, the older the woman, the faster is the rate of growth of cervical cancer.[69]

In Polyps

Endometrial polyps in younger women do not appear to be dangerous. However, after 60, they often develop into a cancer. The reasons for the bleed can be manifold,[118] but there is a lack of consistent experimental studies to define the cause of the bleedings. Nonetheless, bleeding is generally halted by removing the polyps—provided tht one does not cut a large pedical and thereby create a large exposed surface area.

Endocrine Factors

A variety of endocrine factors can stimulate aberrant uterine bleeding. These include hypothyroidism as well as unopposed estrogen that occurs either naturally in anovulatory cases where little progesterone is secreted, or through prescribed estrogen replacement therapies. The unopposed estrogen can lead to a pattern of endometrial growth that eventually may outgrow the local blood supply and become necrotic; it can also lead to breakdowns in patchy areas and subsequently to bleeding. Such a condition, while distressing to the patient, carries no true malignant potential and should be distinguished from the cancers.[118]

PROLAPSE

Prolapse of the uterus appears most often in the sixth decade[25] and is more common in women who have borne many than in those who have borne fewer children.[118] While not necessarily causing abnormal uterine bleeding, the condition is so distressing that some other form of treatment, usually hysterectomy, is indicated.

Other prolapsed structures, *i.e.*, bladder or bowel, create a variety of pathologic conditions whose surgical correction also should be considered at any age at which they are revealed. The use of pessaries is usually a temporizing measure that inadequately manages these "hernia-like" variations. They are best corrected surgically.

MORPHOLOGICAL FEATURES

A consensus among pathologists describing the morphological picture of the various gynecologic conditions supports the view that the varied and often confusing morphological patterns reflect the capacity of uterine smooth muscle and stroma to undergo alterations in different locations with wide variation with respect to each other.[103,118,132] Therefore a cautious attitude in the diagnosis of any localized region is warranted. Smooth muscle uterine tumors themselves are generally not cancerous. Unless there is increased cellularity mitotic activity, or atypia, they are rarely cause for concern.[19,118] Myoma, fibromyoma or fibroids are the most common sites for uterine neoplasms. The gross appearance, of uterine neoplasms varies widely in size, shape, and location and may appear singly or in clusters. The firmer ones contain more fibrous elements. In contrast, degeneration secondary to interference with blood supply leads to soft tumors unless calcification of the older fatty degeneration occurs. Cancerous or sarcomatous degeneration is rare: it occurs in fewer than 5% of all uterine malignancies. Occasionally it arises from the myometrium itself and not from alterations in a myoma. This malignancy is comprised of fusiform cells with a preponderance of large nuclei with numerous mitoses.

The mitotic index appears to be a useful criterion for determining malignancy; the minimum criterion for malignant behavior in smooth muscle tumors is a mitotic index of

5 mitotic figures per 10 high-power fields in the most active areas.[19,35,103] Where there are at least 10 mitotic figures per 10 high-power fields, the prognosis for the patient living through the next five years is poor. These criteria have been found to be particularly useful in predicting metastasis of smooth muscle tumors of the uterus.[35]

Other observations not helpful in defining prognosis include intranuclear cytoplasmic inclusions, the location of the tumor in a particular part of the uterine wall the maximum tumor diameter, and the presence of other leiomyomas.[19] For further discussion of the endometrial pathology, the reader is referred to Chapter 5.

STEROID MILIEU

The clinical science of reproductive endocrinology is in its infancy. With rapid appreciation of the complexity of this magnificent physiology and thanks to the availability of the technology that affords us this opportunity, continued rapid development is inevitable. Indications are that, with improved assay availability, much information will become available about the neoplastic process by evaluating the plasma levels of both androgens and estrogens or other endocrine related parameters.[22,23,171] The reader is referred to Chapter 5 for the previous discussion. In addition, a few examples follow here. Comparing women with endometrial cancer to age-matched controls, cancer patients have been found to have significantly higher levels of plasma androstenedione,[22] serum total dehydroepiandrosterone,[23] and serum estrone.[22,23] Ovarian vein elevations of testosterone, not appreciated in antecubital veins, were also noted in adenocarcinoma patients.[13] Marked elevations of testosterone into the male range or higher are suggestive of a neoplastic process.[171] Testosterone elevations of two- to threefold can express polycystic ovarian disease, hyperthecosis, or a tumor. These endocrine observations are of increasing interest. Hopefully, the technology and our understanding of their interplay will become clearer in the future.

Other endocrine factors that are reflective of uterine pathology include hypo-thyroidism, which is one of the associates of hyperplasia, as well as unopposed stimulation by estrogens that lead to an endometrial growth that may eventually outgrow the blood supply. Such reasoning may explain the local areas of necrosis that break down and produce bleeding. No definitive statements of exact estrogen levels for such a condition exist, but the continuous estrogen stimulation of the perimenopausal anovulatory ovary is considered to contribute to this[118] as is the unopposed estrogen replacement therapy regimens so common before the advisability of progestin opposition to it became better understood.[57] Sudden reductions in endogenous estrogen level, possibly in the 50% range, can produce endometrial changes that result in bleeding.

Such observations are equivalent to the bleeding seen after exogenous estrogen withdrawal. In the postoophorectomized woman with an intact uterus who has been placed on low-dose replacement of estrogen, sampling of the endometrium 48 hours after withdrawal of estrogen will reveal subnuclear vacuolization in a proliferative endometrium reminiscent of the early postovulatory changes. These estrogen withdrawal effects precede the endometrial breakdown that is seen when bleeding occurs. They are reminiscent of the midcycle bleeding that occurs after ovulation in some women. Breakthrough bleeding probably reflects a similar mechanism but relates to the endogenous metabolism aiding and abetting the interaction of estrogen or progestin on the target organ. Changes in the endocrine histology reflective of estrogen or progestin effects can be quite varied.

GYNECOLOGIC PATHOLOGY—DIAGNOSIS AND MANAGEMENT

PATIENT HISTORY AND EXAMINATION

Recalling the earlier discussions of the normal variation in menstrual patterns at the perimenopause reveals how often the "abnormal bleeding" may actually be normal. Merrill has suggested that a careful history and thorough examination, especially of the endometrium, are most definitely required; even in the presence of a malignant lesion of the cervix, one is cautioned to evaluate the endometrium as well, for it, too, may be harboring malignancy.[107,118] One should not underestimate the importance of the clinician taking time and offering dedicated patience to his or her patients.

It is through such dedicated efforts that the clinician can evaluate the details of a specific patient, *i.e.*, by combining the physical findings with a better appreciation of the general emotional framework of the patient. The clinician should be perceptive of the patient's ability to accurately recall and present her history.

INVESTIGATIVE APPROACHES

A detailed gynecologic examination, whether for postmenopausal bleeding or in an attempt to define whether the patient is a good candidate for hormone replacement therapy, is essential. Inherently included as part of this examination should be cytological diagnosis. In the presence of abnormal bleeding, endometrial biopsy, dilation and curettage and/or hysteroscopy should form the basis for the identification of the pathologic condition. Each has its benefits as well as its risks.

One should be aware that all of the methods for endometrial and uterine assessment are uncomfortable. This is an often overlooked point. For example, Moore, while evaluating pain during hysterosalpingography, concluded that 32% experienced moderate or more severe pain upon placing the tenaculum or the cervix.[109] In addition, if proper application of the tenaculum and careful manipulation are not adhered to, varying degrees of cervical laceration can be experienced. Hamou reminds us of the frequency of these side-effects and points out that commonly these are not even mentioned.[70] Moreover, one should be aware that the cervical os region has a neural innervation pattern that changes as a function of age. Women in their menopausal years are less likely to experience pain because the neural network has diminished greatly. Nonetheless, sensitivity of the gynecologist is essential.

Cytology

Cytology for the diagnosis of endometrial carcinoma is not adequate. The degree of accuracy is complicated by the subtle variations between cancerous and hyperplastic tissue.[107] Moreover the sampling difficulties can pose a problem. Some have attempted to compare the diagnostic accuracy of different forms of cell samplings, and all techniques were judged to be less than satisfactory.[107,151] Anderson and colleagues, evaluating cytological diagnoses of endometrial cancer, compared four cytological techniques on over 2500 specimens in a hospital setting. Misdiagnosis rates (evaluated at subsequent D & C) of 22% to 35% occurred for all four methods: saline irrigation, endometrial brush biopsy, vacuum aspiration, and Gravelly jet washer.[4] It was therefore concluded that, as routine medical care, cytological diagnosis of endometrial cancer leaves much to be desired. There is some ambiguity in the literature. In the hands of Hutton and colleagues, endometrial assessment with the Isaacs Cell Sampler appeared to be considerably more accurate.[76]

Cervical Biopsies

Patients with abnormal cytologic patterns or with abnormal or nonreactive Schiller or Lugol staining of the cervical and vaginal epithelium should have colposcopy-directed biopsies of the abnormal areas. Careful mapping of these areas is helpful in pursuing an accurate diagnosis. Conization, while often considered a compromise to the detailed multiple bunch biopsies of the exocervix, may have greater advantages in accurately appraising the endocervical involvements. The endocervical area should be curetted carefully; endophytic lesions may be difficult to assess.

Endometrial Sampling

In contrast, the endometrial biopsies that use suction appear to be consistently effective. Weinstein and co-workers reported on diagnostic vacuum aspiration curettage in 300 clinic and private patients as carried out by house staff or physicians.[168] All were performed for vaginal bleeding abnormalities; most patients were over the age of 40.

The approach for endometrial biopsy sampling is presented here for those who may find it useful.

> After insertion of the bivalve speculum, cervix and vagina are cleansed with either hypochlorite or betadyne solution. A tenaculum is used to grasp the anterior lip of cervix. The aspiration cannula is gently inserted through the endocervical canal without prior dilatation and generally without need for analagesics. A thin proper curvature of the instrument such as that of the Garcia-Rock endometrial aspirator allows for the introduction of the instrument with minimal discomfort. The AR modification, for the Antiflexed or Retroflexed configuration, has a great curvature that conforms to the patient's angulated uterine cavity. This set of instruments is available from V. Mueller of Chicago. A 20-cc syringe can be used to create a vacuum. Several strokes with a general up and down motion along the anterior, posterior, and lateral walls will provide an adequate specimen that can be blown onto a Telfa pad. The endometrial tissue can thus be isolated from blood before placement in the fixative solution.

Another variance is the Vabra suction that uses a pressure suction pump. Again several strokes with the instrument reaching the higher endometrium will permit the specimen to reach the tissue chamber trap. Depending on the analgesics used and the reactions of the patient after the procedure, it is often advisable to require the patient to rest before she departs. Some 10% may profit from paracervical anesthesia.

With the Vabra, the diagnostic accuracy was excellent and the authors concluded that the advantage of this form of endometrial assay was that it did not require the use of general anesthetics. However, there is some discomfort; some patients tolerate it better than others, the discomfort of the cannula being chief source. It is noteworthy that the instruments that conform to the uterine curvature create less discomfort. Another disadvantage is the fact that polyps cannot be easily removed as they can be with the hysteroscope.

Contraindications for the use of suction curettage include the following:[168]

profuse uterine bleeding
cervical obstruction (tumor, leiomyoma, or trauma)
pelvic infection
intrauterine gestation (except for pregnancy termination)
an anxious patient who cannot remain still while on the examining table

Although the danger of perforation of the uterus is real, this is so only if it is not recognized. Hathcock and co-workers reported generally similar results from a study of 1800 aspiration curettages of the endometrium.[71] The authors concluded that aspiration curettage is effective and does not compromise the safety of the patient. In only 29 cases of the 1800 was a more serious lesion subsequently found, 19 by repeat aspiration when symptoms returned (usually 1 or 2 years later).[71] The authors were convinced that the therapeutic outcome was never compromised in any of these patients and recommended that a mild analgesic combined with a careful, patient explanation to the patients leads to high acceptance of the procedure.[71] The success with the method is not universal [51] and appears to require a high degree of competence and training.[107]

Dilation and Curettage

Dilation and curettage (D & C) has been compared to suction curettage in diagnosing aberrant and abnormal bleeding. In competent hands the diagnostic accuracy seems equivalent. D & C allows for general anesthesia for the anxious patient or the one with a stenotic cervical canal, in whom suction curettage may be more hazardous. Correlations greater than 95% are generally reported.[4,43,95] Cytological procedures are generally less accurate[4,107,151] but there are exceptions.[76]

The frequency with which a D & C misses a diagnosis has been reported to vary between about 10% and 40%.[95] Furthermore, the accuracy with which D & C can be used to diagnose endometrial cancer has not been empirically determined. However, it appears to be fallible, although only a small percentage of the time.[107] Small focal lesions could easily be missed by D & C or by other sampling procedures. Repeat evaluation may be necessary.

Hysteroscopy

The hysteroscope has begun to obtain a more widespread favor in the literature.[41,53,64,163] DeCherney and Polan point out that, when appropriate, the procedure offers a low complication rate and a shorter hospital stay and may obviate the need for more aggressive approaches.[41] Its diagnostic capacity is excellent.[74] There is some controversy as to the appropriate indications and contraindications for its use, most of which revolve around its safety.

Indications for its use have been described by a number of investigators. Hyperplasia of the endometrium, polyps, and submucous fibroids were easily recognizable as early as 1957 with the hysteroscope.[53] By 1960 it was noted that polyps, normal thick endometrial stalks, submucous myomas, intramural myomas, and the general condition of the endometrium could be well characterized through the view allowed by the hysteroscope.[64] Although much can be seen, it is noted that chronic endometritis cannot be distinguished from a normal endometrium.[53]

Several investigators have suggested that hysteroscopy is appropriately indicated for all women with unexplained abnormal recurrent bleeding after recent curettage.[18,74,114] Others suggest that hysteroscopy is appropriately indicated for the investigation of endocervical and intrauterine neoplasms and that these would be an important indication for its use.[100] The issue is far from resolved.

Valle and Sciarra suggested contraindications:[165]

- Recent or existing uterine infection
- Profuse uterine bleeding
- Cervical malignancy
- Pregnancy.

The potential danger of dislodging malignant tissue through the oviducts and into the peritoneal cavity with the hysteroscope mandates caution when cancer is suspected. Should a technique for hysteroscopy allow the investigator to avoid such a problem, conceivably this diagnostic tool would be beneficial. It appears to be the most accurate diagnostic tool currently available for evaluating the endometrial cavity and deflecting resident pathology. Compared with hysteroscopy, curettage permits one to sample the endometrium incompletely resulting in an inaccurate diagnosis rate of 25% to 65%.[53,64,114,164] In the best of hands, the yield from curettage is probably at the higher levels, but hysteroscopy appears to have the potential for a more complete and accurate diagnosis.[70] Table 8-2 shows the uterine hysteroscopic findings observed in premenopausal women with abnormal bleeding.

In comparison, among 115 postmenopausal patients with abnormal bleeding, hysteroscopy revealed polyps in 24%, endometrial cancer in 16%, and endometrial atrophy in 10%.[70]

Perhaps the most significant advantage offered by hysteroscopy is its ability to permit accurate diagnoses of uterine pathologic conditions that may obviate the need for a hysterectomy.[18] Burnett, in reviewing the literature, concluded that endometrial polyps

TABLE 8-2. Hysteroscopic findings in four series of premenopausal patients with premenopausal abnormal uterine bleeding

Findings	Hamou	Siegler	Sciarra	Barbot
Total number of cases	164	36	104	213
Normal cavity	9	15	30	30
Polyps	15	10	42	34
Submucous myomata	49	6	18	44
Endometrial hyperplasia	39	0	4	42
Endometrial atrophy	24	0	0	3
Vascular dystrophy	12	0	0	0
Adenomyosis	3	0	0	3
Synechiae	0	1	2	0
Adenocarcinoma	1	0	0	1
Cervical carcinoma	0	0	0	2
Septum	0	1	4	0
Cesarean section scar	2	0	4	0
Endometritis	10	0	0	0
Placental polyp	29	0	0	0
Decidua (ectopic pregnancy)	3	0	0	0
Other	22	0	0	0

occur in about 3% to 9% of aberrant bleeding problems that were not detected by curettage. Hysterectomy would have been unnecessary with a more appropriate technique for the visualization and removal of the polyps.[18] Table 8–2 shows a range from 10% to 42% of polyps detected by hysteroscopy in patients with abnormal uterine bleeding.[70] The hysteroscope and resectoscope have frequently been used safely to remove the polyps and correct recurrent bleeding.[41] Greater clinical experience should provide more accurate statistics in the future.

Summary and Conclusions

A number of different techniques for evaluating uterine pathology are available, each with its potential value and risk. The hysteroscope holds the promise of greatly increasing the accuracy of the information that can be obtained for diagnosis. In the pre- and perimenopausal woman, hysteroscopy during the early proliferative phase may maximize accuracy since the thin endometrium would be less likely to hinder the view.[64] A word of caution in its use is necessary, however. It is generally agreed that when using the hysteroscope for operative procedures, a simultaneous laparoscopy needs to be performed with two "scopers" communicating back and forth to reduce the possibility of perforation of the uterus. The hysteroscope transillumination through the myometrium heralds the location of the scope. Moreover, blanching of the tissue is observed when excessive pressure is applied and perforation is imminent.[41] Although laparoscopy during the luteal phase has been claimed to be more valuable since the corpus luteum can be visualized to assess that ovulation has occurred,[70] we now know that a corpus can, on occasion, retain its egg and thus mislead the viewer. Moreover, visualization during this phase, particularly with adhesions, can be a detriment because of its inherent fragility leading to ovarian disruption during the probing for visualization. Thus the proliferative phase is best for both laparoscopy and hysteroscopy.

The D & C has long been known to improve aberrant bleeding problems but its method of action remains unclear.[118] The aspiration biopsies, in competent hands, can provide a great deal of information.

HYPERPLASIA

Hyperplasia is closely associated with abnormal uterine bleeding. Unopposed estrogen stimulation by an anovulatory perimenopausal ovary promotes a tendency to produce hyperplasias, as can unopposed estrogen replacement therapies. It has long been known that progestin can correct (reverse) this condition. Thus hyperplasia appears to be preventable, and once discovered it is frequently reversible with progestin therapies. The critical questions revolve around appropriate doses and their schedules.

Gambrell and colleagues have described the efficiency with which The Progestin Challenge Test reduces the risk of endometrial cancer.[57,58,60] Although this test has been reviewed in the earlier chapters, certain salient features are highlighted here. The effective use of progestin therapy in endometrial hyperplasia has been documented, albeit we look forward to larger-scale studies in the future.[169] Progestin therapy in two studies reversed fully the adenomatous and atypical hyperplasia in both premenopausal and postmenopausal women who were diagnosed as having hyperactive endometria.[169] Dosages administered at that time were 100 mg dimethisterone per day for 6 weeks followed by frequent curettings or biopsies. There was no recurrence in any of the 110 patients studied with follow-up durations of 1 to 5 years. In addition to the 100-mg dimethisterone dose, 20 mg of oral megesterol acetate appeared to be equally effective.

Although the authors of that study concluded that young women should be treated with progestins and older ones with hysterectomy, their own demonstration that both groups responded favorably, combined with preliminary new information suggesting an unfavorable aftermath of hysterectomy, should propose a reevaluation of that perspective. It would be prudent to expect that hysterectomy should be avoided when other therapeutic modalities are available. The risk in waiting appears to be minimal.[172] In their review of up to 8 years after bleeding, Woodruff and co-workers found only 1 of the 333 cases had been a missed malignancy initially and her ultimate hysterectomy provided adequate therapy. They concluded that there is little harm in waiting when malignancy is not found and, by waiting, much needless surgery is avoided.

GENITAL CANCERS

Endometrial cancer accounts for 50% of all genital cancers in women, and the cervical cancer rate closely equals that of endometrial cancer. Uterine sarcomas are rare, occurring in fewer than 10% of all uterine body malignancies. They comprise about 1% of all genital malignancies. Although they are infrequent, they are among the most lethal of all uterine malignancies. In the more advanced cases, palliative approaches with radiation and chemotherapy are offered.[12] In the less progressed cases, surgical extirpation and possible radiation and chemotherapy are used. The peak age incidence for uterine cancer is between 55 and 65 years, and it is more common in women who are infertile or who have had children more than 15 years before their menopause.[98,112,156] Its overall 5-year survival rate is slightly more than 60%.[108] Factors that influence survival include the patient's age when discovered and the stage and grade of the tumor.[98] Risk factors include obesity, nulliparity, estrogen secreting tumors, and adenomatous hyperplasia.[66,67,96,98,156] Although late menopause is believed by some to influence the risk of endometrial cancer,[96,156] others have evaluated cancer patients and found that this was not the case.[98] While estrogens generally are contraindicated in genital malignancies, it has been pointed out that the use of estrogen replacement therapy does not appear to influence the survival rate once the disease is contracted.[98]

It is generally agreed that the appropriate treatment for any form of uterine cancer is hysterectomy, but the confirmation of carcinoma requires a microscopic analysis.[118] Its slow growth rate allows the clinician the time to diagnose the lesion without patient compromise.

Endometrial polyps sometimes grow in polypoid fashion and need to be distinguished from carcinomas that also can grow in polypoid fashion.[118] Competent pathological diagnosis is clearly indicated. Moreover, in the presence of uterine malignancy, Mattingly notes no increased risk of subsequent cervical cancer when the cervix is retained at hysterectomy.[102]

The most important risk factors include the stage of the tumor, the status of the pelvic lymph nodes, the depth of myometrial penetration, tumor grade, the cell type, and the patient age.[12] Berman and co-workers have suggested that radiation therapy should follow, not precede, a pelvic operation because of the inherent inaccuracies in attempting to stage the disease preoperatively. More recent evaluations concur.[39]

Ovarian cancer is silent until it is well advanced. More than half the patients have tumors that extend beyond the confines of the pelvis when they are first seen.[156] Case control studies of women with carcinoma of the ovary have established certain risk factors.[111,153,154] Fewer of the cancer patients have married. There are fewer pregnancies, fewer children, a tendency toward a shorter reproductive span—meaning an early menopause and/or late menarche. Menopause, especially before age 45, is common in the group with ovarian cancer. The most common form is the adenocarcinoma, thought to arise from the surface epithelium. Fifty to 60 years of age is the peak age incidence. The survival rate over the next 5 years approximates 85% in those cases where the tumor is confined to one ovary, is discovered early, and is treated with surgery and subsequent chemotherapy.[156] Edmondson and colleagues have shown the survival rates by months after the start of therapy. Figure 8–1 shows the rapid fatality pattern.[51] Such obvious decline in survival rate heralds an extremely fast-growing cancer. In this treatment regimen, either of two treatments was equally ineffective: cyclophosphamide alone (1 g/m²) for 3 weeks or 500 mg/m² plus Adriamycin 4 mg/m² every 3 weeks IV.[51]

The treatment for ovarian malignancy generally employs surgery (tumor debulking with chemotherapy in advanced disease).[49] Progestational agents have been shown to convert a tumor from one that is proliferative in appearance to one showing secretory activity.[156] However, prompt treatment is currently the most critical factor in predicting disease-free individuals 5 years later. Unfortunately, the silent, rapid growth pattern militates against such a benign outcome.

Receptor Levels

The occurrence of multiple steroid hormone receptors in disease free vs. neoplastic human ovary has been studied.[56] Receptor levels do not adequately differentiate healthy from cancerous tissues for use as a diagnostic tool. A comparison of healthy ovarian tissue, malignant tissue, and benign tumors showed that each class of patient had some overlapping percentage of receptors for 17β-estradiol, progesterone, and $5\text{-}\alpha\text{-}$dihydrotestosterone.[56] This 1981 study was the first to detect ovarian estrogen receptors and progesterone receptors, and we await further investigations of this subject.

Likewise, because it is generally accepted that uterine myomas originate from muscle tissues, it was suggested that ovarian steroids might be controlling their growth.[155] Again the search revealed no insights. Androgen receptors were not found in uterine myometrium or myoma, but estrogen and progesterone receptors were found in both. Although the myoma cell samples contained more estrogen receptors than did myometrium, there was no difference in estradiol uptake between the two tissues. Therefore receptor levels do not appear to provide a critical influence on tumor formation, and other mechanisms in the nucleus were presumed to be involved in the growth of the cancers.[155]

POLYPS

Endometrial polyps with abnormal bleeding are characterized by insidious, persistent, and scant bleeding that becomes heavier only after a long developmental progression. Most frequently, they occur in the late childbearing age. Neither estrogen nor progestin treatment alters the pattern.[18] Because endometrial polyps in older (over 60) women may progress to a cancer, there is some concern about the appropriateness of removing them. Some 3% to 24% of the aberrant bleeding problems derive from polyps, and simple curettage may be inadequate treatment.[18,70] However, controlled curettage with the hysteroscope allows for the successful removal of the polyps and can thereby prevent inappropriate treatment.[18,70]

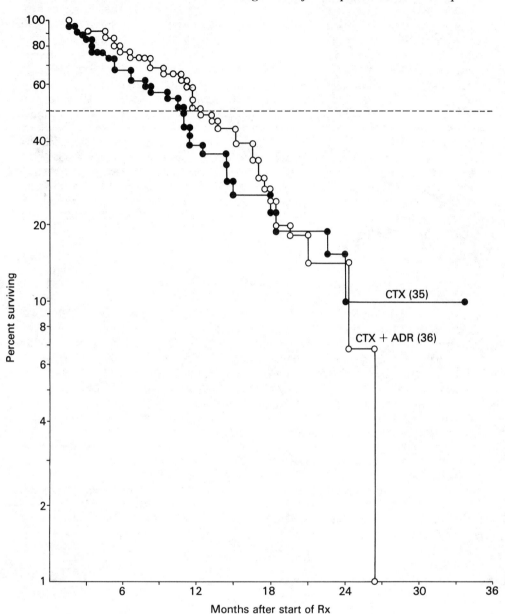

FIG. 8-1. Ovarian cancer survival rates for advanced-disease group (Edmondson J, Fleming TR, Decker DG, Malkasian GD, et al, 1979, Cancer Treatment Rep 63:241–247)

RECURRENT BLEEDING

The problems of recurrent bleeding (frequency, cause, and significance) have not really been resolved in the literature. Hysterectomies for undiagnosed recurrent bleeding are common, but an analysis of the uteri from such hysterectomies shows a high rate of normal organs, suggesting that a repeat D & C or hysteroscopy rather than hysterectomy would have been the preferred treatment.[107] One exception appears to be obesity. When recurrent bleeding occurs in the presence of obesity, the potential for malignancy is high. Some feel that a hysterectomy may be more warranted in obese bleeders since carcinomas are more easily missed.[83,172] However, the proper use of the hysteroscope should eliminate this concern.

Since the critical concern of recurrent bleeding is the potential for malignancy, it is noteworthy that postmenopausal bleeding is coincident with a malignancy in less than 15% of the cases.[107] One prognostic risk factor for malignancy is the length of the clear (no-bleed) span. The longer it lasts before a subsequent bleed, the greater the incidence of malignancy.[120] Malignancy was twice as common after a clear span of more than 24 months than in the shorter clear spans; malignancy occurred in 33% of the less-than-24-month clear spans.[120] Again, properly used, hysteroscopy would have allowed for earlier diagnosis.

Recurrent bleeding is not likely to be associated with malignancy[120,172] and is relatively uncommon. For women with undiagnosed initial postmenopausal bleeding, subsequent recurring bleeding occurred in fewer than 10% of the patients in one report[120] and in 22% of a different sample.[172] In both cases, the authors concluded that the appearance of recurrent bleeding by itself was probably *not* cause for immediate alarm nor did it signal the need for hysterectomy. Although the bleeding is distressing to the patient and worthy of further investigation, the prognosis is generally good.

HYSTERECTOMY

In the United States, an alarming rise in the incidence of hysterectomy over the last 25 years has been reported.[26,27,94,97,136,148,159] Few data are available to explain such a rise. Moreover, variations in the incidence of hysterectomy from one part of the nation to another have been reported by the Centers for Disease Control (Fig. 8–2).

In 1966, demographic surveys suggested that 35% of menopausal women had a surgically induced menopause.[97] Nine years later this rate reached 40%.[148] The overall incidence in the United States accelerated 40% in 7 years: from 300,000 (1970) to 442,000 (1977).[27] The number of hysterectomies performed in the United States increased approximately 60% between 1965 and 1973—far in excess of the population growth.[94] Between 1970 and 1978, more than 35 million women aged 15 to 44 underwent nonradical hysterectomy.[47] The lifetime estimate for the likelihood of having a hysterectomy by age 70 hovers between 52% and 62%, according to demographic analyses.[136] Perhaps the most revealing was a prospective study by Treloar. Data collected from 1935 to 1981 followed women from their menarche to their menopause. From the 769 involved, 31% had a hysterectomy before reaching their natural menopause and all had been part of a healthy college-age population when they entered the study.[159] Just recently, the Centers for Disease Control have indicated a declining hysterectomy rate in the 15- to 44-year-old age group.[27a] The rate per thousand in 1979 was 8.0, in 1980, 7.6. These data contrast with 9.1, 9.0, and 9.1 for 1973, 1974, and 1975.

What remains unanswered is whether there has been an unusual rise in the incidence of uterine pathology. The most common pathologic condition leading to hysterectomy appears to be fibroid tumors (32%). Dysfunctional uterine bleeding accounts for 26%.[29] Uterine prolapse or malposition also accounts for a large proportion of hysterectomies in women aged 15 to 44.[81]

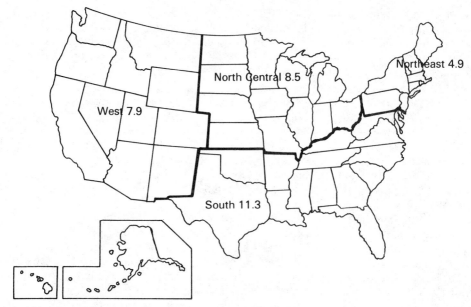

FIG. 8-2. Geographic distribution by region of incidence of hysterectomy in women aged 15 to 44 in the United States from 1976 to 1978. U.S. Department of Health and Human Services, Morbidity and Mortality Weekly Report, April 24, 1981, Vol. 30, No. 5.

In the quest of curing the pathologic problem, the effects of hysterectomy often are dwarfed. Evidence suggests that there are significant aftereffects. Currently available data are inadequate to define the appropriateness of the medical indications for any surgery including hysterectomy.[16,36,55] Although tissue committee and other regulatory mechanisms sincerely aim to assure quality control, their data are not readily available—probably owing to medical-legal reasons. Nonetheless, there have been suggestions that some are done for birth control, for cancer prevention, or to improve the quality of life.[16,116] The latter practices should not be condoned.

Other studies support an increased longevity and reduction in rates of certain diseases after a hysterectomy when it is combined with hormone replacement therapy. This serious issue is complex and requires much more detailed attention before it can be resolved. In the management of the problem presented by the patient, specific details must be stressed.

There are clear problems with hysterectomy, both in the immediate aftermath and in the likelihood for certain long-term consequences. There may also be profound benefits. In determining an appropriate course of treatment, all of these factors must be balanced.

IMMEDIATE POSTSURGICAL AFTERMATH

Most cancers of the endometrium can be treated by simple extrafascial hysterectomy if diagnosed early enough. This avoids the need for radical hysterectomy. Radical hysterectomy is associated with some immediate alterations in bladder physiology: decreased and altered awareness of vesical distention, prolonged postoperative urinary retention, stress incontinence, and hypertonic cystometric findings.[54] Satisfactory voiding occurred significantly earlier (day 20 vs. day 51) in those who had an incomplete transsection of the sympathetic nerves because of division of the cardinal ligaments.[54]

Although castration predictably leads to rapid steroid declines and frequent hot flashes,[6,40] hysterectomy without oophorectomy also frequently is followed by a transient occurrence of hot flashes associated with significant drops in sex steroids.[78,150] This transient, posthysterectomy hot flash appears to be independent of anesthesia, gonadotropin alterations, and prolactin changes.[150] It could be a local interruption of the ovarian blood supply that, in time, returns to normal.

The structures that are particularly sensitive to operative trauma include the pelvic blood vessels and, the rectum, bladder, and ureters.[50,87] There is some variation in postsurgical aftermath depending on whether the vaginal or abdominal route is employed.

When abdominal and vaginal hysterectomies are equally appropriate, the potential aftermath merits consideration. Both vaginal and abdominal approaches yield higher rates of postoperative trauma in clinic patients than in private patients—a situation attributed to the inexperience of the surgeons in such clinics.[170] Wound infections and transfusion rates appear to be more common in abdominal procedures.[170] However, overall postoperative morbidity is generally much higher with vaginal than with abdominal approaches—usually a short-term fever with or without urinary infections.[47,89]

Prophylactic antibiotics are suggested for use with vaginal hysterectomy because they substantially reduce the complication rate.[47] Moreover, vaginal cuff infections are more controlled by meticulous surgical technique than by attempts at prophylactic measures.[52,172] There is some question about the propriety of prophylactic antibiotics in abdominal operations—at least one large study concluded its value was not demonstrable.[47] The excessive cost of postoperative infection was estimated at $1800 for vaginal hysterectomy. For abdominal hysterectomy, a lower figure of $700 was calculated due to the lower incidence of postoperative infection.[143] The costs of specific prophylactic microbials were studied, and a cost benefit analysis showed that the average net benefit for cephazolin sodium (3 doses) was sufficient to make it worthwhile.[143] However, these authors noted that these benefits would be eroded by the newer, more expensive cephalosporins unless they were considerably more effective—a phenomenon that has not been demonstrated.

The potential inconveniences associated with the recovery from surgery should be discussed with the patient as well as the long-term risks. Several potential long-term consequences of hysterectomy that are only now becoming more apparent should be better understood. These include depression, sexual deficits, increased risk of coronary heart disease, and subsequent patient dissatisfaction in an increasingly litiginous world.

LONG-TERM CONSEQUENCES OF HYSTERECTOMY

Depression

There appear to be relationships between hysterectomy and depression. The issues are still unclear and additional research is necessary to clarify and refine our understanding.[38,84,138] Studies have recorded an incidence of hysterectomy-related depression of 7% to 70%.[9,92,101,137] The role of ovariectomy in predisposing the patient to postoperative depression has not been appropriately studied and may prove to be relevant. Recent findings of the role of ovariectomy in reducing β-endorphin levels in female monkeys[167] support the potential of the role of β-endorphin in well-being and depression.

Factors predisposing one to depression have been studied and appear to include the following:[122]

Previous history of psychiatric problems
A medically unnecessary operation
Marital interruption
Very young patient
Lack of any preoperative anxiety
Inadequate preparation for the operation

Any of these can herald a future posthysterectomy depression. It is especially important that the clinician take time to prepare the patient emotionally for her operation as well as to counsel her afterward while she's experiencing the to-be-expected feelings of being damaged.[92] The time-course of convalescence, by self-report, was three times longer for hysterectomized women than for other postsurgical controls.[137] However, other investigators concluded that hysterectomy was no more traumatic than cholecystectomy.[105] Patients who experience a delayed return of energy seem to be the ones particularly likely to become depressed. This is especially so because the depression that does develop tends to appear late in the postoperative period. For example, although most patients followed up for the first 6 postoperative weeks appear not to report depression,[9] those who were followed for 3 years were different. Significantly higher, *i.e.*, 70%, rates of posthysterectomy depression emerged.[137] The majority of depressions occur preoperatively.[110]

Posthysterectomy depression may represent a different problem. Former psychiatric patients are the women most at risk for postoperative depression. By 18 months after the operation, the majority of women who had been psychiatrically treated before surgery were now severely depressed. This finding was compared with one-fourth this incidence among prehysterectomized nonpsychiatric controls.[61] The peak period for postoperative depression occurs 2 years after surgery and begins to decline about 1 year later.[9] After surgery younger women are more likely to be depressed than older ones,[110] a finding not surprising considering the loss of potential childbearing that these younger women endure. No relationship with marital status was observed in one study that investigated this factor.[110]

Effective treatment of postoperative hysterectomy depression depends on its cause and the time at which it is revealed. Estrogen depletion depressions are most properly treated by estrogen replacement therapy,[33] although placebos are as effective as estrogens in the short term when compared with no treatment. Psychiatrically disturbed patients also appear to be at higher risk of undergoing hysterectomy.[3,61] However, women with dysfunctional uterine bleeding were no more psychiatrically disturbed than those with a demonstrable uterine pathologic condition.[61]

We are thus faced with some apparent ambiguities in the literature, all of which suggest that hysterectomy plays some role in postoperative depression and that emotion plays some role in stimulating the potential for hysterectomy. For these reasons, the clinician is alerted and advised to do the following:

1. Establish whether there are preoperative depressions and, if there are, consider carefully whether the excess bleeding report coming from the patient is more a reflection of her depressive state than of any demonstrable pathologic condition
2. Be alert to the potential of a slowly developing depression following hysterectomy and urge that the patient be followed for at least 3 years after surgery, or

3. See that the patient is referred postoperatively to someone alert to the potential for a slowly developing postoperative depression
4. Be sure that the patient is aware of the importance of continuing postoperative care to detect not only the potential of slowly developing postoperative depression but also other deviations from the norm, *i.e.*, pelvic masses
5. Do not overlook the inestimable value that hormonal replacement therapy represents for the woman. Estrogen with progestin opposition should be the prime underlying endocrine theme of her therapy.

Sexual Alterations

The potential for a cervicouterine orgasm was described in Chapter 3. Hysterectomy will necessarily remove the structures that might be involved in such an orgasmic response. There appear to be two distinct neural pathways, carried independently by the pudendal and the pelvic nerves, which transmit afferent stimuli from the genital region in women. However, most of the evidence is drawn from studies in lower mammals. In female rats, the recent discovery of a cervically stimulable neural pathway that terminates in the arcuate nucleus has been firmly established. A summary of the works arriving at this conclusion can be found in a recent review.[37] The arcuate nucleus is particularly pertinent because recent efforts clearly demonstrate that it secretes beta endorphins into the pituitary stalk blood of certain primates. When these primates are ovariectomized and hysterectomized, the pituitary stalk beta endorphin secretion is diminished to nondetectable levels.[167] Subsequent hormone replacement therapy (estrogen and progesterone) to mimic physiologic levels yields a return of the prehysterectomy beta endorphin levels in the pituitary stalk blood.[37] Adequate beta endorphins appear to be necessary for gonadotropin surges.[37] Thus, in at least some mammals (particularly the primates), there may be a neurohormonal network involving cervicouterine tissue that could originate in the cervix and terminate in the pituitary secretion of gonadotropin. Hysterectomy would disrupt such a reflex pathway. Recently, Kilkku and co-workers reported a significantly greater loss of orgasmic capacity in their 107 consecutive posthysterectomy patients as compared with those 105 who underwent supravaginal uterine amputation, a procedure that retained the proximal vagina and cervix.[86]

Clinically, Zussman and co-workers considered the cervix and/or uterus important and quoted articulate comments of women who complained plaintively of the loss of their more profound cervical (or uterine) orgasm after hysterectomy.[176] They stated that the percentage of women for whom the cervix was important was unknown because this issue had not yet been studied. Some preliminary data to that end were collected by Cutler and Garcia in both young college women and perimenopausal women; these data support the contention that 40% of sexually active women have a clear preference for deep penetration at coitus—the coincident percentage to those who lost libido after surgery. Moreover, it was noted that those women who have a definite sexual preference for deep penetration at coitus were the ones most likely to experience a reduction in coital frequency after hysterectomy. It is probable that women with such a deep penetration preference might be the ones particularly at risk for a loss of libido after hysterectomy.

At any rate there is now a sufficient body of information in the literature to suggest that not all is known about the potential for sexual deficits after hysterectomy.[2,34,44,45,88,160,161] Accordingly, the clinician should be aware and share this with the patient.

Coronary Heart Disease

The influence of hysterectomy on coronary heart disease is ambiguous in the literature because, although it is clear that hysterectomy combined with bilateral oophorectomy does increase the risk of coronary heart disease, the question of the role of hysterectomy alone is currently unresolved. Centerwall reviewed a number of studies and concluded that there was a three- to five-times increased incidence of coronary heart disease among women who had sustained a hysterectomy than among intact age-matched controls.[28] He concluded that the results of a number of studies that he reviewed showed the same risk regardless of ovarian retention. Rosenberg and co-workers concluded there was an average increased risk for bilateral oophorectomy combined with hysterectomy of 2.9 for a myocardial infarction with a lesser (1.6 increase) risk for those having only a hysterectomy.[141] Furthermore, the increased risk of bilateral oophorectomy on the predisposition for myocardial infarction was inversely proportional to age. Bilateral oophorectomy before the age of 35 increased the risk to 7.2 times that of premenopausal age-matched women.[141] There is no association of natural menopause with risk of myocardial infarction. These findings of various relationships between hysterectomy with and without oophorectomy and subsequent heart disease are, therefore, suggestive of some role of the reproductive organs in the prevention of coronary heart disease even after the hormone depletions characteristic of the aging ovary have followed their course.

In Chapter 1, the data available demonstrating sex hormone levels following oophorectomy were reviewed. The results revealed, as would be expected, a greater diminution in ovariectomized younger women in comparison to their older counterparts. These data are reflective of the increased risk of myocardial infarction in age-matched postovariectomized younger women when compared with their older counterparts.

Lipids have also been evaluated. Plasma studies after bilateral oophorectomy show acute increases in triglycerides that return to baseline by 6 months; they also show no changes in cholesterol and no changes in phospholipids.[127] After bilateral oophorectomy, plasma renin activity and daily urinary excretion of aldosterone do not show any particular effects of the surgery.[126] The use of replacement therapy appears benign because no changes in cholesterol or serum triglyceride levels were noted in women who were given either estradiol valerate or estriol succinate (2 mg/day of either).[128] However, both estrogens did result in increases in the phospholipid concentration, the effects of which were considered minimal over the 3 years studied.[128]

The incidence and severity of atherosclerosis have also been studied using autopsy records.[139,173] Results are consistent with the risk factors described previously. A significant increase in coronary atherosclerosis among untreated castrated females occurs with a concomitantly significantly decreased incidence of this atherosclerotic condition in the vessels of patients who had endured hyperestrogenic states (certain cancers).[139] Moreover, when the hearts of bilaterally oophorectomized (during childbearing years) women were examined 2 to 42 years later, those who had been oophorectomized exhibited a tendency toward more advanced atherosclerosis than the intact controls.[173] The site of predilection for the development of severe atherosclerosis appears to be the anterior descending branch of the left coronary artery.[173]

It therefore becomes clear that oophorectomy has profound influences on coronary heart disease and that hysterectomy itself is potentially an etiologic factor in the subsequent development of the disease process. Hormone replacement therapies adequately reverse these risks.

There is one apparent exception in the literature that has been widely cited.[79,80] Although the investigators reported an increased risk of myocardial infarction in women who took menopausal hormone therapies, a close look at the data reveals that it is not the hormone therapies, but the artificially induced menopause in premenopausal women that most adequately explains the risk. Details of this widely cited study are appropriately mentioned at this point. There were 14 cases of myocardial infarction in the age group 39 to 45 years. Of the 14, 50% were estrogen users. This was contrasted with 19% of age-matched controls who were estrogen users. Although the 50% figure seemed to indicate a higher use of estrogen among myocardial infarction victims, a closer look at the data revealed that 12 of these 14 had been hysterectomized. Thus, although this widely cited study claimed to show, in opposition to the other studies in the literature, that estrogen replacement therapy increased the risk of coronary heart disease, a closer look showed hysterectomy to be the more likely etiologic determinant. None the less, the mechanisms involved remain unclear. Punnonen and Rauramo, evaluating the effect of castration and oral estrogen therapy on serum lipids, noted that untreated controls tended to show increases in cholesterol whereas those taking estrogen therapy did not.[128] One clue perhaps can be gleaned from two classic studies evaluating autopsy records described above. A significant increase in coronary atherosclerosis in untreated castrated females with a significant decrease below normal for atherosclerosis in cancer patients who were presumably hyperestrogenic was noted.[139,173]

The impact of long-term estrogen support after hysterectomy provided clear evidence of a marked drop in deaths from all causes, 80% of expected death rates, due mainly to reduced heart attack and cancer mortality.[17,21]

The evidence is therefore consistent in showing the sensible, perhaps mandatory, requirement for estrogen replacement therapy in women who are hysterectomized with or without oophorectomy.

Patient Dissatisfaction

In our increasingly litiginous society, and with women's developing awareness that hysterectomy may be altering their sexual response, sense of well-being, and risk of coronary heart disease, it behooves the clinician to discuss carefully these issues with his patient when seeking informed consent for hysterectomy. In 1957, Dalton discussed the long-term aftermath of hysterectomy in her 10-year follow-up study of her post-hysterectomy patients.[38] She reported that the patient's perception of her well-being changed sharply with time: Less than 1 year after the operation, 83% were satisfied, but between 1 and 5 years, only 41% were satisfied with the results of their surgery. At 6 to 10 years, 33% were satisfied, and this figure began to rise again to 50% satisfaction rate after 10 years. She noted that the sequela leading to patient dissatisfaction often began after the last postsurgical medical visit so that the reported incidences of morbidity are disproportionately low compared to reality. The conservative caring clinician should be appropriately forewarned.

THE CASE FOR HYSTERECTOMY

Decreased All-Cause Mortality if Hormone Replacement Therapy is Added After Hysterectomy

Clear indication of reduced incidence of all-cause mortality was recently reported after hysterectomy in women using hormonal replacement therapy.[20] Compared with age-matched controls not using estrogens, the relative risk of death in estrogen therapy users was 0.54 in gynecologically intact, 0.34 in hysterectomized women, and 0.12 in bilaterally oophorectomized women. These results show a profound health benefit attributed to hormone replacement therapy when added to the postsurgical milieu; for these reasons a potential benefit in longevity accrues to the postsurgical patient. Likewise the studies of Burch and Byrd provide similar conclusions.[17,21] A word of caution is in order. Although the facts reveal reduced mortality, they do not permit evaluation of the relative well-being or sexual satisfaction of the people involved—two critical components to be considered in the decision process for or against hysterectomy.

Elimination of Pathology

Clearly, hysterectomy can permanently eliminate certain pathologic conditions. Although malignancy appears to be appropriately treated this way, given current available therapeutic modalities, the case is less clear for the other conditions that can often be treated with less invasive methods. These are usually to be preferred.

OVARIECTOMY

Perspectives are changing on the propriety of ovariectomy when no ovarian disease exists. As shown in Chapter 1, in many cases old ovaries continue to secrete critical hormones that contribute to the well-being and general health of the older woman. On the other hand, the gynecologist is concerned with the potential of malignant transformation—a deadly prospect. The question of propriety is best evaluated from two perspectives: the review of future function of retained ovaries and a consideration of current data on ovariectomy.

RETAINING THE OVARIES

The incidence of retention of ovarian cyclicity after hysterectomy remains unclear. The majority of posthysterectomy patients under age 48 continue to show an ovarian cycle according to any of several criteria: bioassay of weekly urine samples,[11] cyclic records of premenstrual tension phenomenon,[7] plasma hormone evaluation,[134] and studies of vaginal smears.[42] However, the phenomenon appears to be less than universal. Ranney and co-workers evaluated the future function and control of ovarian tissue that is retained *in vivo* during hysterectomy and concluded that approximately 50% of their large sample continued to show clinical signs of ovarian hormone production (*i.e.*, vaginal tissue maintenance) but the other 50% did not.[131] This was the only study of the ones just described that sampled very large groups of women, and these results, therefore, suggest that some women stop showing ovarian cyclicity shortly after hysterectomy. The influence of an intact uterus on ovarian function is currently unresolved but with the recent discovery of uterine secretions of large quantities of prostaglandins there is reason to study the issue.[30] The reduction in prostaglandin after hysterectomy could potentially be a factor in the loss of ovarian cyclicity. Alternatively, the loss of the putative reflex pathway from cervix to pituitary could also be responsible.

RISK OF OVARIAN CANCER

The incidence of ovarian cancer varies markedly with age.[147] Figure 8–3 shows the epithelial cancer rates of the ovary at the M.D. Anderson Hospital in its review of over 2000 cases. One notes that the peak years for this cancer occur between ages 40 and 70 paralleling the times during which estrogen levels are declining most precipitously.

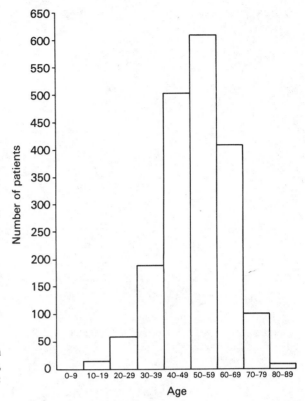

FIG. 8-3. Incidence of ovarian cancer by age (Smith JP, Day TG, 1979, Am J Obstet Gynecol 135: 984–993)

Ninety percent of the cancers of the ovary in this sample were epithelial, and the most important prognostic factors included higher stage or grade of tumor and the presence of ascites. The wealthy did worse on survival, perhaps due to the excess fat in their diet. Postoperative radiation was better able to improve the survival rate than postoperative chemotherapy in that report.[147] As therapeutic techniques change, re-evaluation will, no doubt, alter this perspective. The size of the largest remaining cancer mass in the body was more predictive of survival than the number of focal malignant sites. Interestingly enough, despite the present consensus to the contrary, the spillage of cystic contents of the mass at surgery did not lower the survival rate. Five-year survival rates also varied considerably as a function of age. Figure 8–4 shows the decreasing survival rate with increasing age. The fact that ovarian cancer is so resistant to treatment led to the routine removal of perfectly healthy ovaries under the assumption that such action would prevent potential ovarian cancers. However, the presently available data do not support the logic of this course. In fact, it makes more sense to retain healthy ovaries.

The risk of ovarian cancer in women with uterine disease has now been studied in two different ways. One can look at the ovarian cancer patients and compare them to patients who have not had prior ovarian ablation. One can ask what the hysterectomy rate was for each population. If it were dangerous to retain the ovaries after a hysterectomy, one would expect to find a higher frequency of formerly hysterectomized women among ovarian cancer patients than among those without ovarian cancer. The opposite is true. Studies have consistently shown that ovarian cancer patients have a much *lower* rate of

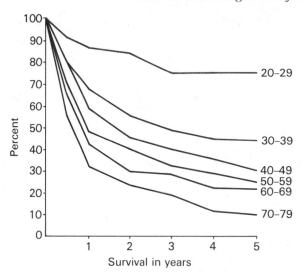

FIG. 8-4. Survival by age with ovarian cancer (Smith JP, Day TG, 1979, Am J Obstet Gynecol 135:984–993)

hysterectomy than is found in the general population. For example, Annegers and co-workers reported a 5% prior hysterectomy rate in ovarian cancer patients compared with a 23% hysterectomy rate in age-matched women who have not had prior ovariectomy.[5] Two other studies published in the 1950s showed a similar 4%[146] and a 4.5%[32] rate of hysterectomy among the ovarian cancer patients. Unfortunately, even though these data clearly show that hysterectomy in ovarian cancer patients is disproportionately lower, misleading logic has been applied to form the reverse conclusion, *i.e.,* that ovaries should be removed at hysterectomy.[65] This incorrect conclusion has been widely cited and, thereby, a false premise perpetuated. Nonetheless, lest it be concluded that extirpative surgery be preventive of ovarian cancer, the reader should be aware of the extremely low incidence of this deadly disease.

Another line of investigation also supports the safety of retaining the ovaries at hysterectomy. Prospective rates of ovarian cancer in retained ovaries after hysterectomy also support the absence of a risk.[130] A cohort study following 900 hysterectomized women for 20 years showed an overall rate of subsequent ovarian cancer at 0.2% in the sample.[130] The women who had both ovaries preserved showed a much lower (0.01%) rate of subsequent cancer than those who had only one ovary preserved (0.3%). There is, therefore, a consistent and clear picture when we analyze the data rather than the published conclusions. The surgical prevention of ovarian cancer should not lead to the decision for ovariectomy at hysterectomy. In fact, in 1982, a report of intra-abdominal carcinomatosis after prophylactic oophorectomy in ovarian cancer-prone families showed the futility of such a course.[158] Oophorectomies were performed "prophylactically" on 28 members of 16 families that were at high risk of ovarian carcinoma. Three of these women subsequently developed disseminated intra-abdominal malignancy anyway. The authors concluded that "the development of intra-abdominal carinomatis in oophorectomized women from ovarian cancer prone families suggests that genetic susceptibility is not limited to ovarian carcinoma but extends to cancers arising in tissues embryologically related to the ovary."[158] There is therefore no apparent advantage to be gained by the routine removal of healthy ovaries at hysterectomy.

OVARIAN TUMORS

Varying types of ovarian tumors may be encountered each having its distinct anatomical and clinical properties.[8,133,140,149] A knowledge of gross anatomical pathology aided by the histologic prowess of the pathologist particularly by frozen section may be most helpful in deciding whether oophorectomy or simple resection of the pathologic portion, *e.g.*, endometriosis, benign cystic teratomas, is sufficient. Ovarian benign cystic teratomas as large as the normal ovary in postmenopausal women have also been reported.[62]

Although the occurrence of ovarian tumors has been occasionally reported in the literature, there has been no attempt to relate them to a need for hysterectomy. Moreover, recent experimental manipulations in primates have shown a potential for embryo transfer into ovariectomized primates.[72] The implications support once again the need for uterine retention.

OVARIAN REMNANT SYNDROME

Symmonds and Pettit described two cases of intense pelvic pain after oophorectomy.[152] Ovarian remnants were found. These are usually embedded within adhesions. It was noted that the pain tended to be cyclic, perhaps corresponding to an ovarian cycle. More often this syndrome is likely to occur when oophorectomy is carried out under difficult conditions such as extensive severe pelvic inflammatory disease.

OVARIECTOMY—CURRENT INCIDENCE AT HYSTERECTOMY

In spite of what appears to be a clear case against routine ovariectomy during hysterectomy, current surgical practice has been different. Using data from the National Center for Health Statistics, Dicker and colleagues evaluated women aged 25 to 44 from 1970 to 1977.[48] They reported that ovariectomy during hysterectomy was occurring about 25% of the time and did not change throughout the years the data were collected. Older women, the group from 40 to 44, had approximately a 50% rate of ovariectomy at hysterectomy. In light of the currently available knowledge demonstrating hormone secretion by ovaries in the 40s, 50s and 60s (see Chap. 1) such routine practice should be discontinued. Despite decline in estrogen secretion by the ovary, there is a parallel rise in androgen secretion that provides a major source of the androgens that are peripherally converted to estrogens. Although those who have an inadequate source of androgen or peripheral conversion capacity may benefit from hormonal replacement, there remains a significant (15%) number who do not require hormonal support. The evidence continues to suggest that ovaries should be retained unless they are diseased.

ENDOCRINE CHANGES FOLLOWING OVARIECTOMY

The results of studies of ovariectomized women before, immediately after, and at various intervals after surgery are generally consistent. Both gonadotropins predictably show a rapid rise that by 3 weeks, can easily have reached 10 times the preoperative levels.[166,175] Likewise, within 3 hours, estrogen drops to 60% of the presurgical level,[10] reaching a nadir by 5 days post operation,[75] and leveling off thereafter at the new lower values.

Hormone replacement therapy does reduce these gonadotropin steroid levels. FSH more closely approaches its preoperative levels.[162,166] In one study, LH changes required combination estrogen and progestin hormone therapy.[166] Estradiol levels in plasma increase to preoperative levels when estrogen replacement therapies are sufficiently concentrated.[102] However, no estrogen dose is able to equilibrate both the gonado-tropins and the steroids at the preoperative equivalency in women 45 to 53 years old. To reduce gonadotropins to preoperative levels, one must produce a hyperestrogenic state.[102] The ovarian hormones then probably include other substances that are not replaced by estrogen or progestins.

Oophorectomized women frequently experience hot flushes, and studies have shown that those women who do flush postoperatively have significantly lower andro-stenedione levels than those women who do not,[10] which is another reflection of the value of preservating the ovaries.

Also noteworthy is the significant decline in epidermal thickness that follows oophorectomy at any age.[129] This epidermal thickness can be restored, or the decline prevented, by a weak estrogen (estriol succinate 2 mg/day) whereas stronger estrogen (estradiol valerate, 2 mg/day) sometimes produces the opposite effect.[125]

It is therefore apparent that oophorectomy affects steroid levels, symptomatology, and, inevitably, osteoporotic potential. For a fuller review of the osteoporotic results after surgery, the reader is referred to Chapter 2.

CONCLUSIONS—OVARIECTOMY

Because oophorectomy has such profound influences at every age and because there are no meaningful data in the literature to support the value of routine oophorectomy, oophorectomy should only be performed when the ovaries are diseased. One exception might be the case of familial ovarian carcinoma syndrome.[8,93,121,158] In such an instance the patient should be properly informed and given the option despite the possibility of subsequent disseminated peritoneal carcinomatosis in some.

CONCLUSIONS—PERIMENOPAUSAL BLEEDING AND HYSTERECTOMY

Bleeding must be investigated when it is unexpected. Several kinds of bleeding are expected; these include aberrant patterns during the 7 premenopausal years, withdrawal bleeding when hormone therapies induce them, and vaginal bleeding after coitus in women with atrophied tissue. Aberrant bleeding patterns during the 7 premenopausal years can offer a dilemma.[8,93,121,158] These patients must be properly diagnosed to assure that neoplastic disease is not overlooked. Failure to diagnose the cause of the bleeding is common. However, routine hysterectomy in such a case is not recommended.

Malignancy is rare, generally occurring in less than 15% of unexpected bleeding cases. The time course is slow, allowing time for subsequent diagnosis and treatment.

The uterus and the ovaries of aging women are valuable organs, potentially sexually as well as in limiting the risks of coronary heart disease and osteoporosis. These reproductive organs should only be removed for cause.

REFERENCES

1. Abramson D, Driscoll SG (1966) Endometrial aspiration biopsy. *Obstet Gynecol* 27:381–391.
2. Amias AG (1975) Sexual life after gynaecological operations—I. *Br Med J* 2:5971:608–609.
3. Ananth J (1978) Hysterectomy and depression. *Obstet Gynecol* 52:724–730.
4. Anderson DC, Eaton CJ, Galinkin LJ, Newton CW, Haines JP, Miller NF (1976) The cytologic diagnosis of endometrial cancer. *Am J Obstet Gynecol* 125:376–383.

5. Annegers JF, Strom H, Decker DG, Dockerty MB, O'Fallon WM (1979) Ovarian cancer: incidence and case-control study. *Cancer* 43:2:723–729.

6. Askel S, Schomberg DW, Tyrey L, Hamond CB (1976) Vasomotor symptoms, serum estrogens, and gonadotropin levels in surgical menopause. *Am J Obstet Gynecol* 126:165–169.

7. Backstrom CT, Boyle H (1981) Persistence of premenstrual tension symptoms in hysterectomized women. *Br J Obstet Gynaecol* 88:530–536.

8. Barber HRK (1982) *Ovarian Carcinoma*, 2nd Edition. Masson Publishing USA. New York.

9. Barker MG (1968) Psychiatric illness after hysterectomy. *Br Med J* 2:91–95.

10. Barlow DH, Macnaughton MC, Mowat J, Coutts JRT (1981) Hormone profiles in the menopause. In: *Functional Morphology of the Human Ovary.* Coutts RT (ed). Baltimore, University Park Press.

11. Beavis ELG, Brown JB, Smith MA (1969) Ovarian function after hysterectomy with conservation of the ovaries in premenopausal women. *J Obstet Gynecol Br Commonwealth* 76:969–978.

12. Berman MI, Ballon SC, Lagasse DL, Watring WG (1980) Prognosis and treatment of endometrial cancer. *Am J Obstet Gynecol* 136:679–688.

13. Botella-Llusia J, Oriol-Bosch A, Sanchez-Garrido F, Tresguerres J (1980) Testosterone and 17B estradiol secretion of the human ovary. *Maturitas* 2:1–7.

14. Brewer JI, Miller WH (1954) Postmenopausal uterine bleeding. *Am J Obstet Gynecol* 67:988–1013.

15. Buchman MI, Kramer E, Feldman GB (1978) Aspiration curettage for asymptomatic patients receiving estrogen. *Obstet Gynecol* 51:339–341.

16. Bunker JP (1976) Elective hysterectomy: pro and con: public-health rounds at the Harvard School of Public Health. *N Engl J Med* 295:264–268.

17. Burch JC, Byrd BF, Vaughn WK (1975) The effects of long-term estrogen administration following hysterectomy. *Front Horm Res* 3:208–214.

18. Burnett JE (1964) Hysteroscopy—controlled curettage for endometrial polyps. *Obstet Gynecol* 24:621–625.

19. Burns B, Curry R, Bell MEA (1979) Morphologic features of prognostic significance in uterine smooth muscle tumors: a review of eighty-four cases. *Am J Obstet Gynecol* 135:109–114.

20. Bush TL, Cowan LD, Barrett-Connor E, Criqui MH, Karon JM, Wallace RB, Tyroler HA, Rifkind BM (1983) Estrogen use and all-cause mortality. *JAMA* 249:903–906.

21. Byrd BF, Burch JC, Vaughn W (1977) The impact of long term estrogen support after hysterectomy. *Ann Surg* 185:574–580.

22. Calanog A, Sall S, Gordon G, Southren AL (1977) Androstenedione metabolism in patients with endometrial cancer. *Am J Obstet Gynecol* 129:553–556.

23. Carlstrom K, Damber M, Furuhjelm M, Joelsson I, Lunell N, von Schoultz B (1979) Serum levels of total dehydroepiandrosterone and total estrone in postmenopausal women with special regard to carcinoma of the uterine corpus. *Acta Obstet Gynecol Scand* 58:179–181.

24. Caspi E, Perpinial S, Reif A (1977) Incidence of malignancy in Jewish women with postmenopausal bleeding. *Isr J Med Sci* 13:299–304.

25. Centaro A, Ceci G, de Laurentis G, de Salvia D (1974) Epidemiologic studies of postmenopausal endometrial adenocarcinoma. In: *The Menopausal Syndrome,* pp 133–138. Greenblatt RB, Mahesh VB, McDonough PG (eds). New York, Medome Press.

26. Centers for Disease Control Surgical Sterilization Surveillance. Hysterectomy in women aged 15–44. (1981) US Department of Health and Human Services, Centers for Disease Control, Center for Health Promotion and Education, Family Planning Evaluation Division, Atlanta.

27. Centers for Disease Control, US Department of Health and Human Services Morbidity and Mortality Weekly Report, April 24, 1981. Vol 30, No 15. Hysterectomy in women aged 15–44, United States, 1970–1978.

27a. Hysterectomy among women of reproductive age. U.S. Update for 1979–1980 in *CDC Surveilance Summaries* (published quarterly). Aug 1983:32(Suppl. 3):1ss–7ss.

28. Centerwall BS (1981) Premenopausal hysterectomy and cardiovascular disease. *Am J Obstet Gynecol* 139:58–61.

29. Chakravarti S, Collins WP, Newton JR, Oram DH, Studd JWW (1977) Endocrine changes and symptomatology after oophorectomy in premenopausal women. *Br J Obstet Gynaecol* 84:769–775.

30. Charbonnel B, Kremer M, Gerozissis K, Dray F (1982) Human cervical mucus contains large amounts of prostaglandins. *Fertil Steril* 38:109–111.

31. Cheek DB, Davis JE (1946) Pathologic findings in genital bleeding two or one year after spontaneous cessation of menstruation. *Am J Obstet Gynecol* 52:756–764.

32. Counseller VS, Hunt W, Haigler FH (1955) Carcinoma of the ovary following hysterectomy. *Am J Obstet Gynecol* 69:538–542.

33. Coppen A, Bishop M, Beard RJ, Barnard GJR, Collins WP (1981) Hysterectomy, hormones, and behavior. *Lancet* Jan 17:126–128.

34. Craig GA, Jackson P (1975) Letter: sexual life after vaginal hysterectomy. *Br Med J* 3:5975:97.

35. Cramer SF, Meyer JS, Kraner JF, Camel M, Mazur MT, Tenenbaum MS (1980) Metastasizing leiomyoma of the uterus: S-phase fraction, estrogen receptor and ultrastructure. *Cancer* 45:932–937.

36. Cutler WB (1982) Premenopausal hysterectomy and cardiovascular disease. *Am J Obstet Gynecol* 141:849.

37. Cutler WB, Garcia CR (1980) The psychoneuroendocrinology of the ovulatory cycle of woman. *Psychoneuroendocrinology* 5:89–111.

38. Dalton K (1957) Discussion on the aftermath of hysterectomy and oophorectomy. In: Section of General Practice, Proc R Soc Med 50:415–418.

39. Danoff B (1983) An overview of radiation therapy in gynecology. *Present Concepts in Obstetrics and Gynecology,* pp 17–23. University of Pennsylvania Course Syllabus.

40. Daw E (1974) Luteinising hormone changes in women undergoing artificial menopause. *Curr Med Res Opin* 2:256–259.

41. DeCherney A, Polan ML (1983) Hysteroscopic management of intrauterine lesions and intractable uterine bleeding. *Obstet Gynecol* 61:392–396.

42. DeNeef JC, Hollenbeck ZJR (1966) The fate of ovaries preserved at the time of hysterectomy. *Am J Obstet Gynecol* 96:1088–1097.

43. Denis R, Barnett JM, Forbes SE (1973) Diagnostic suction currettage. *Obstet Gynecol* 42:301–303.

44. Dennerstein L, Burrows G, Wood C, Hyman G (1980) Hormones and sexuality: effect of estrogen and progestogen. *Obstet Gynecol* 56:316–322.

45. Dennerstein L, Wood D, Burrows G (1977) Sexual response following hysterectomy and oophorectomy. *Obstet Gynecol* 49:92–96.

46. Dewhurst J (1983) Postmenopausal bleeding from benign causes. *Clin Obstet Gynecol* 26:769–776.

47. Dicker R, Greenspan J, Strauss L, Cowart M, Scally M, Peterson H, DeStefano F, Rubin G, Ory H (1982) Complications of abdominal and vaginal hysterectomy among women of reproductive age in the United States. *Am J Obstet Gynecol* 144:841–848.

48. Dicker RC, Scally MJ, Greenspan JR, Layde PM, Maze JM (1982) Hysterectomy among women of reproductive age. *JAMA* 248:323–327.

49. Di Sai PJ, Creasman WT (1981) *Clinical Gynecologic Oncology* 312–313 CV Mosby, St. Louis

50. Donahue VC (1976) Elective hysterectomy: pro and con. *N Engl J Med* 295:264.

51. Edmonson J, Fleming TR, Decker DG, Malkasian GD, Jorgensen EO, Jefferies JA, Webb MJ, Kvols LK (1979) Different chemotherapeutic sensitivities and host factors affecting prognosis in advanced ovarian carcinoma versus minimal residual disease. *Cancer Treat Rep* 63:241–247.

52. England GT, Randall HW, Graves W (1983) Impairment of tissue defenses by vasoconstrictors in vaginal hysterectomies. *Obstet Gynecol* 61:271–274.

53. Englund S, Ingelman-Sundberg A, Westin B (1957) Hysteroscopy in diagnosis and treatment of uterine bleeding. *Gynaecologica* 143:217–222.

54. Forney JP (1980) The effect of radical hysterectomy on bladder physiology. *Am J Obstet Gynecol* 138:374–382.

55. Fribourg S (1982) Hysterectomy among women of reproductive age. *JAMA* 249:9.

56. Galli MC, DeGlovanni C, Nicoletti G, Grilli S, Nanni P, Prodi G, Gola G, Rocchetta R, Orlandi CC (1981) The occurrence of multiple steroid hormone receptors in disease-free and neoplastic human ovary. *Cancer* 47:6:1297–1302.

57. Gambrell RD (1977) Postmenopausal bleeding. *Clin Obstet Gynecol* 4:129–143.

58. Gambrell RD Jr. (1981) Preventing endometrial Ca with progestin. *Contemp Obstet Gynecol* 17:133–143.

59. Gambrell RD, Castaneda TA, Ricci CA (1978) Management of postmenopausal bleeding to prevent endometrial cancer. *Maturitas* 1:99–106.

60. Gambrell RD Jr., Massery FM, Castaneda TA, Ugenas AJ, Ricci CA, Wright JM (1980) Use of progestogen challenge test to reduce the risk of endometrial cancer. *Obstet Gynecol* 55:732–738.

61. Gath DH (1980) Psychiatric aspects of hysterectomy. In: *The Social Consequences of Psychiatric Illness.* Robins L (ed). New York, Brunner/Mazel.

62. Gordon A, Rosenstein N, Parmley T, Bhagavan B (1980) Benign cystic teratomas in postmenopausal women. *Am J Obstet Gynecol* 138:8:1120–1123.

63. Greenberg M (1981) Letter: hysterectomy, hormones and behavior. *Lancet* Feb 21:449.

64. Gribb JJ (1960) Hysteroscopy an aid in gynecologic diagnosis. *Obstet Gynecol* 15:593–601.

65. Grogan RH (1967) Reappraisal of residual ovaries. *Am J Obstet Gynecol* 97:124–129.

66. Gusberg SB (1976) The individual at high risk for endometrial carcinoma *Am J Obstet Gynecol* 126:535–542.

67. Gusberg SB (1975) A strategy for the control of endometrial cancer. *Proc R Med* 68:163–168.

68. Gusburg SB, Kaplan AL (1963) Adenomatous hyperplasia as Stage O carcinoma of the endometrium. *Am J Obstet Gynecol* 87:662–678.

69. Hakama M (1981) Components of cervical cancer. *Lancet* July 11:90–91.

70. Hamou J, Taylor PJ (1982) Panoramic, contact and microcolpohysteroscopy in gynecologic practice. *Curr Probl Obstet Gynecol* 1–71.

71. Hathcock FW, Williams GA, Englehardt SM, Murphy AL (1974) Office aspiration curettage of the endometrium. *Am J Obstet Gynecol* 120:205–213.

72. Hodgen GD (1983) Surrogate embryo transfer combined with estrogen-progesterone therapy in monkeys. *JAMA* 250:16:2167–2171.

73. Hormeister FJ, Barbo DM (1964) Cancer detection in private gynecologic practice: a concluding study. *Obstet Gynecol* 23:386–391.

74. Hofmeister FJ (1974) Endometrial biopsy: another look. *Am J Obstet Gynecol* 119:773–777.

75. Hunter DJ, Julier D, Franklin M, Green E (1977) Plasma levels of estrogen, luteinizing hormone, and follicle-stimulating hormone following castration and estradiol implant. *Obstet Gynecol* 49:2:180–185.

76. Hutton JD, Morse AR, Anderson MC, Beard RW (1978) Endometrial assessment with Isaacs cell sampler. *Br Med J* 1:947–949.

77. Inglis RM, Weir JH (1976) Endometrial suction biopsy: appraisal of a new instrument. *Am J Obstet Gynecol* 125:1070–1072.

78. Janson PO, Jansson I (1977) The acute effect of hysterectomy on ovarian blood flow. *Am J Obstet Gynecol* 127:4:349–352.

79. Jick H, Dinan B, Rothman K (1978) Noncontraceptive estrogens and non fatal myocardial infarctions. *JAMA* 239:1407–1408.

80. Jick H, Dinan B, Herman R, Rothman K (1978) Myocardial infarction and other vascular diseases in young women. *JAMA* 240:2548–2552.

81. Johnson J (1982) Tubal sterilization and hysterectomy. *Fam Plan Perspect* 14:28–30.

82. Jordan JA (1980) Is death from cervical cancer avoidable? *R Soc Health J* 100:6:231–233.

83. Kaplan E (1977) Recurrent postmenopausal bleeding. *S Afr Med J* 52:1121–1123.

84. Kav-Venaki S, Zakham L (1983) Psychological effects of hysterectomy in premenopausal women. *J Psychosom Obstet Gynecol* 2:76–80.

85. Keirse MJNC (1973) Aetiology of post menopausal bleeding. *Postgrad Med J* 49:344–348.

86. Kilkku P, Gronroos M, Hirvonen T, Rauramo L (1983) Supravaginal uterine amputation vs. hysterectomy: Effects on libido and orgasm. *Acta Obstet Gynecol Scand* 62:147–152.

87. Knapp RC, Donahue VC, Friedman FA (1973) Dissection of paravesical and pararectal spaces in pelvic operations. *Surg Gynecol Obstet* 137:758–762.

88. Krueger JC, Hessell J, Goggins DB, Ishimatsu T, Publico MR, Tuttle FJ (1979) Relationship between nurse counseling and sexual adjustment after hysterectomy. *Nurs Res* 28:3:145–150.

89. Laros RK, Work BA (1975) Female sterilization III. Vaginal hysterectomy. *Am J Obstet Gynecol* 122:693–697.

90. Lauritzen C (1973) The management of the premenopausal and the postmenopausal patient. *Front Horm Res* 2:2–21.

91. Levin DL, Devesa SS, Godwin JDII, Silverman DT (1964) Cancer rates and risks, p 13. Washington, Department of Health, Education and Welfare.

92. Lewis E, Bourne S (1981) Letter: hysterectomy, hormones and behavior. *Lancet* Feb 7:324–325.

93. Lynch H, Albano W, Lynch J, Lynch P, Campbell A (1982) Surveillance and management of patients at high genetic risk for ovarian carcinoma. *Obstet Gynecol* 59:5:589–596.

94. Lyon LJ, Gardner JW (1977) The rising frequency of hysterectomy: its effect on uterine cancer rates. *Am J Epidemiol* 105:439–443.

95. MacKenzie IZ, Bibby JG (1978) Critical assessment of dilatation and curettage in 1029 females. *Lancet* 2:566–568.

96. MacMahon B (1974) Risk factors for endometrial cancer. *Gynecol Oncol* 2:122–129.

97. MacMahon B, Worcester J (1966) National Center for Health Statistics. Age at menopause, US 1960–1962. Washington, DC, USPHS Publication 1000, Series 11, No 19.

98. Malkasian GD, Annegers JF, Fountains KS (1980) Carcinoma of the endometrium: Stage 1. *Am J Obstet Gynecol* 136:872–888.

99. Mantalenakis SJ, Papapostolon MG (1977) Genital bleeding in females aged 50 and over. *Int Surg* 62:103–105.

100. March CM (1983) Hysteroscopy—the womb revisited. *Fertil Steril* 39:4:455–457.

101. Martin RL, Roberts WV, Clayton PJ, Wetzel R (1977) Psychiatric illness and noncancer hysterectomy. *Dis Nervous System* 38:11:974–980.

102. Mattingly R (1977) Myomata Uteri. In: *TeLinde's Operative Gynecology*, 5th Edition. Philadelphia, JB Lippincott.

103. Mazur MT, Kraus FT (1980) Histogenesis of morphologic variations in tumors of the uterine wall. *Am J Surg Pathol* 4:59–74.

104. McBride JM (1959) Pre-menopausal cystic glandular hyperplasia and endometrial carcinoma. *J Obstet Gynecol Br Commonwealth* 66:288–296.

105. Meikle S, Brody H, Pysh F (1977) An investigation into the psychological effects of hysterectomy. *J Nerv Ment Dis* 164:36–41.

106. Menczer J, Modan M, Ezra D, Serr DM (1980) Prognosis in pre- and postmenopausal patients with endometrial adenocarcinoma. *Maturitas* 2:37–44.

107. Merrill JA (1981) Management of postmenopausal bleeding. *Clin Obstet Gynecol* 24:285–299.

108. Mickal A, Torres J (1974) Adenocarcinoma of endometrium. In: *The Menopausal Syndrome*, pp 139–142. Greenblatt RB, Mahesh VB, McDonough PG (eds). New York, Medcom Press.

109. Moore DE (1982) Pain associated with hysterosalpingography: Ethiodol versus salpix media. *Fertil Steril* 38:629–631.

110. Moore J, Tolley D (1976) Depression following hysterectomy. *Psychosomatics* 17:2:86–89.

111. Newhouse ML, Pearson RM, Fullerton JM, Boesen EAM, Shannon HS (1977) A case control study of carcinoma of the ovary. *Br J Prev Soc Med* 31:148–153.

112. Ng ABP, Reagan JW (1970) Incidence and prognosis of endometrial carcinoma by histologic grade and extent. *Obstet Gynecol* 35:437–442.

113. Ng ABP, Reagan JW, Storaasli JP, Wentz WB (1973) Mixed adenosquamous carcinoma of the endometrium. *Am J Clin Pathol* 59:765–781.

114. Norment WB (1956) The hysteroscope. *Am J Obstet Gynecol* 71:426–432.

115. Novak E, Richardson EH (1941) Proliferative changes in the senile endometrium. *Am J Obstet Gynecol* 42:564.

116. Osterholzer HO, Grillow D, Kruger PS, Dunnihoo DR (1977) The effect of oral contraceptive steroids on branches of the uterine artery. *Obstet Gynecol* 49:227–232.

117. Panda S, Panda SN, Sarangi RK, Habeebullah S (1977) Postmenopausal bleeding. *J Indian Med Assoc* 68:185–188.

118. Parsons L, Sommers SC (1962) *Gynecology*, pp 629–649. Philadelphia, WB Saunders.

119. Paterson MEL, Wade-Evans T, Sturdee DW, Thom MH, Studd JWW (1980) Endometrial disease after treatment with oestrogens and progestogens in the climacteric. *Br Med J* 96:1–8.

120. Payne FL, Wright RC, Getterman HH (1959) Postmenopausal bleeding. *Am J Obstet Gynecol* 77:1216–1227.

121. Piver MS, Barlow JJ, Sawyer DM (1982) Familial ovarian cancer: increasing in frequency? *Obstet Gynecol* 60:3:397–401.

122. Polivy J (1974) Psychological reactions to hysterectomy. *Am J Obstet Gynecol* 118:417–426.

123. Population Reports (1982) Oral contraceptives in the 1980's. Series A, No 6, *Population Information Program*. Johns Hopkins University, Baltimore.

124. Procope BJ (1971) Aetiology of postmenopausal bleeding. *Acta Obstet Gynecol Scand* 50:311–313.

125. Punnonen R (1972) Effect of castration and peroral estrogen therapy on the skin. *Acta Obstet Gynecol Scand* 21:1–44.

126. Punnonen R, Lammintausta R, Erkkola R, Rauramo L (1980) Estradiol valerate therapy and the renin-aldosterone system in castrated women. *Maturitas* 2:91–94.

127. Punnonen R, Rauramo L (1976) Effect of bilateral oophorectomy and peroral estradiol valerate therapy on serum lipids. *Int J Gynaecol Obstet* 14:13–16.

128. Punnonen R, Rauramo L (1976) The effect of castration and oral estrogen therapy on serum lipids. In *Concensus on Menopause Research.* van Keep PA, Greenblatt RB, Albeaux-Fernet M (eds). Proc First International Congress on the Menopause Help in France. Baltimore, University Park Press.

129. Punnonen R, Rauramo L (1977) The effect of long-term oral oestriol succinate therapy on the skin of castrated women. *Ann Chir Gynaecol* 66:4:214–215.

130. Randall CL (1963) Ovarian conservation. In *Progress in Gynecology.* Meigs JV, Sturgis SH (eds). New York, Grune and Stratton.

131. Ranney B, Abu-Ghazaleh S (1977) The future function and control of ovarian tissue which is retained in vivo during hysterectomy. *Am J Obstet Gynecol* 128:626–634.

132. Reagan JW, Ng ABP (1973) *The Cells of Uterine Adenocarcinoma,* 2nd Edition, Basel, Karger.

133. Reed MJ, Hutton JD, Beard RW, Jacobs HS, James VH (1979) Plasma hormone levels and oestrogen production in a postmenopausal woman with endometrial carcinoma and an ovarian thecoma. *Clin Endocrinol (Oxf)* 11:2:141–150.

134. Reynoso RL, Aznar RR, Bedolla TN, Cortes-Gallegos V (1975) Cyclic concentration of estradiol and progesterone in hysterectomized women. *Reproduction* 2:1:45–49.

135. Richard EM (1979) The debate over screening for endometrial cancer. *Contemp Obstet Gynecol* 4:100–131.

136. Richards BC (1978) Hysterectomy: from women to women. *Am J Obstet Gynecol* 131:446–449.

137. Richards DH (1974) A post hysterectomy syndrome. *Lancet* 2:983–985.

138. Richards DH (1973) Depression after hysterectomy. *Lancet* 2:430–433.

139. Rivin AU, Dimitroff SP (1954) The incidence and severity of atherosclerosis in estrogen-treated males and in females with a hypoestrogenic or hyperestrogenic state. *Circulation* 9:533–539.

140. Rome RM, Fortune DW, Quinn MA, Brown JB (1981) Functioning ovarian tumors in postmenopausal women. *Obstet Gynecol* 57:6:705–710.

141. Rosenberg L, Hennekens CH, Rosner B, Belanger C, Rothman KJ, Speizer RE (1981) Early menopause and the risk of myocardial infarction. *Am J Obstet Gynecol* 139:47–51.

142. Scheckler W (1983) Editorial—the cost of prevention: common sense and decision trees. *JAMA* 249:10:1328.

143. Shapiro M, Schoenbaum S, Tager I, Munoz A, Polk F (1983) Benefit-cost analysis of antimicrobial prophylaxis in abdominal and vaginal hysterectomy. *JAMA* 249:10:1290–1294.

144. Sharma SP, Misra SD, Mittal VP (1979) Endometrial changes—a criterion for the diagnosis of submucous uterine leiomyoma. *Indian J Pathol Microbiol* 22:33–36.

145. Sherman AI, Brown S (1979) The precursors of endometrial carcinoma. *Am J Obstet Gynecol* 135:947–956.

146. Smith GV (1958) Ovarian tumors. *Am J Surg* 95:336–340.

147. Smith JP, Day TG (1979) Review of ovarian cancer at the University of Texas Systems Cancer Center MD Anderson Hospital and Tumor Institute. *Am J Obstet Gynecol* 135:984–993.

148. Stadel BV, Weiss N (1975) Characteristics of menopausal women: a survey of King and Pierce Counties in Washington, 1973–1974. *Am J Epidemiol* 102:3:209–216.

149. Sternberg WH (1947) The morphology, androgenic function, hyperplasia, and tumors of the human ovarian hilus cells. *Am J Pathol* 25:493–521.

150. Stone SC, Dickey RP, Mickal A (1975) The acute effect of hysterectomy of ovarian function. *Am J Obstet Gynecol* 121:2:193–197.

151. Swingler GR, Cane DG, Mitchard P (1979) Diagnostic accuracy of Mimark endometrial cell sampler in 101 patients with postmenopausal bleeding. *Br J Obstet Gynaecol* 86:816–818.

152. Symmonds RE, Pettit PDM (1979) Ovarian remnant syndrome. *Obstet Gynecol* 54:174–177.

153. Szamborski J, Czerwinski W, Gadomska H, Kowalski M, Wacker-Pujdak B (1981) Case control study of high-risk factors in ovarian carcinomas. *Gynecol Oncol* 11:1:8–16.

154. Szamborski J, Czerwinski W (1980) Serous verus endometrioid ovarian cancer: clinical characteristics and risk factors. *Ginekol Pol* 51:7:629–636.
155. Tamaya T, Motoyama T, Ohono Y, Ide N, Tsurusaki T, Okada H (1979) Estradiol-1/B-progesterone and 5a-dihydrotestosterone receptors of uterine myometrium and myoma in the human subject. *J Steroid Biochem* 10:615–622.
156. Taylor RW (1979) Gynecological malignancy. *Practicioner* 222:1328:195–201.
157. TeLinde RW (1930) A clinical and pathologic study of postmenopausal bleeding. *South Med J* 23:571–579.
158. Tobachman JK, Tucker MA, Kase R, et al (1982) Intra abdominal carcinomatosis after prophylactic oophorectomy in ovarian cancer prone families. *Lancet* October 8:795–797.
159. Treloar AE (1981) Menstrual cyclicity and the premenopause. *Maturitas* 3:249–264.
160. Utian WHS (1972) The true clinical features of postmenopause and oophorectomy and their response to oestrogen therapy. *S Afr Med J* 46:732–737.
161. Utian WH (1975) Effect of hysterectomy, oophorectomy and estrogen therapy on libido. *Int J Obstet Gynecol* 13:97–100.
162. Utian W, Katz M, Davey D, Carr P (1978) Effect of premenopausal castration and incremental dosages of conjugated equine estrogens on plasma follicle-stimulating hormone, luteinizing hormone and estradiol. *Am J Obstet Gynecol* 132:297–302.
163. Valle R (1978) Hysteroscopy: diagnostic and therapeutic application. *J Reprod Med* 20:115–118.
164. Valle RF (1981) Hysteroscopic evaluation of patients with abnormal uterine bleeding. *Surg Gynecol Obstet* 153:521–526.
165. Valle RF, Sciarra JJ (1979) Current status of hysteroscopy in gynecologic practice. *Fertil Steril* 32:619–632.
166. Wallach EE, Root AW, Garcia CR (1970) Serum gonadotropin responses to estrogen and progestogen in recently castrated human females. *J Clin Endocrinol Metab* 31:376–381.
167. Wardlaw SL, Wehrenberg WB, Ferin M, Antunes JL, Frantz AG (1982) Effect of sex steroids on B-endorphin in hypophyseal portal blood. *J Clin Endocrinol Metab* 55:877–881.
168. Weinstein H, Slenker L, Porges RF (1977) Diagnostic vacuum aspiration curettage. *NY State J Med* 77:373–376.
169. Wentz WB (1974) Progestin therapy in endometrial hyperplasia. *Gynecol Oncol* 2:362–367.
170. White SC, Wartel LJ, Wade ME (1971) Comparison of abdominal and vaginal hysterectomies: a review of 600 operations. *Obstet Gynecol* 37:530–537.
171. Wiebe RH, Herbert X, Morris CV (1983) Testosterone, androstenedione ratio in the evaluation of women with ovarian androgen excess. *Obstet Gynecol* 61:279–284.
172. Woodruff JD, Prystowsky H, Telinde RW (1966) Postmenopausal bleeding. *South Med J* 51:302–305.
173. Wuest JH, Dry TJ, Edwards JE (1953) The degree of atherosclerosis in bilaterally oophorectomized women. *Circulation* 7:801–809.
174. Wynder EL, Escher GC, Mantel N (1966) An epidemiological investigation of cancer of the endometrium. *Cancer* 19:489–520.
175. Yen SSC, Tsai CC (1971) The effect of ovariectomy on gonadotropin release. *J Clin Invest* 50:1149–1153.
176. Zussman L, Zussman S, Sunley R, Bjornson E (1981) Sexual response after hysterectomy-oophorectomy: recent evidence and reconsideration of psychogenesis. *Am J Obstet Gynecol* 140:725–729.

9

Common Problems and Available Solutions

GENERAL ISSUES

Are the terms "menopause" and "climacteric" synonymous?

"Menopause" means a specific point in time at which menses have stopped and can only be confirmed in retrospect. The "climacteric" includes a much longer period of time during which a woman moves from a reproductive to a nonreproductive phase. "Climacteric" is synonymous with perimenopause and generally spans about 7 years.

When should one begin to treat the climacterium?

Therapy should begin whenever there are indications of estrogen depletion. Ideally, the aware gynecologist is on the alert for perimenopausal symptomatology in women age 35 to 45. On the average, the symptoms of estrogen deprivation begin at about age 42, but there is a wide variation from average.

What areas of the body does menopausal care encompass?

In theory, the totality of the patient's health care needs should be considered when one is managing the patient who is either estrogen deficient or under care for prehysterectomy and posthysterectomy evaluation. The endocrine alterations have profound influences on all of the systems, *i.e.,* bones, cardiovascular fitness, emotional lability, and sexual function. Therefore, appropriate care should encompass all. Consultation with the subspecialists should be sought when indicated.

Can a perimenopausal woman become pregnant?

Yes. Contraception in the perimenopause period other than the oral contraceptive is advisable because the risk of pregnancy continues. Ovulation and subsequent ovarian alterations become less able to support a pregnancy but not completely unable. With increasing age, the incidence of pregnancy declines.

Do women continue to make estrogen after menopause?

They do, but with varying degrees of efficiency. The ovary continues to produce a small amount of androstenedione, and the adrenal glands produce larger amounts of this androgenic hormone. The androstenedione is converted peripherally first to estrone and then to estradiol. An obese postmenopausal woman would convert much more androstenedione to estrogen than a slender woman (see Chapter 1).

SYMPTOMS

My patients in their 40s complain about extreme mood swings, especially depression or anxiety, in the last 6 or 7 days before menstruation begins. Is this related to the menopausal transition?

Probably. The postovulatory estrogen levels decline with time whereas the preovulatory estrogen levels increase with time. Consequently, the swings from high to low estrogen levels become more pronounced with the passing years (see pages 11–13). Estrogen depletion has been associated with depression (see pages 130–132); estrogen replacement, with increased well-being (see pages 128–129). In theory, one might want to consider estrogen therapy in the week preceding menses in patients so troubled. However, careful follow-up and variations in treatment including supplementation with calcium and addition of progestin should be considered.

Is the vasomotor flush a psychosomatic or physical (real) response?

It is real. Changes in skin resistance, skin temperature, core temperature, and pulse rate can be measured at the time subjective symptoms occur.

What are the indications for estrogen replacement therapy for a perimenopausal or postmenopausal woman?

Indications for estrogen replacement include vasomotor instability, *i.e.,* hot flashes, vaginal and urinary tract symptoms, psychosomatic symptoms such as anxiety and irritability in conjunction with evidence of approaching menopause, and low back pain with subsequent bone fractures. Evidence of osteoporosis usually presents late in this sequence even though the progression of the disease began simultaneously with the appearance of the hot flashes—often 10 or more years earlier.

The patient presents with irregular menstrual cycles. She is in her late 30s to late 40s. Is this necessarily an abnormal pattern and what should the physician do?

Although irregular menstrual bleeding can be the expected component of the transition years, one must not be beguiled and overlook a potential pathologic condition. An endometrial biopsy is indicated. See Chapter 1 for information showing the normal variation in menstrual habit during the climacteric and Chapter 8 for a discussion of pathology.

PRESCRIBING HORMONAL REPLACEMENT THERAPY

When should hormonal replacement therapy begin?

Hormonal replacement therapy should begin when symptoms of estrogen or calcium deficiency appear, often in the perimenopausal years. These symptoms include those of vasomotor instability, vaginal complaints secondary to atrophy, as well as low back aches and other skeletal complaints. Women exhibiting these symptoms should be screened by densitometry. Hot flashes at any time, premenopause or postmenopause, are suggestive of ovarian failure. The patient should be evaluated and treated accordingly. A declining stature is indicative of bone loss. Vaginal atrophy is most commonly encountered after the menopause is well progressed.

Is it unnecessary to give progestins to a woman taking estrogen replacement therapy?

Progestogens are the safest and most effective way of balancing the valued effects of estrogen while protecting against the unopposed effects of estrogen on the endometrium and probably the breasts.

Is it always necessary to give progestogens to a woman taking estrogen replacement therapy?

The evidence is mounting that low-dose progestogen enhances the physiology of the menopausal woman. The most current information supports the idea that there is protection against breast carcinoma as well as enhancement of bone deposition when progestogen is appropriately opposed to estrogen. See Chapters 2 and 4.

What regimen do you prescribe for postmenopausal women with, and without, a uterus?

The same, since the trend of information in the literature supports the view that estrogen low-dose progestogen in opposition maximizes bone, minimizes the risks of carcinogenic transformation in the breast and uterus, if present, and reduces the risk of death from heart disease.

Because progestins do relieve flushes and do not increase the risk of endometrial cancer, why not simply prescribe progestins for relief from flushes?

This is a regimen that treats only the hot flashes. The progestins have antiestrogenic influences that may potentially create other problems. For example, they are likely to accelerate vaginal atrophy, to increase the risk of arterial disease, and to have negative influences on well-being. Estrogen replacement therapy is the approach of choice. Details of the studies appear in Chapters 1, 4, and 6.

Are synthetic hormones acceptable?

For the present, one must conclude that the natural hormones are preferable since they have less risk of adverse effects (see Chapters 6 and 7).

Are the hepatic effects of oral hormonal replacement therapy (HRT) regimens all bad?

Probably they are not. It is too soon to know for certain. What is clear is that the reported increase in the beneficial HDL-Ch, in contrast to the absence of such cnanges by the percutaneous route, offers at least one potential benefit for oral estrogen replacement therapy. For specific details, the reader should refer to Chapter 6 on HRT and coronary health factors.

Why are there no natural progesterones available from US pharmaceutical companies?

Drug companies must prove efficacy and safety in order to obtain FDA approval for any natural progesterone in its vehicle. They cannot patent these naturally occurring substances and would have to spend more research dollars than would be cost effective. Natural progesterone can be compounded locally by a pharmacist in a cocoa butter base or other media (see page 210), but the cost to the patient is high. The pharmaceutical houses probably could do similarly for less if the FDA regulations were less restrictive.

What hormone replacement treatment schedule do you recommend for a menopausal woman?

First, it is recommended that the clinician understand the influences of hormones (see Chapter 1) in order to discern the general endocrine state of the patient. See Chapter 7 for details of specific dosages, routes of administration, and forms of steroids.

Is a hormone-free week necessary in hormonal replacement therapy regimens? My patients report discomfort when they are off hormones.

Continuous estrogen with intermittent monthly courses of progestogen is probably preferable. For a full discussion, see pages 207–210.

UTERINE FACTORS

How can one prevent endometrial cancer in the patient who is taking replacement therapy?

There is no approach to prevent cancer in all cases. One must recognize that there is some, albeit low, incidence of endometrial cancer in all populations of women that have been studied. Those who are on appropriately dosed hormone regimens appear to experience an even lower incidence than those who take no hormones (see pages

151–154). Both endometrial biopsy and the Progestin Challenge Test have been reported to be reliable approaches for preventing and/or reversing endometrial hyperplasias, which are the first warning signs of a subsequent, potential developing carcinoma.

How often is it necessary to check the endometrium in a woman taking hormone replacement therapy?

With a progestin opposition to estrogen hormonal replacement therapy (Chapter 7) and without unexplained bleeding, endometrium sampling has not been shown to be essential. Certainly, with unexplained bleeding, an endometrial cancer screen is essential.

How does one manage breakthrough bleeding?

If patient compliance is assured (no omission from hormone replacement therapy regimen schedule), first check for a pathologic condition by an endometrial cancer screen. If there is persistent bleeding, a hysteroscopy/laparascopy evaluation is recommended.

Endometriosis and myomata uteri appear to respond to the analogs of gonadotropin releasing hormone (GnRH). Does this form of therapy lead to a down-regulation of endogenous gonadotropins with subsequent ovarian suppression? If so, would this not predispose one to perimenopausal and menopausal-like vaginal and bone symptomatology? Would not osteoporosis ensue?

The down-regulation with GnRH analogs yields estrogen deprivation by suppressing ovarian function. This is essential if the desired effects on endometriosis and myomata uteri are to be achieved. Whether this approach can be fine-tuned enough (1) to reduce estrogen to a level sufficient to affect the endometriosis or the fibroids while simultaneously (2) not causing vaginal atrophy or even osteoporosis remains to be shown.

With what frequency do you recommend that we screen for endometrial cancer?

In the perimenopause, only those with unexplained uterine bleeding should be screened for endometrial cancer. Postmenopausal women, particularly after age 60, are the prime candidates for screening. If they are on a recommended estrogen and progestogen routine (see Chapter 7), then screening would be limited to unexplained bleeding.

Is it necessary to perform a D & C after a cytological sample indicates a possible pathologic pattern?

If you have a uterine cytological sample with an abnormality detected, then the possibility of a pathologic condition must be pursued. If a repeat cytological sample is negative AND the symptom does not persist, then it is reasonable to omit the D & C. However, careful follow-up of the patient is essential.

Is it ever recommended to treat a patient on the basis of a cytological sample?

No, never, because one still needs a diagnosis. Thus, one should always expect a tissue confirmation after a screening procedure reflects an abnormality.

A patient presents with bleeding more than 1 year after her last menstrual period. What is the likely cause?

The likely cause is not neoplasia. However, one must rule out this eventuality. See Chapter 8 for the conditions most commonly associated with unexplained bleeding.

OSTEOPOROSIS AND ITS PATHOPHYSIOLOGIC IMPLICATIONS

What is meant by the term "osteopenia"? How does it differ from osteoporosis?

Osteopenia is commonly used to denote any loss of bone mass to levels below normal. Osteoporosis is the abnormal rarefaction of bone in response to reduced levels of estrogen, calcium, and/or vitamin D. It is the most common disease entity of the menopause. See Chapter 2.

Who is at risk for osteoporosis?

Any woman who has estrogen or calcium deficiencies is at risk. Particularly at risk is the woman small in stature or excessively thin, with fair complexion, who is nulliparous, a smoker, or experiencing an early menopause.

How can one diagnose bone status?

The status of bone density can be assessed by CT scan. Although it is the most sensitive method, it is costly and potentially delivers unacceptable doses of radiation. Dual photon absorptiometry is not only expensive, but is also of low precision. Single photon absorptiometry currently is the most economic and acceptable method available. See Chapter 2.

Is a 1% loss of bone per year normal? Acceptable?

A 1% loss of bone per year is so common that it is often accepted as normal. Nonetheless, the end result of this bone loss is unacceptable because it is preventable.

I have heard that the bulk of bone loss occurs within the first 3 years post oophorectomy. Is this true? Is there any point in prescribing estrogen for bone loss if the patient arrives more than 3 years post oophorectomy?

Yes. In the first 3 years, annual rates of bone loss average about 3%; they subsequently decelerate to about 1% per year. Nonetheless, whenever appropriate therapy is begun, further decline is reversed. In some women, it may take 3 years of therapy before these effects are noted. See Chapters 2 and 7.

What does one do for the patient who continues to have bony loss and fractures in the face of estrogen and calcium therapies?

First, one must screen for other bone diseases. If the findings are negative, it is advisable to increase the dose of estrogen and progestogen and to recheck for adequate vitamin D (400 IU per day) and adequate dietary or supplemental calcium ingestion (1000–1500 mg/day).

Can calcium prevent osteoporosis?

It cannot do it alone unless it is given in such large doses (2 g/day) that the risk of renal calculi outweighs the benefits. This has been shown in studies at the Mayo Clinic. Calcium seems to act synergistically with estrogen, and a postmenopausal woman taking estrogen replacement therapy usually requires about 1 g calcium/day.

What is the relationship between exercise and osteoporosis?

This relationship is extremely complex. Fitness levels of exercise do not appear to alter bone mass except potentially at the stress points of the exercise. The overall skeletal mass does not change. Nonetheless, the increased muscle tonus helps reinforce and support bone and minimize the risks of fracture. Extreme levels of exercise (*i.e.,* long-distance running) have been associated with amenorrhea, reduced estrogen levels, and loss of bone mass. Moderation in exercise therefore appears to be the ideal practice. It should be emphasized that older individuals unused to exercise should start with walking or stationary bicycle riding and should increase the heart rate to 110 to 120 beats/minute for 15 or more minutes. More intense physical exertion may lead to injury in the uninitiated.

SPECIAL ISSUES

Do obese patients require special care during menopause?

Yes. Because they are at increased risk for endometrial cancer, routine follow-up should be scheduled more frequently than for the non-obese patient. Obese patients have a higher peripheral conversion of androstenedione to estrone as well as a tendency to store estrogen in their fat depot. An obese patient should probably be seen every 3 months and a weight reduction plan begun. If the patient understands the increased propensity for endometrial and breast cancer associated with excess weight, she may consider weight loss a more essential goal.

Does maintaining a thin body protect against atherosclerosis in oophorectomized patients?

No. Hormones do. See Chapter 6.

Does it matter what time of day the patient gives blood for plasma analysis?

This depends on the specific endocrine parameters under investigation. Often it does matter. Moreover, multiple samples (4 spaced at 15-minute intervals) are highly desirable to form a reliable evaluation of estrogen in the perimenopausal and postmenopausal years in order to account for the pulsatile variations (see Chapter 1).

Does taking corticosteroids influence the patient's endocrine condition?

Yes. Her estrogen levels can be expected to be extremely deficient. As a consequence, bone loss would be expected. Hot flashes are also frequently observed.

How should vulvar itching in the aging woman be treated?

It's treated in two ways: (1) Examine the patient and make sure there is no problem other than atrophic vaginitis. (2) Use a hanging drop to see what the vaginal flora presents that might be contributing as an irritant.

If there is a causative condition, it obviously should be treated first. Depending on the findings—usually both are negative—the therapy is estrogen hormonal replacement with topical vaginal creams used initially. Concomitant antibiotic or antibacterial chemotherapeutic approaches can be combined with estrogen vaginal cream in the elderly patient. It should be recalled that in the era before antibiotics, estrogen vaginal cream was the treatment of choice for bacterial vaginitis and was very effective.

How can I achieve patient compliance in following the correct dietary (high-calcium) and hormonal regimens?

There are many approaches. One optimal way is by involving the patient in her own management; for example, if you show her the photon absorptiometry readings that you have been collecting every 6 months, she can see whether there is bone loss. The graphs will help convince the patient of her progress.

How do you deal with patients who "improve" (modify) the regimen that has been prescribed?

One must document this in the file and impress upon the patient that failure to adhere to the regimen will not protect or benefit her health and welfare.

How should one manage a patient who develops elevated blood pressure while on hormonal replacement therapy at minimal doses?

A careful review of the patient's activities, diet, and severity of symptoms is necessary. If simple measures, such as sodium and dietary restriction, are not effective, medication should be discontinued to evaluate its effect on the blood pressure.

How can the clinician optimize the use of his or her time in working with the menopausal woman?

Time can be optimized by encouraging the patient to become informed about her own body and about the risks and benefits of the available treatment approaches. With the litiginous climate of medical practice in the 1970s and 1980s, it behooves every physician to share with the patient the responsibility in choosing treatment. This requires informed consent and can only be achieved through education.

The book, *Menopause: A Guide for Women and the Men who Love Them*, published in 1983 by W.W. Norton Co., written by us together with Dr. David Edwards, is intended to serve women in becoming more knowledgeable about their maturing systems. We believe that not only the doctor but also the patient would benefit from its availability to the woman. Women appreciate the fact that it is not feasible to cover all of this information during the span of an office visit. The knowledgeble patient becomes a better patient.

Index